DSM-IV Diagnosis	Medication	
Panic disorder	Tricyclic antidepressants	(p. 142)
	Alprazolam	(p. 142)
	Clonazepam	(p. 213)
Pervasive developmental disorders	Haloperidol	(pp. 103–104)
	Fluphenazine	(p. 108)
	Naltrexone	(pp. 233–235)
	Fenfluramine	(p. 76)
	Clomipramine	(pp. 162–163)
	Buspirone	(p. 219)
	Clonidine	(p. 246)
Posttraumatic stress disorder (acute)	Propranolol	(p. 238)
Schizophrenia	Antipsychotics	(pp. 78–120)
Selective mutism	Fluoxetine	(pp. 173–174)
Separation anxiety disorder	Imipramine	(p. 122, 140–142)
	Chlordiazepoxide	(p. 209)
	Fluoxetine	(pp. 170–171)
	Alprazolam	(pp. 142, 213)
	Buspirone	(pp. 217–218)
	Clomipramine	(pp. 163–164)
	Clonazepam	(p. 214)
Sleep disorders		
Primary insomnia	Benzodiazepines	(pp. 202–203, 207t)
	Diphenhydramine	(pp. 221–222)
	Hydroxyzine	(p. 223)
Circadian Rhythm Sleep disorder	Benzodiazepines	(pp. 201–204)
	Diphenhydramine	(pp. 221–222)
	Hydroxyzine	(pp. 222–223)
Sleep terror disorder	Benzodiazepines	(p. 211)
	Imipramine	(p. 142)
	Carbamazepine	(p. 227)
Sleepwalking disorder	Benzodiazepines	(p. 211)
	Imipramine	(p. 142)
Tourette's disorder	Haloperidol	(p. 79)
	Pimozide	(pp. 109–110)
	Clonidine	(pp. 246–249)
	Desipramine	(pp. 156–157)
	Guanfacine	(pp. 250–251)
	Nortriptyline	(pp. 146–147)
	Fluoxetine	(pp. 170–171)

Child and Adolescent Clinical Psychopharmacology

SECOND EDITION

Related Titles in Psychiatry by Williams & Wilkins

William S. Appleton: *Practical Clinical Psychopharmacology*, Third Edition (1988/224 pages/12 illustrations/#0-683-00239-2)

Domenic A. Ciraulo, Richard I. Shader, David J. Greenblatt, Wayne Creelman: *Drug Interactions in Psychiatry, Second Edition* (1995/352 pages/16 illustrations/#0-683-01944-9)

Lindsay C. DeVane: *Fundamentals of Monitoring Psychoactive Drug Therapy* (1990/298 pages/45 illustrations/#0-683-02452-3)

Philip G. Janicak, John M. Davis, Sheldon H. Preskorn, Frank J. Ayd, Jr: *Principles and Practice of Psychopharmacotherapy* (1993/608 pages/28 illustrations/#0-683-04373-0)

Harold I. Kaplan, Benjamin J. Sadock: *Pocket Handbook of Psychiatric Drug Treatment* (1993/288 pages/29 illustrations/#0-683-04538-5)

Lloyd I. Sederer, Barbara Dickey: *The Clinician's Guide to Outcomes Research in Psychiatry* (1995/352 pages/6 illustrations/#0-683-07630-2)

Call to order 1-800-638-0672

Child and Adolescent Clinical Psychopharmacology

SECOND EDITION

WAYNE HUGO GREEN, M.D.

Associate Professor of Clinical Psychiatry
Department of Psychiatry
and
Director of Training and Education
Division of Child and Adolescent Psychiatry
New York University School of Medicine

Director, Child and Adolescent Psychiatric Clinic
Bellevue Medical Center
New York, New York

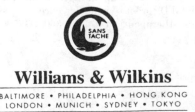

Williams & Wilkins

BALTIMORE • PHILADELPHIA • HONG KONG
LONDON • MUNICH • SYDNEY • TOKYO

A WAVERLY COMPANY

Editor: David C. Retford
Managing Editor: Kathleen Courtney Millet
Production Coordinator: Barbara J. Felton
Copy Editor: Lois Shipway
Designer: Norman W. Och
Cover Designer: Wilma E. Rosenberger

Copyright © 1995
Williams & Wilkins
351 West Camden Street
Baltimore, Maryland 21201-2436 USA

Accurate indications, adverse reactions, and dosage schedules for drugs are provided in this book, but it is possible that they may change. The reader is urged to review the package information data of the manufacturers of the medications mentioned.

Printed in the United States of America

First Edition 1991

Library of Congress Cataloging-in-Publication Data

Green, Wayne H.
    Child and adolescent clinical psychopharmacology / Wayne Hugo Green. —
2nd ed.
        p. cm.
    Includes bibliographical references and index.
    ISBN 0-683-03767-6 (pbk.)
    1. Pediatric psychopharmacology. I. Title.
    [DNLM: 1. Mental Disorders—drug therapy. 2. Mental Disorders—in infancy
& childhood. 3. Mental Disorders—in adolescence. 4. Psychopharmacology.
5. Psychotropic Drugs—therapeutic use. WS 350.2 G798c 1995]
RJ504.7.G74 1995
615′.78′083—dc20
DNLM/DLC
for Library of Congress   95-10273
                                                                    CIP
                                            95 96 97 98 99
                                        2 3 4 5 6 7 8 9 10

To my parents,
Albert George Green
and
Mildred Hugo Green,
and my uncle and aunt,
Alfred John Green
and
Ada May Green

FOREWORD

Building on the well-deserved success of the First Edition, Wayne Hugo Green has again provided us with the up-to-date and practical information that the thoughtful clinician needs for the careful and wise administration of psychopharmacological agents in the treatment of children and adolescents. This Second Edition uses DSM-IV nomenclature throughout and draws on the scientific literature through early 1995. More than 100 new references are cited, including recent finding on specific serotonin uptake reinhibitors (SSRIs) and new material on clozapine and risperidone.

Dr. Green is not only extremely knowledgeable about new and established individual drugs, but he is also fully aware of the recent trend to make use of multiple drugs. Dr. Green's discussion on the use of polypharmacy is masterful. He notes the clinical and theoretical advantages of such usage, but also offers wise and cautious recommendations regarding their combined use. Dr. Green keeps in mind that the treatment of children and adolescents with psychiatric disorders is almost always multimodal and may include individual, family, or other kinds of psychotherapeutic interventions as well as the use of medications, singly or in combination. Dr. Green rightly cautions the clinician against believing that multiple medication regimens alone can solve all problems in the child and family.

The burgeoning research on these issues in the scientific literature, together with the rapidly accumulating clinical experience of seasoned clinicians, augers well for the future comprehensive psychiatric treatment of children and adolescents.

Wayne Hugo Green, in this Second Edition, has steered us in the right direction and has given us ample information to enable us to practice state-of-the-art child and adolescent psychiatry. As both a skilled clinician and a leading expert on pharmacological intervention, Dr. Green's truly comprehensive mastery shines through in every page of this Second Edition. This is an excellent book.

Melvin Lewis, MBBS, FRCPsych, DCH

PREFACE

Much has happened in child and adolescent psychopharmacology since the First Edition was published 4 years ago. Three different areas stand out: (a) new information about drugs already in use, (b) the introduction of new drugs, and (c) an increase in the use of polypharmacy. Although there is much cause for optimism in that significant advances are being made, there is also an increasing need for caution.

New Information About Drugs Already in Use

For example, the reports of sudden death in children and younger adolescents taking tricyclic antidepressants, especially desipramine, have resulted in many papers concerned with untoward cardiovascular effects of the tricyclic antidepressants. As no specific cardiac finding has any known predictive value when recommended ECG and serum drug and metabolite parameters are followed, some clinicians are increasingly reluctant to prescribe tricyclic antidepressants in this age group.

Geller et al. (1993) caution that the use of tricyclic antidepressants in depressed 6- to 12-year-olds may precipitate switching to mania and hasten the onset of bipolarity and perhaps increase later rapid cycling. They urge the clinician to consider these possibilities and discuss them with the family and patients as appropriate in formulating a treatment plan.

Introduction of New Drugs

There has been a remarkable increase in the use of the specific serotonin uptake reinhibitors (SSRIs) and the atypical antipsychotics, clozapine and risperidone, over the last few years. Although their FDA approval was based on studies including at most a few older adolescents and they are not approved for use in children, clinicians have rapidly appropriated these drugs in treating child and adolescent psychiatric disorders. There are good reasons physicians treating children and adolescents were eager to embrace these new medications. Only one double-blind placebo-controlled study has found that tricylcic antidepressants were more effective than placebo in treating children or adolescents diagnosed with MDD and that study controlled plasma levels (Preskorn et al., 1987) while several found no significant difference between drug and placebo. In addition, much has been written about cardiotoxicity and sudden deaths in children and adolescents treated with tricyclic antidepressants, especially desipramine. The rapidity with which the SSRIs have displaced tricyclic antidepressants in treating depression in adults and the initial preponderance of glowingly positive reports in the press over the negative have undoubtedly been influential as well. However, in using any new medications for off-label indications in children and adolescents it is essential to remain vigilant and cautious and to remember that, for any given drug, because of maturational/developmental factors, e.g., potentially significantly different pharmacokinetic and pharmacodynamic factors, less mature central nervous systems, and differing psychological factors, children and younger adolescents may react differently than adults do. When first introduced, fluoxetine was available only in 20-mg capsules. Experience found this was often not only too high an initial dose and but exceeded the optimal daily dose of 5 to 10 mg for some children and adolescents. The subsequent introduction of a 10-mg capsule has been helpful in titrating dosage of fluoxetine. Unexpected untoward effects may also occur. Recently for example, Bangs et al. (1994) documented fluoxetine-induced memory impairment in an adolescent which improved significantly on 3 WISC-R scales after fluoxetine was discontinued. Whether this is a rare side effect or a particularly severe example of an untoward effect which occurs more frequently but at a lower level of intensity is unknown but potentially important.

Increased Use of Polypharmacy

There are increasing numbers of reports in the literature concerning the simultaneous use of more than one medication in treating psychiatric disorders in children and adolescents. In some reports, only one drug is focused upon, whereas many subjects are simultaneously taking one or a variety of other drugs, which potentially confounds results. The impression from colleagues is that polypharmacy is not rare in treatment-resistant cases when clinically significant symptoms remain after trials of the usual medications and when comorbid diagnoses are present.

For example, Zito et al. (1994) reported that 64 (40%) of 131 children and adolescents hospitalized in four New York State Psychiatric facilities who were treated with neuroleptics were receiving two or more drugs with strong anticholinergic action. Kaplan et al. (1994), describing prescribing patterns of child psychiatrists practicing in New York and Ohio, reported that of 49 children diagnosed with ADHD with no comorbid conduct or oppositional disorder, 37 (76%) were treated with a stimulant, 3 (6%) were treated with clonidine, 2 (4%) with a combination of a stimulant and antidepressant, and 1 (2%) each with propanolol and antihistamines; stimulants and antihistamines; stimulants and lithium; clonidine and anticonvulsants; antidepressants only; stimulants and antipsychotics; and antipsychotics only.

Polypharmacy has a rational appeal both because a substantial percentage of patients have comorbid diagnoses and, in some cases, the use of two different medications may permit lower doses of each drug and result in a decrease in number or intensity of untoward effects. In addition, increasing awareness of neurotransmitter specificity and numbers of neurotransmitter subtypes and of the genetic variability of patients also suggests that more than one drug may be necessary to achieve satisfactory amelioration of different target symptoms. Clinically, it is essential, however, to resist the tempting but erroneous notion that the right combination of drugs will solve any problem and to continue to evaluate the impact of the family and psychosocial environment on the child or adolescent. Satisfactory resolution of psychiatric disorders in children and adolescents almost always requires additional individual, family, or other psychotherapeutic interventions.

Wilens et al. (1995) have provided a useful review of the current status of combined pharmacotherapy in treating child and adolescent psychiatric disorders. Walkup (1995) has offered algorithms detailing systematic, sequential trials of drugs, including various combinations of drugs, for children and adolescents diagnosed with ADHD, mood disorders, or psychoses, who are treatment resistant, or who do not respond to pharmacotherapy with single drugs. Green (1995) reviewed the literature on polypharmacy in children and adolescents diagnosed with ADHD only or with comorbid disorders and noted that nonstimulant medications, e.g., tricyclic antidepressants, SSRIs, and clonidine, have been used in combination with stimulants as adjunctive drugs, for their synergistic effects, or to augment partial, but inadequate responses to stimulant medication alone. Research data evaluating the overall safety and efficacy of various combinations of drugs as compared to the use of single agents are only beginning to appear in the literature. It is likely that some individual patients will benefit significantly; however, it remains to be determined which subgroups of patients with comorbid diagnoses or treatment resistance to standard drugs will benefit most from which combinations of drugs.

I am gratified by the positive response to the First Edition and appreciate the many suggestions and comments colleagues have made to update and improve this Second Edition. I hope that I have succeeded.

Wayne Hugo Green

PREFACE TO THE FIRST EDITION

This book is written with the conviction that proper psychiatric treatment of children and adolescents will, on some occasions, necessitate the use of psychopharmacotherapy. It is not intended to suggest that psychopharmacotherapy is warranted for most patients in this age group. Most children and adolescents seen in private practices and in mental hygiene clinics do not require medication. Indeed, medication is not appropriate for many patients of this age group seen on inpatient psychiatric services.

Clinicians who administer psychoactive medication to children and adolescents will almost certainly encounter individuals with strong viewpoints on this treatment. Some are convinced that drugs are the answer to a child's or adolescent's problem. Others are equally certain that drugs are an anathema and ought to be avoided at all costs.

In this second, antidrug group, two lines of reasoning seem to appear with regularity in a significant minority of cases.

Some health and educational professionals working with children and adolescents maintain that in the face of compelling psychological explanations for a mental disorder, or for significant contributions to it, drugs should not be used. This group argues that drugs may have inimical effects and, further, that psychotherapy alone should be able to do the job.

A few professionals, but more often parents and relatives, offer a variation on this theme. They believe drugs should be avoided because they will make their children "zombies" or "dope them up" or "make them become drug addicts later on."

The author's point of view is that the etiology of virtually all psychiatric disorders is multiply determined. Each individual case must be fully assessed and evaluated for the potential benefits and risks of administering a specific medication. In those cases where potential benefits appear to significantly outweigh risks, usually a trial of medication is indicated.

Still, extreme caution is required in employing psychoactive medications. The long-term effects of psychoactive medications on the maturation and development of children and adolescents are at best only partially known, and many of their known untoward effects are potentially harmful.

But when a mental illness is delaying or disrupting the maturation and development of a patient, effective medication may aid considerably in bringing about more normal development and socialization. The medication often will augment the patient's ability to respond to other treatment modalities as well.

The clinician must successfully negotiate among these conflicting viewpoints and objectives in order to undertake a clinical trial of a psychoactive drug in a reasonably favorable or at least dispassionately neutral atmosphere.

Time and reality are two extremely important factors often overlooked by critics of psychopharmacotherapy. In deciding about medication, it is essential to employ a realizable goal, not some unattainable ideal.

For example, a latency-age child is diagnosed with a conduct disorder and attention deficit hyperactivity disorder. School officials threaten to suspend the child, with eventual placement in a special education class for children with behavioral problems.

In many such cases, an argument can be made that the child's problems are primarily psychological, that they could be helped by tutoring and individual and family therapies, and that medication should be withheld.

However, the realities of the case and the time frame for behavior change may call for trying medication. It may be exceedingly difficult to engage and work with the parents and the child. The child's symptoms may not have responded to the initial evaluation and intervention. The attitude of the school officials may be that the child's behavior must improve quickly.

In a situation such as this, if psychopharmacotherapy is likely to significantly hasten the therapeutic response to other treatments, or to prevent the patient from being removed from the regular classroom, the author recommends a trial of medication, unless other compelling factors are involved.

This book provides a framework for making an informed decision to undertake a clinical trial of a psychoactive medication and guides the clinician through the myriad issues involved in that decision.

Wayne Hugo Green

CONTENTS

SECTION TWO
Specific Drug Treatments

LIST OF TABLES AND FIGURES

Tables

Figures

. . . .

Introduction and General Principles of Psychopharmacotherapy with Children and Adolescents

1

Introduction

This book will review selected topics and representative drugs used in child and adolescent psychopharmacology from a practical, clinically oriented perspective and is intended primarily for clinicians actively engaged in treating children and adolescents with psychoactive medication. This includes child psychiatrists, residents in general psychiatry who are treating children and adolescents, residents specializing in child and adolescent psychiatry, pediatric residents, and other physicians who may prescribe drugs to patients in this age range.

In addition, other clinicians and mental health personnel who work with children who are receiving psychoactive medication may wish to review the medications their patients are receiving.

The first part of the book focuses rather intensively on the general principles of psychopharmacotherapy with children and adolescents. The reader is presented with a clinically useful way of thinking about psychopharmacotherapy, beginning with the initial clinical contact and continuing through the psychiatric evaluation, psychodynamic formulation, diagnosis, and development of the treatment plan. For those cases where psychoactive medication is advocated as a part of the treatment plan, the necessary medicolegal responsibilities of the clinician in introducing and explaining the purpose of medication to the patient and relevant caretakers, ways of maximizing the chances of the patient and his or her legal guardians' accepting a trial of the medication and their cooperating with its administration, and the necessary documentation of these facts in the clinical record are reviewed. Following this, the entire process of administering medication is discussed. This begins with consideration of which drug to choose for the initial trial of medication, the necessary documentation of target symptoms and any baseline behavioral ratings that will be useful in assessing clinical response or the development of untoward effects, and which baseline physical and laboratory assessments to select.

This first part of the book ends with a detailed presentation of the principles of administering psychoactive medication from the initial dose, through titration and determining the optimal dose, to maintenance therapy, duration of treatment, and issues in terminating medication. These principles are generalizable and provide clinical guidelines for selecting and administering any psychoactive medication to children and adolescents.

The second portion of the book begins with a brief discussion of the history of child psychopharmacology and some issues concerning psychopharmacological research in children and adolescents. The purpose of this review is to remind the reader of where the information that follows is placed in the history of child psychopharmacology and of the importance of research and a critical assessment of the presented data for informed clinical practice.

After these brief introductory comments, the remainder of Section II of the book focuses on specific psychopharmacological agents that are presently the most important in the clinical practice of child and adolescent psychiatry. These drugs are presented by class. Many specific psychoactive medications are presently used to treat diverse psychiatric disorders or symptoms across psychiatric diagnoses (e.g., lithium's use for its antiaggressive effects), and this method of organization avoids repeating similar information under several diagnoses. Equally important, as we learn more about the etiopathogenesis of psychiatric disorders, it becomes increasingly useful, both scientifically and clinically, to think about how drugs affect basic neurotransmitter and psychoneuroendocrine functioning across diagnoses. A given drug may affect one or more neurotransmitter systems. Likewise, a specific neurotransmitter system may be important in one or more diagnostic categories. For example, there appears to be a relationship between the serotonergic system's functioning and aggressive or violent behavior and self-destructive behavior among various diagnostic groups (Linnoila et al., 1989; Mann et al., 1989). Several books devoted solely to the behavioral pharmacology of serotonin have been published, e.g., Bevan et al., 1989; Coccaro and Murphy, 1990; and Brown and van Praag, 1991.

As might be expected in a clinically oriented book, the standard psychopharmacological treatments established by investigational and clinical studies as both efficacious and safe for use in children and adolescents and approved by the U.S. Food and Drug Administration (FDA) for advertising as such are emphasized.

The literature reviews determining the efficacy of these treatments, however, are kept to a minimum, because comprehensive reviews are readily available elsewhere. (For the interested reader a list of such additional readings is given in the introductory comments to Section II of this book.)

The author emphasizes that no book can substitute for a careful reading of the manufacturer's labeling, which is packaged with drugs and is reprinted verbatim in the current *Physicians' Desk Reference* (PDR) and its supplements, unless, of course, the book itself reprints verbatim the package insert. The FDA-approved labeling (package insert) contains additional information on all FDA-approved medications discussed in this book. No drug should be prescribed without the physician's having read and become familiar with its labeling information; to do so is a disservice to one's patient and renders one vulnerable to professional liability.

In addition to standard treatments, however, selected medications currently prescribed to children and adolescents for unlabeled (non-FDA-approved) indications and medications that have recently been under clinical investigation and with which the clinician should be familiar are reviewed. Medications that appear to be possible candidates for eventual approval as standard treatments (e.g., clomipramine, approved by the FDA for treating symptoms of obsessive-compulsive disorder in persons at least 10 years of age, is still not approved for younger children) or that may be clinically important when patients do not respond to standard treatments are emphasized. Because reviews of these medications are usually less readily available and some studies are very recent, relevant studies are summarized herein. Although this relative emphasis on the literature of studies of drugs used for non-FDA-approved or off-label indications over FDA-approved drugs may seem paradoxical, it is deliberate. This is because, in clinical practice, a major difficulty occurs when a patient does not respond with sufficient amelioration of symptoms to standard pharmacological treatments currently available. When, despite treatment with standard medications, the patient's symptoms prevent him or her from functioning in a psychosocial environment that will facilitate normal growth, maturation, and development, many clinicians will consider the possibility of using FDA-approved drugs for non-FDA-approved indications to treat their patient. Although not proselytizing for the use of medication for non-FDA-approved uses, this book does present the clinician with possible alternative treatments for patients who are resistant to standard pharmacological treatments. In fact, the use of some of these medications for off-label indications is medically accepted in clinical practice.

As with standard treatments, the physician must consider, perhaps even more carefully, the risks versus the potential benefits of using any medication for non-FDA-approved indications. Medicolegal and some practical issues of using nonstandard treatments are considered below in the appropriate sections of the book.

2

General Principles of Psychopharmacotherapy with Children and Adolescents

Psychiatric Diagnosis and Psychopharmacotherapy

Psychopharmacotherapy should always be part of a comprehensive treatment plan arrived at after a thorough psychiatric evaluation that results in a diagnosis, or at minimum a working diagnosis. It is scientifically indefensible to initiate treatment without first attempting to formulate as clear an understanding of the clinical picture as possible. This will enable clinicians to institute the most appropriate and rational treatment(s) available in their therapeutic armamentaria for the situation at hand.

CURRENT PSYCHIATRIC DIAGNOSTIC NOMENCLATURE

A major difficulty with the official American Psychiatric Association (APA) nomenclature, the *Diagnostic and Statistical Manual of Mental Disorders, Fourth Edition* (DSM-IV) (APA, 1994), and indeed with most current psychiatric nomenclatures is that usually etiology is not taken into account in formulating a diagnosis. One reason for this is that, at our present state of knowledge, we do not know the etiologies of many conditions. Hence we are often treating specific constellations of behavioral symptoms without understanding adequately their biological and genetic underpinnings and how they interact with their psychosocial and physical environments. For example, autistic disorder is not etiologically homogeneous but has a multitude of causes.

Theoretically, drugs may be effective for a given psychiatric disorder by correcting the condition(s) leading to it or by influencing events somewhere along the usually complex pathways between the hypothesized abnormality(ies) and its subsequent psychological and/or behavioral consequences. Thus some psychoactive drugs may be effective in several dissimilar disorders because they influence or modify neurotransmitters and psychoneuroendocrine events in the brain along or near the end of these interacting, partially confluent, or final common pathways.

Other psychoactive drugs appear to exert their therapeutic effects through entirely different mechanisms in different diagnostic entities; for example, imipramine in depression, attention deficit hyperactivity disorder (ADHD), and enuresis.

Some patients with a specific diagnosis (e.g., ADHD, autistic disorder, or schizophrenia) will not have a satisfactory clinical response or will be refractory to a specific drug—even one known to be highly effective in statistically significant double-blind studies—or will even have a worsening of symptoms. This may reflect differences in genetic makeup or other biologically determined conditions, psychosocial environments, and/or internalized conflicts and the contributions each makes to the etiopathogenesis of each patient's psychiatric disorder.

Although diagnostic issues are not discussed specifically in this book, it is emphasized that an accurate diagnosis may be of critical importance in choosing the correct medication. For example, Bowden and Sarabia (1980), Carlson and Strober (1978), and Horowitz (1977) reported on a total of 17 adolescents with bipolar manic-depressive disorder who were initially misdiagnosed as having schizophrenia. Most of the patients with bipolar disorder who were diagnosed incorrectly were treated with antipsychotics and failed to show clinical improvement or responded poorly. When subsequently diagnosed correctly as having manic-depressive disorder and treated with lithium carbonate, the patients showed remarkable improvements or complete remissions of their psychoses. Horowitz (1977) noted that the presence of mood disturbance with marked lability and prominent elevations and depressions, grandiosity and flight of ideas, and pressured speech, hyperactivity, and distractibility predicted lithium-responsive manic-depression (bipolar disorder) even when massive alterations of thinking and hallucinations were present. Thus at times the lack of expected clinical response to a medication should suggest to the clinician the possibility of an incorrect diagnosis and that a careful diagnostic reconsideration should be undertaken.

Other unfortunate clinical consequences may result from incorrect diagnoses. For example, antidepressants may precipitate an acute psychotic reaction when given to individuals with schizophrenic disorder. Stimulant medications, too, may precipitate psychosis when given to children or adolescents with borderline personalities or unrecognized schizophrenia.

Wender (1988) noted that clinical experience suggested that some children diagnosed with ADHD who were treated with stimulants and rapidly developed tolerance to them were actually suffering from a major depressive disorder and that they responded to treatment with tricyclic antidepressants with remarkable improvement. Changing diagnostic criteria may also complicate matters. For example, some of the controversy regarding the efficacy of stimulants in the mentally retarded may have resulted from diagnostic issues. Until the publication of the *Diagnostic and Statistical Manual of Mental Disorders, Second Edition* (DSM-II) by the APA in 1968, there was no specific APA diagnosis for what was commonly known as the hyperactive child. There were various labels for this condition including hyperactive child, hyperkinetic syndrome, minimal brain dysfunction, and minimal cerebral dysfunction. One influential definition of minimal brain dysfunction was that of the Minimal Brain Dysfunction National Project on Learning Disabilities in Children in 1966. This report defined minimal brain dysfunction (MBD) to designate

> children of near average, average, or above average general intelligence with certain learning and/or behavioral disabilities ranging from mild to severe, which are associated with deviations of function of the central nervous system. These deviations may manifest themselves by various combinations of impairment in perception, conceptualization, language, memory, and control of attention, impulse, or motor function. These aberrations may arise from genetic variations, biochemical irregularities, perinatal insults or other illnesses or injuries sustained during the years which are critical for the development and maturation of the central nervous system, or from other unknown organic causes (Clements, 1966, p. 53).

Mental retardation was considered evidence of more than "minimal" dysfunction, and the various etiologies were thought to be biological. Because of this concept, children with mental retardation were excluded from the possibility of receiving a codiagnosis of minimal brain dysfunction, hyperactive child, or an equivalent diagnosis, and some clinicians may not have tried stimulant medication in their patients who had even mild mental retardation.

The situation changed with the publication of DSM-II, which noted that "in children, mild brain damage often manifests itself by hyperactivity, short attention span, easy distractibility, and impulsiveness" (APA, 1968, p. 31). It also suggested that unless there are significant interactional factors (e.g., between child and parents) that appear to be responsible for these behaviors, the disorder should be classified as a nonpsychotic organic brain syndrome and not as a behavior disorder such as hyperkinetic reaction of childhood or adolescence. DSM-II conceptualized hyperkinetic reaction of childhood as a reactive disorder secondary to internalization of interpersonal conflicts with resulting characteristic symptoms. There was no other available category for a child or adolescent of normal intelligence who exhibited such symptoms as his or her natural baseline of behavior, unless one assumed some degree of brain damage.

In DSM-III (APA, 1980a), the diagnosis of attention deficit disorder with hyperactivity (ADDH) was based on the presence of a specific constellation of symptoms, and no etiology was hypothesized. Hence children of any intelligence could exhibit such features. DSM-III additionally notes that mild or moderate mental retardation may predispose to the development of ADDH and that the addition of this diagnosis to the severely and profoundly retarded is not clinically useful because these symptoms are often an inherent part of the condition.

DSM-III-R redefines ADDH somewhat, renames it attention-deficit hyperactivity disorder (ADHD), and refines its relationship to mental retardation. It notes that many features of ADHD may be present in mentally retarded persons because of the generalized delays in intellectual development. Both DSM-III-R and DSM-IV (APA, 1994) note that a mentally retarded child or adolescent should be additionally diagnosed with ADHD only if the relevant symptoms significantly exceed those that are compatible with the child's or adolescent's mental age.

Diagnosis and Target Symptoms

In making the decision about which psychoactive medication to select initially, two major issues should be addressed: diagnosis and target symptoms. Both are important and are often interrelated. It is essential to make an accurate diagnosis and to identify and quantify target symptoms in order to choose an efficacious drug and to assess the results of medication. The target symptoms must be of sufficient severity and must interfere so significantly with the child's or adolescent's current functioning and future maturation and development that the potential benefits of the drug will justify the risks concomitant with its administration.

The initial medication may be chosen with respect to either diagnosis or target symptoms or both. Sometimes the decision is not difficult, because the same medication is appropriate for both the target symptoms and the diagnosis. For example, antipsychotics are the drugs of first choice for treating schizophrenia and are also appropriate for most of the significant target symptoms (e.g., hallucinations, thought disorder, and delusions). The symptom "hyperactivity," however, is present in numerous childhood psychiatric disorders, but all hyperactivity is not the same. The clinician should be fully aware of the diagnosis in treating this symptom. Hyperactivity in a youngster with ADHD would be expected to respond favorably to the administration of a stimulant, whereas a schizophrenic youngster who is in relative remission but exhibits marked hyperactivity would have a good chance of having his or her psychotic symptoms reexacerbated if stimulant medication were used. Stimulant drugs, the drugs of choice in ADHD, are considered to be relatively contraindicated in schizophrenia and may cause worsening of psychotic symptoms.

Medication also can be prescribed to treat certain specific diagnoses. Lithium, for example, has a certain specificity for treatment of mania in patients diagnosed with bipolar disorder, manic, but also appears to have an antiaggressive action that cuts across various diagnoses. Lithium has been used effectively to treat aggression directed against others or self-injurious behavior in children and adolescents diagnosed with conduct disorder, mental retardation with disturbance of behavior, and autistic disorder.

Special Aspects of Child Psychopharmacotherapy

MATURATIONAL/DEVELOPMENTAL ISSUES

Physiological Factors:

The relationship of biological developmental issues to psychopharmacotherapy has been emphasized in the 1987 book *Psychiatric Pharmacosciences of Children and Adolescents* (Popper, 1987b). Children and adolescents often require larger doses of psychoactive medication per unit of body weight than adults to attain similar blood levels and therapeutic efficacy. It is usually assumed that two factors explain this situation: more rapid metabolism by the liver and an increased glomerular filtration rate in children compared with that in adults. The latter suggests a greater renal clearance for some drugs, including lithium, which helps to explain the fact that therapeutic dosages of lithium in children usually do not differ from those in adults (Campbell et al., 1984a).

Teicher and Baldessarini (1987) pointed out that children may respond to drugs differently from adults because of pharmacodynamic factors (drug-effector mechanisms) that are caused by developmental changes in neural pathways or their functions (e.g., Geller et al. [1992] reported that prepubescent subjects treated with the tricyclic antidepressant nortriptyline reported almost no anticholinergic untoward effects; especially noteworthy was the lack of any prominent dry mouth frequently reported by adults) or because of pharmacokinetic factors caused by developmental changes in the distribution, metabolism, or excretion of a drug.

Jatlow (1987) has noted that although the rapid rate of drug disposition may decrease gradually throughout childhood, around puberty there may be an abrupt decline. Drug disposition usually reaches adult levels by mid- to late adolescence. Clinically, this would indicate that the clinician should be especially alert to possible changes in pharmacokinetics during the time period around puberty and be ready to adjust dose levels if necessary. When they are available, it may be useful to obtain plasma concentration levels if there appears to be a change in the clinical efficacy of a drug as a child matures into an adolescent.

Puig-Antich (1987) summarized some of the evidence that catecholamine (norepinephrine, epinephrine, and dopamine) systems are not fully anatomically developed and operationally functional until adulthood. The relatively high prevalence of ADHD in younger children and its spontaneous improvement in many children over time may reflect maturational changes in catecholamine function. Interestingly, both the fact that younger children respond to stimulant medication differently from older adolescents and adults with respect to affect or mood and do not report elation, excitation, or euphoria and the fact that mania and euphoria are relatively rare in childhood may also be explained by the immaturity of the catecholamine systems (Puig-Antich, 1987); they also can be considered to result from developmental pharmacodynamic factors.

Similarly, the pharmacokinetics of many drugs change over the course of life. Children and younger adolescents may differ from older adolescents and adults, as the elderly may again differ from middle-aged persons. For example, children and adolescents under 15 years of age treated with clomipramine had significantly lower steady-state plasma concentrations for a given dose than did adults (see package insert). Rivera-Calimlim et al. (1979) reported that children and adolescents 8 to 15 years of age required larger doses of chlorpromazine than adults to attain similar plasma concentrations.

There may also be differences between acute and chronic pharmacokinetics. For example, Sallee et al. (1985) noted in one subject that magnesium pemoline elimination half-time almost doubled from 7.5 hours after an acute dose to 14.3 hours after 3 weeks of treatment with magnesium pemoline. Rivera-Calimlim et al. (1979) reported a decline in plasma chlorpromazine levels in most of their child and adolescent patients who were on a fixed dose and suggested it might be due to autoinduction of metabolic enzymes for chlorpromazine during long-term treatment, as had been reported previously in adults.

A clear relationship between plasma concentrations and clinical response to imipramine was noted for prepubescent subjects and older subjects with endogenous depression but not for adolescents (Burke & Puig-Antich, 1990). The authors hypothesized that the relatively poor clinical efficacy of tricyclic antidepressants in postpubescent adolescents and young adults compared with the clinical response of prepubescent children and older adults is secondary to a negative effect of increased sex hormone levels on the antidepressant action of imipramine. Because of this, monoamine oxidase inhibitors may be of particular use in selected depressed adolescents who do not respond satisfactorily to other antidepressants.

Herskowitz (1987) reviewed the developmental neurotoxicity of pharmacoactive drugs. Developmental neurotoxicity is concerned with stage-specific, drug-induced biochemical or physiological changes, morphological manifestations, and behavioral symptoms. For example, stimulant medication may adversely affect normal increases in height and growth, at least temporarily, in some actively growing children and adolescents. Some psychoactive drugs taken during early pregnancy have significant potential for damaging the fetus (e.g., lithium may cause cardiac malformations).

Cognitive/Psychological/Experiential Factors

The maturation and development of the central nervous system as well as the life experiences accumulating since infancy determine much of the specific level of functioning of a given child or adolescent. Although detailed knowledge of these factors is essential to evaluate psychiatrically any child or adolescent, this book addresses only their specific relevance to psychopharmacotherapy.

In general, the younger the patient, the less verbal facility is available to convey information to the clinician and, reciprocally, the less cognitive ability is available to understand information the clinician wishes to impart. Part of the psychiatric evaluation leading to a decision that psychotropic medication is indicated will provide the clinician with an assessment of the level of the patient's ability to communicate his or her emotional status and of his or her cognitive/linguistic ability to understand the proposed treatment and reliably report the effect of the treatment.

In the very young child or the child with no communicative language, the clinician can only observe behavioral effects of medication directly or learn of them as reported by others. The younger the child, the fewer complaints (or compliments) about beneficial or untoward effects. Also, the young child has less-differentiated emotions and more limited experience with feelings and emotions and with communicating them to others than have older children. In addition, some chronically depressed or anxious children may not have had a sufficiently recent normal emotional baseline to which they can compare their present mood. Such children may experience a depressed mood as their normal, usual state of being and thus do not have a normal baseline frame of reference upon which to draw in describing how they feel.

The younger the child, the less accurate are the time estimates. Until about 10 years of age, concepts of long periods of time are often not easily understood. It can be very useful and at times essential to use concrete markers of time in discussing time concepts and chronology of events with children. For example, the clinician may inquire if something occurred before or after the last birthday, specific holidays (e.g., Christmas, Thanksgiving, or Halloween), specific events, (e.g., separation or divorce of parents, when the family moved to another home, an operation, a relative's death, or the birth of a sibling), the seasons or weather (e.g., winter, snow, cold, or summer, hot), or the school year (e.g., specific teacher's name or grade, or Christmas, spring or Easter, or summer vacation).

Concepts such as concentration, distractibility, and impulsivity may be beyond the understanding of some early latency-age children. Different children may use different words or expressions to mean the same concept. It is important to be certain that a child knows the meaning of a specific word and not assume an understanding because the child responds to a question. If there is any doubt, ask what something means or explain it in another way. It can be very useful to ask the same thing in several different ways.

In the final analysis, once the patient's psychopathology and his or her developmental experiential factors are taken into account, it is the quality of the relationship between the clinician and the child or adolescent that becomes paramount in determining the usefulness of information shared.

RELATIONSHIP TO THE PATIENT'S FAMILY OR CARETAKERS

Diagnosis, Formulation, and Development of the Treatment Plan

A complete psychiatric assessment, including appropriate psychological tests, resulting in a working diagnosis and comprehensive treatment plan; appropriate physical and laboratory examinations; and baseline behavioral measurements should be completed as minimum prerequisites before initiation of psychopharmacotherapy. The treatment plan should be developed in conjunction with both the parents or the primary caretaker and include participation of the child or adolescent as appropriate to his or her understanding. Treatment with psychoactive drugs should always be part of a more comprehensive treatment regimen and rarely, if ever, is appropriate as the sole treatment modality for a child or adolescent.

At variance with this traditional wisdom, however, are the results of several studies comparing treatment of hyperactive children with stimulant medication alone versus stimulant medication combined with other interventions, such as cognitive training, attention control, social reinforcement, and parent training. A review of these studies concluded that "the additional use of various forms of psychotherapies (behavioral treatment, parent training, cognitive therapy) with stimulants has not resulted in superior outcomes than medication alone" (Klein, 1987, p. 1223). One possible factor contributing to this result is that in several studies children who were treated with methylphenidate alone showed improvement in social behavior. Following this course of treatment, adults—both parents and teachers—related to the children more positively (Klein, 1987). It seems clinically unlikely, however, that all of the difficulties of ADHD children are secondary to the target symptoms that improve with methylphenidate. Those difficulties that result from other psychosocial problems, including psychopathological familial interactions and long-standing maladaptive behavioral patterns, would be expected to benefit from additional interventions; until it is possible to differentiate those children whose difficulties arise from their attention deficit per se from children whose symptoms are of multidetermined origin, a comprehensive treatment program is recommended for all children.

The legal guardian and the child or adolescent patient, to the degree appropriate for the patient's age and psychopathology, should participate in formulating the treatment plan. The use of medication, including expected benefits and possible short- and long-term untoward effects, should be reviewed with the parents and patient in understandable terminology. Their informed consent should be obtained and included in the clinical record.

It is essential to assess carefully the attitude and reliability of the persons who will be responsible for administering the medication. Unless there is a positive or at least honestly neutral attitude toward medication and some therapeutic alliance with the parents, it will be difficult or infeasible to make a reliable assessment of drug efficacy and compliance. Likewise, to store and administer medication safely on an outpatient basis requires a responsible adult, especially if there are young children in the home or if the patient is at risk of suicide.

It should be explained to parents that, even if medication helps some biologically determined symptoms (e.g., in some cases of ADHD), the disorder's presence may have caused psychological difficulties in the child or adolescent as well as disturbances in familial and social relationships. Controlling or ameliorating the biological difficulty usually does not immediately correct the long-standing internalized psychological or interpersonal problems. Resolving these difficulties will take time and may often require concomitant individual, group, family, or other therapeutic intervention.

Compliance

Compliance is an issue of particular importance in child and adolescent psychiatry. Because the parents or other caretakers usually are interposed between the physician and patient, compliance is somewhat more complex than in adult psychiatry, in which the patient usually relates directly to the physician.

Obviously, for psychopharmacotherapy to be effective in the disorder for which it is prescribed, the drug must be taken following the prescribed directions. Erratic compliance or running out of medication may cause the patient to undergo what is in effect an abrupt withdrawal of medication. Withdrawal syndromes may sometimes be confused with untoward effects, worsening of the clinical condition, or inadequate medication levels. In some cases, such as when an antipsychotic is used, the patient is at increased risk for an acute dystonic reaction if the physician starts at the optimal dose after the drug has been discontinued for several days or more. In addition, when medication is stopped, it may sometimes require a higher dose of medication to regain the same degree of symptom control. For example, Sleator et al. (1974) found that 7 of 28 hyperactive children who showed clinical worsening during a month-long placebo period after having received methylphenidate for 1 to 2 years required an increase in dose to regain their original clinical improvement. Hence it is very important to emphasize to parents that running out of medication is to be avoided. Many factors may interfere with compliance. Some parents will at times withhold medication if their child appears to be doing well, or, conversely, increase the medication without the physician's approval if behavior worsens, or even administer the drug to the child as a punishment.

When parents or legal guardians seek treatment for their children primarily because of pressure from others such as a school, a child welfare agency, or a court, there may be considerable resistance to both treatment and medication. Some of these parents may delay filling the prescription, lose it, or simply not fill it. Other parents consider it something to be done when convenient, especially if they have to travel any distance to get the prescription filled. If money is involved, even the amount necessary for travel to the pharmacy or to pay for the medication, some families, especially those on public assistance or very limited budgets, may have to delay purchasing the medication for legitimate financial reasons. These issues may come into play each time the prescription is renewed; additionally, it is common in many clinics for parents to miss appointments, including those when medication is to be renewed.

At times, some children and adolescents, both outpatients and inpatients, may actively try to avoid ingesting medication. Their techniques include pretending to place the pill in their mouths and later discarding it, and placing the pill under the tongue or between teeth and the cheek when swallowing and later spitting it out. Compliance in these cases may be improved if the person administering the medication observes it in the mouth and watches the patient swallow it. Crushing the medication may be helpful in some cases, but one must be certain that absorption rates will not be so significantly altered as to cause decreased clinical efficacy or untoward or toxic effects. If available, switching to a liquid form of the drug may be indicated for some patients.

Another factor that influences compliance, particularly in older children and adolescents, is related to untoward effects. For example if they feel "funny" or different or develop a stomachache, they may be more reluctant to take medication. The more responsible a child is for administering his or her own medication, the more likely, in general, that unpleasant, untoward effects will interfere with compliance. Akathisia is a particularly unpleasant untoward effect that Van Putten and Marder (1987) found increased the likelihood of noncompliance in adults receiving antipsychotics. Richardson et al. (1991) reported that children and adolescents who developed parkinsonism while receiving neuroleptics were very aware of the symptoms and described them as "zombie-like" and a reason for noncompliance with outpatient treatment. Sheard (1975) noted that individuals treated for aggressive behavior may tolerate untoward effects poorly and discontinue treatment to avoid them. It is likely that these and other untoward effects would have similar influences on children and adolescents.

Noncompliance may be lessened sometimes if an adequate, understandable explanation of the simple pharmacokinetics of the drug is given to parents and patients when initially discussing medication; for example, the importance of keeping blood levels fairly constant by taking the medication as prescribed can be emphasized and reviewed again if lack of compliance becomes important. Conversely, when parents continue to sabotage treatment either consciously, unconsciously, because of their own psychopathology, or for other reasons, and this behavior seriously interferes with the psychiatric treatment of a child or adolescent, it may be necessary to report the patient to a government agency as a case of medical neglect and request legal intervention. Likewise, it may be necessary to discontinue medication if compliance is very poor or so unacceptably erratic as to be potentially dangerous.

EXPLAINING MEDICATION TO THE CHILD OR ADOLESCENT

The clinician should discuss the medication with the child or adolescent as appropriate to the patient's psychopathology and ability to understand. Giving the patient an opportunity to participate in his or her treatment is helpful for many reasons.

The patient can feel like an active partner in the treatment. This can alleviate feelings of passivity, i.e., that treatment is something over which the patient has no control. Letting the patient know that he or she should pay attention to the effects of the medication in order to report them to the therapist, that the patient will be listened to, and that the information the patient conveys will be considered seriously in regulating the medicine also helps the therapeutic relationship. The patient also can be informed that even though medication may provide some relief or help, it cannot do everything, and he or she still must contribute effort toward reaching the treatment goals. This can be particularly important during adolescence, when issues of autonomy and control over one's own body are normal developmental concerns.

Because the patient is experiencing firsthand the disorder being treated, in many cases valuable information necessary for regulating the medication can be obtained directly. Some quite young children can express whether the medicine makes them feel better, more calm, or quiet; less mad or less like fighting; happier or sadder; less afraid, upset, nervous, or anxious; or worse, sleepy, tired, more bored, madder, or harder to get along with, and so on. Although parents or caretakers can provide much useful information, they may be unaware of some information the patient can provide if time is taken to learn the words or expressions that the child uses to communicate feelings and experiences.

Untoward effects should be explained so that the child or adolescent understands them. The patient's awareness that untoward effects may be transient (e.g., that tolerance for sedation may develop) or reversible with dose reduction may be helpful in gaining cooperation during the titration period. Foreknowledge also increases the sense of control and can decrease fear of some untoward effects. For example, if an acute dystonic reaction is a possibility, it is important to realize how frightening this can be to some patients (and their parents). Discussing beforehand that if this reaction occurs, medicine will help, and the condition will go away can make the experience less frightening. Also, if a rapidly effective oral anticholinergic is made available and patients and parents are aware of what is happening, the medication may be administered earlier in the process, frequently aborting a potentially more severe reaction.

Children who ride bicycles and adolescents who drive a car, motor bike, or motorcycle, or operate potentially dangerous machinery should be cautioned if a medication may cause sedation or other impairment; they should be told to wait until they are sure how they are reacting to the medication before engaging in these activities. Similarly, if an adolescent is likely to use alcohol or other psychoactive drugs, he or she should be warned of possible additive or other adverse effects. Drugs like monoamine oxidase inhibitors cannot be used without very cooperative patients who are able to follow necessary dietary restrictions.

MEDICOLEGAL ASPECTS OF MEDICATING CHILDREN AND ADOLESCENTS

Medicolegal issues usually involve concerns about the clinician's clinical competence. Although it may be obvious, these issues arise primarily when something goes wrong. Incidentally, that "wrong something" may have nothing to do with the clinician's specific treatment or competence but may, for example, be an outcome that displeases the patient or guardian. Even then, for a medicolegal issue to arise, someone who has become aware of it has to decide to pursue the matter legally.

The importance of these issues is that the clinician's relationship with the patient and his or her family or caretakers can either increase or decrease the likelihood of legal proceedings. As a general rule, the better the quality of the relationship and rapport between the physician and the patient and his or her family, the less likelihood there is for legal proceedings to occur. Parents who are angry at their child's physician, who feel neglected or not cared about, are more likely to institute legal proceedings. Taking time to explain what the medicine may and may not do is important; no medication can be guaranteed to be clinically effective and safe for every patient.

If there is a risk a depressed patient may attempt suicide but the patient is not hospitalized, this should be discussed with all concerned parties. The patient may be asked to commit verbally or in writing to a contract to contact the clinician before any attempt to take his or her own life. Legal guardians should be informed of and concur with the decision that their child or ward will not be hospitalized and that, although there is a risk, the degree of risk is acceptable to avoid hospitalization. The guardians should be asked to provide more formal supervision until the depression improves sufficiently. If such measures are carried out and documented and a working rapport established, the risk of legal action and/or liability will be lessened should a suicide attempt be successful or otherwise occur.

The clinician should make a genuine effort to establish a working rapport with parents who have consented under duress to the treatment of their child or adolescent (e.g., because a governmental agency has placed legal pressure on them to comply with treatment), although this is frequently difficult.

Holzer (1989) noted that most if not all malpractice claims occur in cases with either an unexpected clinical outcome or an event that is perceived by the patient (or parents) as avoidable or preventable. The aspects of psychopharmacotherapy that have potential for medicolegal implications parallel this book's entire section on general principles of psychopharmacotherapy. Lawsuits are most frequently brought if something is omitted or if something goes wrong that could reasonably have been prevented. It should be emphasized that proper documentation in the clinical record is essential. If this is not done, the clinician's position is precarious if legal difficulties arise. Particular areas of concern are discussed below.

For a comprehensive overview of malpractice issues in psychiatric practice, the chapter on "Malpractice" in Nurcombe and Partlett's (1994) *Child Mental Health and the Law* is recommended.

Issues Concerning Diagnosis and Implications for Drug Choice and Premedication Work-up

The areas of major concern are making a correct psychiatric diagnosis and being aware of any coexisting medical conditions. Taking accurate medical and psychiatric histories, including previous medications and the patient's response to them, as well as untoward effects and allergic reactions, is essential. Nurcombe (1991) notes that if adverse reactions to a drug or drug interactions occur that could have been predicted by taking an accurate and adequate history, the physician may be held liable. History taking must be followed by a proper premedication work-up; if the patient has a medical condition, the physician must consider how the psychotropic medication would affect that condition and whether there may be interactions with other medications the patient is taking. Some examples of this include: (*a*) making an incorrect diagnosis and prescribing the wrong medication, or failing to detect or recognize coexisting conditions that would contraindicate the chosen medication; (*b*) prescribing a drug that will interact adversely with another medication the patient is taking, or prescribing a drug to which the patient has previously been allergic; or (*c*) failing to perform a baseline and serial ECGs when tricyclics are used because of possible cardiotoxicity.

Issues Concerning Informed Consent

The treatment plan should be discussed and agreed to by the legal guardian and the patient as appropriate for his or her age and understanding. The diagnosis, risks, and benefits of the proposed treatment and alternative treatment possibilities should be reviewed. To give informed consent, a patient (or legal guardian) must be mentally competent, have sufficient information available to make an informed decision, and not be coerced. Adolescents 12 years of age and older should participate formally in developing their treatment plans and in giving informed consent. If this is not possible, it should be so stated in the clinical record. It is wise to have both the legal guardian and, when appropriate, the patient sign the treatment plan and/or an informed consent for medication. If this is not done, at a minimum the clinician must document the discussion of the treatment plan and the response of the patient and legal guardian in the clinical record.

Nurcombe (1991) recommends that the following be discussed:

a. The nature of the condition that requires treatment.
b. The nature and purpose of the proposed treatment and the probability that it will succeed.
c. The risks and consequences of the proposed treatment.
d. Alternatives to the proposed treatment and their attendant risks and consequences.
e. Prognosis with and without the proposed treatment (p. 1132).

Popper (1987a) adds that it should be stated explicitly that there may be unknown risks to taking the medication, especially when using novel psychopharmacological treatments or treatments in which risks versus benefits are uncertain.

Involuntary medication of patients occurs primarily in emergency rooms and on inpatient wards. This is usually permissible in a true emergency, but Nurcombe (1991) cautions that even involuntary commitment to a hospital for psychiatric treatment permits involuntary medication only in narrowly defined circumstances. Administering medication forcibly without judicial approval in a nonemergency situation may be considered battery. Physicians should become thoroughly familiar with their state laws and local hospital policies governing these matters.

Issues Concerning the Administration of Medication

These issues include justification for the decision to use medication in treating the psychiatric condition (risks versus benefits), rationale for the initial drug chosen, and administration of the drug by the appropriate route (orally, intramuscularly, or intravenously) and in a clinically efficacious dose. If a patient is suicidal, the prescribing physician should ascertain to the best of his or her ability and document that sublethal amounts of medication are accessible to the patient and that the supply of medication has been used completely or nearly so before more is prescribed. The clinician must monitor the medication adequately for the duration of the therapy and should either discontinue the medication or attempt to do so at appropriate intervals, or document in the clinical record the reasons for the decision not to follow this protocol.

Examples of behavior that may increase medicolegal risk include failing to prescribe medication for a condition for which most practitioners would prescribe medication, prescribing an inappropriate drug for the diagnosis, using an unsatisfactory rationale to justify the choice of drug, administering an inappropriate dosage for the disorder (e.g., subtherapeutic levels of a tricyclic), or administering medication by an inappropriate route (e.g., continuing to give medication intramuscularly when it is no longer indicated or necessary). A patient's use of prescribed medication to attempt or successfully complete a suicide may also result in legal action.

Deviating from a Manufacturer's Labeling of a Drug

This book discusses many uses of psychoactive medications that are different from those formally recommended by the manufacturer or approved by the FDA for advertising as safe and effective. Many of these off-label uses are medically accepted, but others are not yet common medical practice. Deviating from usual clinical practice increases the risk of legal action. Although legally permissible, using FDA-approved drugs for non-FDA-approved indications and using FDA-approved drugs for approved indications in children below the age limit for which they are approved may increase the potential for liability. Similarly, not adhering to the recommendations of the drug manufacturer (in the package insert or as reprinted in the PDR)—for example, exceeding recommended dosages—should alert the clinician to document carefully the rationale for doing so. In general, however, clinicians are on solid ground if they have assessed the risk/benefit ratio for prescribing a medication for a non-FDA-approved indication and have documented a scientifically reasonable rationale for choosing a particular drug over other possible treatments in the medical record.

In clinical practice, standard treatments and off-label (non-FDA-approved) but clinically accepted treatments that may be efficacious with less risk almost always should be tried before less clinically accepted or riskier medications. Concurrence of a consultant and appropriate psychopharmacological references supporting such use may be helpful when the off-label use is not commonly accepted (Nurcombe, 1991). As a general principle, the more novel the treatment or uncertain the risk/benefit ratio, the more severely disabling should be the condition for which it is used.

Issues Concerned with Documenting Ongoing Appropriate Attention to Medication and Related Matters in the Clinical Record

The patient's clinical record should reflect continued appropriate monitoring of the medication's efficacy, presence or absence of untoward effects, results of laboratory tests or other procedures (e.g., ECG) used to monitor untoward effects, justifications for increases or decreases in dosage or changes in times of administration, decisions to employ a drug holiday or discontinue medication, and the consequences of discontinuing medication, including any change in symptomatology, reexacerbation of symptoms, rebound effects, or withdrawal syndromes such as a withdrawal dyskinesia.

When patients are hospitalized, it is important for the clinician to address in the medical record not only his or her own observations of the patient but also those of other professionals who have reported or recorded behaviors or symptoms that may indicate untoward effects of medication (e.g., unsteadiness of gait reported by a nurse or falling asleep in class reported by a teacher).

Most authorities recommend that children and adolescents who are receiving psychoactive medication should have it discontinued or at least tapered down periodically, typically within 6 months to at most 1 year, to ascertain whether it is still needed or whether a lower dose might be sufficient. That this has been done should be documented in the chart, and if the clinician delays this tapering excessively, the reason should be clearly explained in the chart (e.g., the previous attempt resulted in a severe relapse of symptoms that were difficult to control in a schizophrenic adolescent, or a clinical decision has been reached to delay an attempt to lower or discontinue medication until the completion of the school year because functioning has been marginal even though somewhat improved with medication). Decisions such as these should also be discussed with the parents and the patient and their consent obtained.

Nurcombe's (1991) and Nurcombe and Partlett's (1994) reviews of medicolegal aspects of the entire practice of child and adolescent psychiatry, including specific court cases and decisions, are recommended to the interested reader. Popper (1987a) has written an interesting chapter on ethical considerations of the relationship between obtaining consent for the use of medication from parents and children and adolescents and incomplete or unknown medical knowledge of the risks and long-term effects of psychoactive medication used during childhood and adolescence.

Baseline Assessments Prior to Initiation of Medication

All patients should have a complete medical history and physical and neurological examinations. These examinations are essential to identify any organic factors contributing to the psychiatric symptomatology and any coexisting medical abnormalities. In addition, all drugs may cause untoward physical and psychological effects; hence a baseline examination prior to initiation of psychopharmacotherapy should be mandatory. Relatively little information is available concerning the long-term untoward effects of psychoactive drugs on the growth and development of children and adolescents. Because of this fact as well as the potential medicolegal ramifications, particularly when drugs are used for non-FDA-approved indications, it is recommended that the premedication work-up should be reasonably comprehensive. The reader who wishes a more detailed review of laboratory tests and diagnostic procedures applicable to general psychiatry than that provided below is referred to the helpful book by Rosse et al. (1989).

PHYSICAL EXAMINATION

The physical examination should include recording baseline temperature, pulse and respiration rates, and blood pressure. Height and weight should be entered on standardized growth charts, such as the National Center for Health Statistics Growth Charts (Hamill et al., 1976), so that serial measurements and percentiles may be plotted over time. A pregnancy test should be considered for any adolescent who might be pregnant, because drugs may have known or unknown adverse effects on the developing fetus. As a related issue, if an adolescent is considered to be at significant risk for becoming pregnant despite birth control counseling, certain medications (e.g., lithium) should not be prescribed if at all possible.

LABORATORY TESTS AND DIAGNOSTIC PROCEDURES

The following are frequently recommended premedication laboratory tests and diagnostic procedures. Some of these tests may already have been done as a part of the pediatric/medical evaluation that should be a part of any comprehensive psychiatric evaluation. These tests will be addressed more specifically under each class of medications or, if appropriate, for specific drugs when they are discussed. Obviously, the premedication work-up will be influenced by and should be modified to accommodate any particular abnormal findings in the medical history or examination, such as renal, thyroid, and cardiac abnormalities, or by any initial abnormal laboratory results themselves.

Laboratory tests routinely or frequently recommended as part of a comprehensive, complete, pediatric examination and/or premedication work-up include the following:

1. Complete blood cell count (CBC), differential, and hematocrit
2. Urinalysis
3. Blood urea nitrogen (BUN) level
4. Serum electrolyte levels for sodium (Na+), potassium (K+), chloride (Cl−), calcium (Ca++), and phosphate (PO$_4$−−−) and carbon dioxide (CO$_2$) content.
5. Liver function tests: aspartate aminotransferase (AST) or serum glutamic oxaloacetic transaminase (SGOT), alanine aminotransferase (ALT) or serum glutamic pyruvic transaminase (SGPT), alkaline phosphatase, lactic dehydrogenase (LDH), and bilirubin (total and indirect)
6. Serum lead level determination in children under 7 years of age and in older children when indicated.

Other laboratory tests are often recommended prior to using specific psychoactive medications.

Thyroid Function Tests

Thyroid function tests (thyroxine [T$_4$], triiodothyronine resin uptake [T$_3$RU], and thyroid-stimulating hormone [TSH] or thyrotropin) are recommended prior to the use of tricyclic antidepressants and lithium. Abnormal thyroid function can aggravate cardiac arrhythmias that may occur as an untoward effect of tricyclic antidepressants (PDR, 1995). Lithium has been reported to cause hypothyroidism with lower T$_3$ and T$_4$ levels and elevated I$_{131}$ uptake.

Kidney Function Tests

Because of reported untoward effects of lithium carbonate on the kidney, baseline evaluation of kidney function should be determined. Jefferson et al. (1987) suggest that a baseline serum creatinine and urinalysis are usually adequate and that more extensive testing (e.g., creatinine clearance, 24-hour urine volume, and maximal urine osmolality) is not practical or necessary for most patients.

SPECIAL TESTS

Electrocardiogram

A baseline ECG should be recorded prior to the administration of tricyclic antidepressants to determine any preexisting conduction or other cardiac abnormality because clinically important cardiotoxicity may occur, especially at higher serum levels. The ECG should be monitored with dose increases and periodically thereafter if tricyclics are used (see below under "Tricyclic Antidepressants and Cardiotoxicity").

Lithium may also cause cardiac abnormalities, and an ECG is recommended prior to initiating therapy. Although the ECG may be considered optional in young, healthy subjects, it should be mandatory in any person with a history of or clinical findings suggestive of cardiovascular disease.

Electroencephalogram

An EEG may be considered for patients to whom antipsychotics, tricyclic antidepressants, or lithium will be administered, because all of these drugs have been associated with either lowered threshold for seizures or other EEG changes. This group would include patients who have a history of seizure disorder, who are on an antiepileptic drug for a seizure disorder, or who may be at risk for seizures (e.g., following brain surgery or head injury).

Blanz and Schmidt (1993) reported a significant increase in pathological EEG findings (short biphasic waves) in child and adolescent patients receiving clozapine. Similarly, Remschmidt et al. (1994) reported EEG changes in 16 (44%) of 36 adolescents being treated with clozapine. Baseline EEG and periodic monitoring of EEG while on clozapine should be mandatory.

BASELINE BEHAVIORAL ASSESSMENT

Clinical Observations

Baseline observations and careful characterizations of both behavior and target symptoms must be recorded in the clinical record. These should include direct observations by the clinician in the waiting room, office, playroom, and/or on the ward, as well as those reported by other reliable observers in other locations, such as the home and school. It is important to include usual eating and sleeping patterns, because these may be altered by many drugs. These observations should be described both qualitatively and quantitatively (amplitude and frequency) and the circumstances in which they occur noted in the clinical record.

It is also essential to record an accurate baseline rating in the clinical record before beginning psychopharmacotherapy in children or adolescents who have existing abnormal movements or who are at risk for developing them (e.g., patients diagnosed with autistic disorder or severe mental retardation and/or patients who will be treated with antipsychotics). This documentation is necessary both to follow the patient's clinical course and to be able to differentiate among recrudescence of preexisting involuntary movements, stereotypies, and mannerisms and any subsequent withdrawal dyskinesias or new stereotypies that may occur when medication, particularly an antipsychotic, is discontinued. The availability of these longitudinal data becomes even more critical if the treating physician changes. Although the baseline data can be documented in the clinician's records, the use of a rating scale such as the Abnormal Involuntary Movement Scale (AIMS) ("Rating Scales," 1985) that assesses abnormal movements is strongly recommended.

To be able to assess the efficacy of a specific medication, a baseline observation period, with reasonably stable or worsening target symptoms, is necessary. Other than in emergency situations (e.g., a violent, physically assaultive, and/or severely psychotic individual), observation of the patient for a minimum of 7 to 10 days is recommended before initiating pharmacotherapy. For inpatients, this will permit assessment of the combined effects of hospitalization and a therapeutic milieu and the removal of the identified patient from his or her living situation on the patient's psychopathology and symptoms. For outpatients, this observation period will give the clinician an opportunity to see the effect of the clinical contact and assessment on the symptom expression of the patient and the psychodynamic equilibrium of the family. During this observation period, many children and adolescents, both inpatients and outpatients, will improve sufficiently so that psychopharmacotherapy will no longer be indicated.

Rating Scales

Rating scales are an essential component of psychopharmacological research. They provide a means of recording serial qualitative and quantitative measurements of behaviors, and their interrater reliability can be determined. Two of the most influential publications concerning rating scales and psychopharmacological research in children are the *Psychopharmacology Bulletin's* special issue *Pharmacotherapy of Children* (1973) and its 1985 issue featuring "Rating Scales and Assessment Instruments for Use in Pediatric Psychopharmacology Research" ("Rating Scales," 1985).

Although rating scales are valuable in nonresearch settings, they tend to be used less in clinical practice. Perhaps those most frequently used are the various Conners rating instruments: Conners Teacher Questionnaire (CTQ), Conners Parent-Teacher Questionnaire, Conners Parent Questionnaire (CPQ) (Psychopharmacology Bulletin, 1973). The abbreviated Conners Parent-Teacher Questionnaire (CAPTQ), reproduced as Figure 2.1, is useful in helping to

DEPARTMENT OF HEALTH, EDUCATION, AND WELFARE
HEALTH SERVICES AND MENTAL HEALTH ADMINISTRATION
NATIONAL INSTITUTE OF MENTAL HEALTH

CONNERS PARENT-TEACHER QUESTIONNAIRE

INSTRUCTIONS: Listed below are items concerning children's behavior or the problems they sometimes have. Read each item carefully and decide how much you think this child has been bothered by this problem *at this time:* NOT AT ALL, JUST A LITTLE, PRETTY MUCH, or VERY MUCH. Indicate your choice by circling the number in the appropriate column to the right of each item.

ANSWER ALL ITEMS	Not at All	Just a Little	Pretty Much	Very Much
1. Restless (overactive)	0	1	2	3
2. Excitable, impulsive	0	1	2	3
3. Disturbs other children	0	1	2	3
4. Fails to finish things he starts (short attention span)	0	1	2	3
5. Fidgeting	0	1	2	3
6. Inattentive, distractable	0	1	2	3
7. Demands must be met immediately; frustrated	0	1	2	3
8. Cries	0	1	2	3
9. Mood changes quickly	0	1	2	3
10. Temper outbursts (explosive and unpredictable behavior)	0	1	2	3

	None	Minor	Moderate	Severe
How serious a problem do you think this child has at this time?	0	1	2	3

Figure 2.1. Conners Parent-Teacher Questionnaire. (Modified from Department of Health, Education, and Welfare, Health Services and Mental Health Administration, National Institutes of Health.)

identify patients who have ADHD and to record serial ratings that provide good periodic estimates of the clinical efficacy of medication in the classroom and home environments. The CAPTQ can be completed in a short time because it has only 11 items. The first 10 items are common to the CTQ and the CPQ; the 11th item is an overall estimate of the degree of seriousness of the child's problem at the time of the rating; that item is not included in the following discussion of scoring. A total score of 15 on the first 10 items has been used widely in research as the cut-off for 2 standard deviations (SD) above the mean, and subjects scoring 15 or more points have been considered hyperactive (Sleator, 1986). The mean value of the 10 items of the CAPTQ yields a score comparable to Factor IV, the hyperactivity index, of the CTQ, and a 0.5-point or more decrease in the mean (or a decrease of 5 points in the total score on the first 10 items of the CAPTQ) generally indicates that medication is effecting a meaningful improvement (Greenhill, 1990.)

The AIMS (Fig. 2.2) is a 12-item scale designed to record in detail the occurrence of dyskinetic movements. Abnormal involuntary movements are rated on a 5-point scale from 0 to 4, with 0 being none, 1 being minimal or extreme normal, 2 being mild, 3 being moderate, and 4 being severe. If a procedure is used to activate the movements (e.g., having the patient tap his or her thumb with each finger as rapidly as possible for 10 to 15 seconds separately with the right and then the left hand), movements are rated 1 point lower than those occurring spontaneously. Seven of the items rate abnormal involuntary movements in specific topographies: 4 items concern facial and oral movements, 2 items concern extremity movements, and 1 item concerns trunk movements. Three items are global ratings: 2 by the clinician concern the overall severity of the abnormal movements and the estimated degree of incapacity from them, and a third records the patient's own degree of awareness of the abnormal movements. Using the AIMS will also make it less likely that an area that should be assessed will be omitted inadvertently and will also provide quantitative ratings for following the clinical course. Having a baseline and subsequent AIMS ratings available is most helpful to the initial treating physician in assessing any changes in baseline abnormal involuntary movements increases, decrements, or changes in topography during the course of active treatment with psychoactive medication, as well as during periods of withdrawal from medication. These ratings are often essential to differentiate pre-

existing abnormal involuntary movements from withdrawal dyskinesias. Such ratings are even more helpful when other physicians
may assume the treatment of the patient at a future time.

MEDICATING THE PATIENT: SELECTING THE INITIAL MEDICATION

In general, it is recommended that an FDA-approved standard medication for the patient's age, diagnosis, and target symptoms be chosen initially whenever it is likely to be clinically efficacious. Factors such as selecting the drug with the least risk of serious untoward effects; known previous response(s) of the patient to
psychotropic medication; the responses of siblings, parents, and
other relatives with psychiatric illnesses to psychotropic medication; family history (e.g., a history of Tourette's disorder); and the
clinician's previous experience in using the medication should also
be weighed in choosing the initial and, if necessary, subsequent
drugs.

Generic Versus Trade Preparations

There has been controversy in the literature on the merits of
brand-name drugs, usually the initial, patented preparations of a
medication, and generic preparations that typically enter the market after exclusive patent rights expire and cost considerably less
than the brand-name product. Although the active ingredients in
the various preparations should be pharmaceutically equivalent,
the inert ingredients and the manufacturing processes may vary
and hence the bioavailability of a drug may be significantly different among various preparations.

Many states now permit substitution of generic drugs for drugs
prescribed by brand name under specified conditions. New York
state, for example, requires all prescription forms to have imprinted
on them "This prescription will be filled generically unless pre-
scriber writes 'daw' [dispense as written] in the box below." New
York state publishes a book, *Safe, Effective and Therapeutically
Equivalent Prescription Drugs*, listing approved preparations of various prescription drugs. Pharmacists are directed to "substitute a
less expensive drug product containing the same active ingredients,
dosage form and strength" as the drug originally prescribed, if available (New York State Department of Health, 1988, p. iii). The book
recognizes differences in bioavailability among products. For example, for chlorpromazine it does not authorize substitution of oral

DEPARTMENT OF HEALTH, EDUCATION, AND WELFARE
PUBLIC HEALTH SERVICE
ALCOHOL, DRUG ABUSE, AND MENTAL HEALTH ADMINISTRATION
NATIONAL INSTITUTE OF MENTAL HEALTH

ABNORMAL INVOLUNTARY
MOVEMENT SCALE
(AIMS)

INSTRUCTIONS: Complete Examination Procedure   Code: 0 = None
before making ratings.   1 = Minimal, may be
MOVEMENT RATINGS: Rate highest   extreme normal
severity observed. Rate movements   2 = Mild
that occur upon activation one *less*   3 = Moderate
than those observed spontaneously.   4 = Severe

		(Circle One)
FACIAL AND ORAL MOVEMENTS:	**1. Muscles of Facial Expression** e.g., movements of forehead, eyebrows, periorbital area, cheeks; include frowning, blinking, smiling, grimacing	0 1 2 3 4
	2. Lips and Perioral Area e.g., puckering, pouting, smacking	0 1 2 3 4
	3. Jaw e.g., biting, clenching, chewing, mouth opening, lateral movement	0 1 2 3 4
	4. Tongue Rate only increase in movement both in and out of mouth, NOT inability to sustain movement	0 1 2 3 4
EXTREMITY MOVEMENTS:	**5. Upper** (arms, wrists, hands, fingers) Include choreic movements (i.e., rapid, objectively purposeless, irregular, spontaneous), athetoid movements, (i.e., slow, irregular, complex, serpentine). Do NOT include tremor (i.e., repetitive, regular, rhythmic).	0 1 2 3 4
	6. Lower (legs, knees, ankles, toes) e.g., lateral knee movement, foot tapping, heel dropping, foot squirming, inversion and eversion of foot	0 1 2 3 4
TRUNK MOVEMENTS:	**7. Neck, shoulders, hips** e.g., rocking, twisting, squirming, pelvic gyrations	0 1 2 3 4
GLOBAL JUDGMENTS:	**8. Severity of abnormal movements** None, normal 0 Minimal 1 Mild 2 Moderate 3 Severe 4	

(continues)

Figure 2.2.   Abnormal Involuntary Movement Scale (AIMS). (Modified from Department of Health, Education, and Welfare, Public Health Service, Alcohol, Drug Abuse, and Mental Health Administration, National Institute of Mental Health.)

	9. Incapacitation due to abnormal movements	None, normal	0
	Rate only patient's report	Minimal	1
		Mild	2
GLOBAL		Moderate	3
JUDGMENTS:		Severe	4
	10. Patient's awareness of	No awareness	0
	abnormal movements	Aware, no distress	1
	Rate only patient's report	Aware, mild distress	2
		Aware, moderate distress	3
		Aware, severe distress	4
DENTAL	**11. Current problems with teeth**	No	0
STATUS:	**and/or dentures**	Yes	1
	12. Does patient usually wear	No	0
	dentures?	Yes	1

EXAMINATION PROCEDURE

Either before or after completing the Examination Procedure observe the patient unobtrusively, at rest (e.g., in waiting room).

The chair to be used in this examination should be a hard, firm one without arms.

1. Ask patient whether there is anything in his/her mouth (i.e., gum, candy, etc.) and if there is, to remove it.
2. Ask patient about the *current* condition of his/her teeth. Ask patients if he/she wears dentures. Do teeth or dentures bother patient *now*?
3. Ask patient whether he/she notices any movements in mouth, face, hands, or feet. If yes, ask to describe and to what extent they *currently* bother patient or interfere with his/her activities.
4. Have patient sit in chair with hands on knees, legs slightly apart, and feet flat on floor. (Look at entire body for movements while in this position.)
5. Ask patient to sit with hands hanging unsupported. If male, between legs, if female and wearing a dress, hanging over knees. (Observe hands and other body areas.)
6. Ask patient to open mouth. (Observe tongue at rest within mouth.) Do this twice.
7. Ask patient protrude tongue. (Observe abnormalities of tongue movement.) Do this twice.
■ 8. Ask patient to tap thumb, with each finger, as rapidly as possible for 10–15 seconds; separately with right hand, then with left hand. (Observe facial and leg movements.)
9. Flex and extend patient's left and right arms (one at a time). (Note any rigidity and rate on DOTES.)
10. Ask patient to stand up. (Observe in profile. Observe all body areas again, hips included.)
■ 11. Ask patient to extend both arms outstretched in front with palms down. (Observe trunk, legs, and mouth.)
■ 12. Have patient walk a few paces, turn, and walk back to chair. (Observe hands and gait.) Do this twice.

Activated movements

Figure 2.2. Abnormal Involuntary Movement Scale (continued).

solid immediate-release products because of potential bioequivalence problems.

The FDA Center for Drug Evaluation and Research publishes a book, *Approved Drug Products with Therapeutic Equivalence Evaluations* (the "Orange Book"), which lists drugs, both prescription and nonprescription, approved by the FDA on the basis of safety and effectiveness. The list gives the FDA's evaluations of the therapeutic equivalence of prescription drugs that are available from multiple sources. It classifies drug preparations into two basic categories: A ratings, which are given to drug products that the FDA considers to be therapeutically equivalent to other pharmaceutically equivalent products, for which there are no known or suspected bioequivalence problems or actual or potential problems are thought to have been satisfactorily resolved; and B ratings, which are drug products that the FDA does not at this time consider to be therapeutically equivalent to other pharmaceutically equivalent products.

The 1988 FDA "Orange Book," for example, rates preparations of chlorpromazine for oral administration as "BP," indicating that there are potential bioequivalence problems among these preparations. Oral preparations of nortriptyline are rated "BD," indicating that there have been documented bioequivalence problems when a pharmaceutically equivalent drug from another source was substituted. Dubovsky (1987) reported a case of severe nortriptyline intoxication due to changing from a generic to a trade preparation, which seemed to result from the significantly greater bioavailability of the trade preparation.

These comments are not a recommendation for any preparation over any other but are meant to inform the clinician that different preparations of the same medication of the same strength may have different bioavailabilities, and that when they are substituted for one another, there is a potential for significant clinical repercussions. If prescriptions are written that may be filled with various generic preparations, it is prudent for the physician to inform the patient or responsible adult that if the medication is different when refilled to inform him or her and to note any changes in symptoms or feelings after switching to a new preparation. Although changes in manufacturer may occur at times even when prescriptions are filled at the same pharmacy, the likelihood of a change in manufacturer increases when different pharmacies are used. If a patient runs out of medication while traveling and must obtain the drug(s) from a new source, a change of manufacturer may be more likely. Hence it is worthwhile to remember to ascertain that a patient has sufficient medication before going to summer camp or traveling.

Standard and Nonstandard Treatments

In this book, standard treatments will be considered those treatments that have been approved by the FDA for advertising and interstate commerce. This implies that the drug has demonstrated clinical efficacy and that its use is substantially safe. The FDA's legal authority over how marketed drugs are used, the dosages employed, and related matters is limited to regulating what the manufacturer may recommend and must disclose in the package insert or labeling. "The prescription of a drug for an unlabeled (off-label) indication is entirely proper if the proposed use is based on rational scientific theory, expert medical opinion, or controlled clinical studies" (American Medical Association, 1993, p. 14).

Over the past 2 decades, a substantial body of clinical and investigational data has accumulated on using FDA-approved drugs to treat children below the recommended age (e.g., imipramine to treat major depressive disorder in children under 12 years of age), using FDA-approved drugs to treat children and adolescents for non-FDA-approved (off-label) indications (e.g., lithium to treat aggressive conduct disorder in any age group and tricyclic antidepressants to treat ADHD), and using drugs before they were approved by the FDA for any indication (investigational drugs) to treat psychiatric disorders in children and adolescents (e.g., clomipramine and fluvoxamine maleate).

Lithium and tricyclic and SSRI antidepressants are, at present, the most clinically important of the FDA-approved drugs used for nonapproved (off-label) indications in children and adolescents. There appears to be a growing consensus among child psychiatrists that the risks of using lithium and tricyclic and SSRI antidepressants for non-FDA-approved indications are often preferable to using antipsychotics that increase the risks of impairing cognitive functioning and carry significant risk of producing tardive dyskinesia. This will be discussed in more detail in the specific drug section of the book.

DRUG INTERACTIONS

Many psychoactive drugs have significant interactions with other medications. It is essential to be aware of any medication, prescription or otherwise, that the patient may be taking concurrently and to evaluate the potential interaction.

As part of the medical history, inquiries should be made about all medications, including those prescribed by other physicians, over-the-counter preparations used even occasionally by the patient, and, as appropriate, alcohol and illicit or recreational drug use. Parents or caretakers and patients, as appropriate to their age and mental abilities, should be instructed to inform any physicians who may treat them of the psychoactive medication(s) currently being taken. Similarly, patients the clinician is treating with psychoactive medication should be instructed to report at the next appointment if another physician prescribes any other medication for them or if they take any other drugs, over the counter or illicit, on their own initiative.

If substance abuse is known or suspected, screening of urine and/or blood for toxic substances may be indicated.

Drug interactions are discussed for each of the classes of psychoactive drugs. An attempt has been made to emphasize the most important interactions and those interactions most likely to be encountered by the physician who is treating psychiatrically disturbed children and adolescents.

It is beyond the scope of this book to review all possible drug interactions. It is the prescribing physician's responsibility to attempt to determine any other drugs his or her patient is taking and to assess any potentially adverse interactions of the medications before prescribing a new medication. The package insert, current PDR (1995), current *Drug Interactions and Side Effects Index* (1995), *Drug Facts and Comparisons* (1995), *Drug Interactions in Psychiatry* (Ciraulo et al., 1989), or other suitable reference should be consulted. When appropriate and with the patient's consent, any other physicians treating the patient should be contacted so that a comprehensive treatment regimen that addresses safely both the psychiatric and the medical disorders of the patient may be mutually developed.

REGULATING THE MEDICATION

Selecting the Initial Dosage

It is recommended that the treating physician initially prescribe a low dose, which will be either ineffective or inadequate for most patients. Although this cautious approach may lengthen the time necessary to reach a therapeutic dose, it is worthwhile for several reasons. First, pharmacokinetics vary not only among various age groups but also among individuals of a specific age. For genetic and other reasons, some individuals may be highly sensitive and responsive to a given medication or slow metabolizers, whereas others may be relatively resistant or nonresponsive. By beginning with a low dose, the physician will avoid starting at a dose that is already in excess of the optimal therapeutic dose for a few patients, and those children and adolescents who are good responders at low dosages of medication will not be missed.

If the initial dose is too high, the therapeutic range for these low-dose responders will not be explored and only untoward effects, which may at times even be confused with worsening of target symptoms, will be seen. Hence a potentially beneficial medication may be needlessly excluded. For example, with stimulants a worsening of behavior may occur when optimal therapeutic doses for a specific patient have been exceeded. Second, with some drugs (e.g., methylphenidate) there is no significant relationship between serum level and clinical response. Third, excessive initial dosage may also cause behavioral toxicity, particularly in younger children. Behavioral toxicity may occur before other side effects and includes such symptoms as worsening of target symptoms, hyperactivity or hypoactivity, aggressiveness, increased irritability, mood changes, apathy, and decreased verbal productions (Campbell et al., 1985). Fourth, some untoward effects of the drug may be eliminated or minimized; for example, acute dystonic reactions of antipsychotics and some untoward effects of lithium carbonate appear to be related in many cases to both serum levels and the rapidity of increase in serum level, and sedation may be less of a problem if dosage is increased gradually (Green et al., 1985).

Timing of Drug Administration

Scheduling Dosages.   Times chosen for administration of the drug and the number of times the drug is administered per day should be related to the pharmacokinetics of the drug; for example, stimulants are most frequently given around breakfast and lunch, whereas antipsychotics may initially be given three or four times daily to reduce the risk of sedation and acute dystonic reactions. Once dosage has been stabilized, it may be clinically more convenient and may sometimes increase compliance if medications that have longer half-lives are administered only once or twice daily.

Pharmacokinetics and developmentally determined pharmacodynamic factors must still take precedence over convenience. For example, it may be possible to give the entire daily dose of an antipsychotic at bedtime to children and adolescents, whereas because younger children metabolize tricyclic antidepressants differently than adolescents and adults and they may be more sensitive to car-

diotoxic effects, it is recommended that these drugs continue to be administered to children and younger adolescents in divided doses.
Drug Holidays. Because of the untoward effects of medication and their known and unknown effects on the growth, maturation, and development of children and adolescents, it is universally agreed that it is prudent to use medication in as low a dose and for as short a time as is clinically expedient. For some children, "drug holidays" may be a useful means of minimizing the cumulative amount of medication taken over time. The feasibility and type of drug holidays vary with the diagnosis and the severity of the disorder.

When stimulant medication is needed primarily to improve behavior (increase attention span and decrease hyperactivity and sometimes conduct problems) for classroom functioning, as with some ADHD children, it is often possible to withhold medication on weekends and on school holidays and vacations, including the entire summer. This is particularly important if there appears to be evidence of any suppression of height and weight percentiles, because there may be catch-up or compensatory growth following discontinuation of stimulant medication.

Sometimes parents find that their hyperactive child is not a serious management problem without medication at home but that difficulties arise when the child accompanies them on a shopping excursion or goes to a birthday party. In cases like this, when the parents' judgment can be trusted and medication is not used as a punishment, an understanding with the parents and child that medication may be used occasionally on weekends or vacations in situations that are particularly difficult for the child may be therapeutically indicated.

There is reasonable concern about the possibility of the development of an irreversible tardive dyskinesia in children and adolescents who receive long-term therapy with antipsychotic medication. There is some evidence that the development of tardive dyskinesia may be associated with both the total amount of antipsychotic drug ingested and the duration of treatment, although constitutional vulnerabilities to developing tardive dyskinesia also appear to play an important role (Jeste & Wyatt, 1982). Consequently, possible means of reducing the total amount of an antipsychotic drug ever taken may be clinically important in reducing the likelihood of developing tardive dyskinesia.

Newton et al. (1989) compared 6-week periods of haloperidol daily and 6-week periods of haloperidol with repeated weekly 2-day drug holidays in a crossover experiment with seven older adult schizophrenic patients. Serum haloperidol levels were reduced by about 25% during holiday periods, with no significant change in mental status, severity of psychiatric symptoms, or scores on scales rating movement disorders.

Similarly, Perry et al. (1989) reported on 52 child outpatients aged 2.3 years to 7.9 years diagnosed with infantile autism, full syndrome, who were treated with haloperidol for 6 months. The subjects were assigned on a random basis in a double-blind protocol to receive haloperidol continuously (daily) or discontinuously (5 days per week with 2 contiguous days of placebo). There was no significant clinical difference between the groups, and in both groups children who had symptoms of irritability, angry and labile affect, and uncooperativeness responded best. The incidence of untoward effects, including tardive and withdrawal dyskinesia, did not vary significantly between the two groups.

If additional studies continue to find no significant difference in therapeutic efficacy between antipsychotic drugs administered 7 days versus 5 days per week, this may become the preferred method of long-term maintenance to decrease the total cumulative amount of antipsychotic ingested over time, in the hope of diminishing the incidence of irreversible tardive dyskinesia; it also has the additional benefit of reducing the cost of medication by nearly 30%.

Dosage Increases

Changes in medication level should be based on the clinical response of the patient, and the rationale for each change should be documented in the clinical record. Knowledge of the characteristic time frame of response for a particular drug and diagnosis should influence these decisions. Thus the clinician may increase dosage once or twice weekly in some cases, when using stimulants or neuroleptics. On the other hand, the clinical efficacy of tricyclic antidepressants may not be fully apparent for several weeks when used to treat major depressive disorder. Once-daily dosage has reached a level that is usually associated with clinical response, increasing the dose because of a failure to respond during the first 2 or 3 weeks of treatment is not psychopharmacologically sound practice unless serum drug levels are being monitored and are thought to be in the subtherapeutic range.

Titration of Medication

The goal of the clinician is to achieve meaningful therapeutic benefits for the patient with the fewest possible untoward effects. Here again it is recommended that risks versus benefits be assessed. To do so scientifically, however, it is necessary to explore the dose range of a patient's response. Unless there are extenuating circumstances, it is usually advisable to continue raising the dose level until one of the following events occurs:

1. Entirely adequate symptom control is established.
2. The upper limit of the recommended dosage (or higher level if commonly accepted) has been reached.
3. Untoward effects that preclude a further increase in dose have occurred.
4. After a measurable improvement in target symptoms, a plateau in improvement or a worsening of symptoms occurs with further increases in dose.

Unless this procedure is followed, an injustice may be done to the patient. This occurs most frequently when there is some behavioral improvement and the treating clinician stabilizes the dosage at that point. Further significant improvement that might have occurred had a higher dose been given is missed. It is recommended that the next higher dose or two should be explored. If there is significant additional improvement, the therapist in consultation with the patient and his or her parents can make a judgment regarding whether the benefits outweigh the risks from the additional dosage.

Determining the Optimal Dose

Once the upper limit of the therapeutic dose range has been explored for a specific patient, the lowest possible dose that produces the desired effects should be determined. This is considered the optimal dose for a specific patient. In clinical practice, this may be a compromise, and amelioration of target symptoms to an acceptable degree may occur only when some untoward effects are also present.

In those cases in which either no significant therapeutic benefit occurs or untoward effects prevent employment of a clinically meaningful therapeutic dose, a trial of a different medication must be considered. Clinicians should not continue to prescribe medication in doses that do not result in significant clinical improvement.

UNTOWARD EFFECTS (SIDE EFFECTS)

All drugs, including placebos, have untoward effects or side effects. Actually, if one excludes allergic and idiosyncratic reactions, many untoward effects are as much a characteristic of the pharmacological make-up of a specific drug and are as predictable as the drug's therapeutic effects. Individual patients may vary as much in their development of untoward effects to a drug as in their therapeutic responses to it.

It is sometimes useful to think of untoward effects as the "unwanted effects" of the drug for the specific patient and therapeutic indication. For a different patient and situation, an untoward or side effect will actually become the desired therapeutic action of the drug. For example, sedation, which may be an untoward effect when a benzodiazepine is prescribed for anxiolysis, is the desired result when a benzodiazepine is prescribed as a soporific. Similarly, appetite suppression is usually an undesired effect of stimulants prescribed for ADHD but the action of choice when used in treating exogenous obesity.

Many untoward effects are related to dose or serum levels, but others are not. They may occur almost immediately (e.g., an acute dystonic reaction) or be delayed for years (e.g., tardive dyskinesia). They may be life threatening or fatal, or relatively innocuous. There is also evidence that the untoward effects of a specific drug may differ according to age and/or diagnosis of the subjects. For example, haloperidol produced excessive sedation in hospitalized school-age aggressive-conduct-disordered children on doses of 0.04 to 0.21 mg/kg/day (Campbell et al., 1984b) but not in preschoolers with autistic disorder on doses of 0.019 to 0.217 mg/kg/day (Anderson et al., 1984).

A thorough knowledge of the most important and frequent side effects of the medications considered is essential and will often play a decisive role in which medication is selected and/or which dosage is scheduled. For example, if a schizophrenic youngster has insomnia, the clinician may select a low-potency antipsychotic and adjust the dosage schedule so that any sedation will aid the child in falling asleep. As an added benefit, risk of an acute dystonic reaction is lower than if a high-potency antipsychotic drug had been chosen.

Likewise, the management of unwanted effects is a vital component of pharmacotherapy. In clinical practice, careful attention to unwanted effects and flexibility about the time and amounts of specific doses may enable one to obtain a satisfactory clinical result with a minimal or acceptable level of untoward effects that is not possible if a fixed dosage schedule is used, as in some research protocols. Thus one can adjust medication levels slowly and in small increments, or divide doses unequally over the day (e.g., giving more in the morning or more before bed, or the entire daily dose at bedtime).

The clinician must remember that the ability to understand untoward effects and verbalize unusual sensations, feelings, or discomfort not only varies among individual children but is developmentally determined. Younger children spontaneously report untoward effects less frequently than older children. Hence the younger the child, the more essential it becomes for caretakers to be actively looking for untoward effects and for the physician to ask the patient about untoward effects in language appropriate to the understanding of the child.

It is essential that the clinician examine the patient for the development of untoward effects frequently during the period when the medication is being regulated, at regular intervals during maintenance therapy, and during scheduled periodic withdrawals of the medication. For example, with antipsychotic drugs one should look particularly for sedation and extrapyramidal side effects, the development of abnormal movements, and, during drug withdrawal periods, any evidence of a withdrawal dyskinesia. Completion of the AIMS as described above is recommended as an aid in quantifying and following abnormal movements over time.

MONITORING OF SERUM LEVELS OF DRUGS AND/OR OF THEIR METABOLITES

Morselli et al. (1983) and Gualtieri et al. (1984a) reviewed the pharmacokinetics of psychoactive drugs used in child and adolescent psychiatry and the clinical relevance of determining their serum or blood levels. Determining blood or plasma levels of drugs and/or their metabolites is most useful when accurate measurements of all significant active metabolites of a drug are available and there is a known relationship between the clinical effects of the drug and serum concentration (Gualtieri et al., 1984a).

Clinically, the monitoring of serum levels is useful to verify compliance and to be certain that adequate therapeutic serum levels are available (i.e., that values fall within the therapeutic window) and thus to avoid discontinuing a trial of medication before clinically effective serum levels have been reached or, conversely, to avoid inadvertently reaching toxic serum levels.

School-aged children often have more efficient physiological systems for drug metabolism and excretion than do adults. As a result, doses comparable to those administered to adults, either on a total daily dose or a dose-per-unit-weight basis, may result in subtherapeutic serum levels in children and younger adolescents. This could be one factor contributing to the clinical observation that children with schizophrenia, as a group, appear to show less dramatic clinical improvement than adolescents and adults, when administered neuroleptics (Green, 1989). It will be necessary to measure antipsy-chotic serum levels to determine if this lack of improvement is due to subtherapeutic levels in some cases, because some children may also show clinical improvement at lower serum levels than adults (Rivera-Calimlim et al., 1979).

Meyers et al. (1980) reported the case of a 13-year-old prepubes-cent boy diagnosed as having schizophrenia who required a dose of haloperidol of at least 30 mg/day to reach therapeutic serum neu-roleptic levels. Monitoring serum levels of antipsychotic drugs thus may yield clinical information that is, at times, extremely useful clinically. If a child or adolescent does not have a satisfactory re-sponse to usual doses of antipsychotic drugs, serum neuroleptic lev-els should be determined, if available, before deciding to discontinue the drug.

In addition to age-related differences in pharmacokinetics, re-markable interindividual variations occur. For example, Berg et al. (1974) reported that a 14-year-old girl with bipolar manic-depres-sive disorder required up to 2400 mg of lithium daily to maintain serum lithium levels of 1 mEq/liter. Her father had the same disor-der and also required unusually high doses of lithium to reach ther-apeutic levels.

At the present time regular determinations of serum levels should be considered mandatory when lithium carbonate, anti-epileptic drugs, or tricyclic antidepressants are used in treating chil-dren and adolescents. In current practice, for example, monitoring of drug and metabolite serum levels is of considerable practical im-portance in the use of the tricyclic antidepressants. This monitoring is needed because there is minimal correlation between dose and serum level, and serum levels are correlated significantly with clin-ical response and/or with potentially serious untoward effects (e.g., cardiotoxicity). For example, Puig-Antich et al. (1987) have empha-sized that they found no predictors of total maintenance plasma lev-els, including dosage, in their prepubertal subjects treated with imipramine for major depressive disorder. They also reported that positive therapeutic response to imipramine in prepubertal children was strongly correlated with serum levels over 150 ng/ml.

Similarly, Biederman and colleagues (1989b) reported that de-sipramine serum levels varied an average of 16.5-fold at four differ-ent dose levels in 31 children and adolescents diagnosed with at-tention deficit disorder (ADD). These authors, however, found no significant linear relationship between the total daily dose or weight-corrected (mg/kg) daily dose and the steady-state serum desipramine level and any outcome measure, including clinical improvement. There was a tendency for serum desipramine levels in subjects who were rated very much or much improved on the Clinical Global Improvement scale to average 60.8% higher than in unimproved subjects.

Morselli et al. (1983) also emphasized that monitoring drug plasma levels of haloperidol, chlorpromazine, imipramine, and clomipramine is particularly helpful in optimizing long-term treatment with these agents.

On the other hand, a detailed review of the pharmacokinetics and actions of methylphenidate concluded that "blood MPH [methylphenidate] levels are not statistically related to clinical response, nor are they likely to prove clinically helpful until this lack of correlation is understood" (Patrick et al., 1987, p. 1393).

Serum levels are also mandatory when antiepileptic drugs are being used for control of seizures, although this use is not reviewed in this book. When antiepileptic drugs are used for other psychiatric indications, such as control of aggression or as mood stabilizers, effective serum levels are thought to be in the same range as when they are used to control seizures. Monitoring of serum levels (both drug and significant metabolites) will become increasingly more important for other drugs used in child and adolescent psychiatry as their determinations become more readily available and correlations with clinical efficacy and untoward effects are established.

LENGTH OF TIME TO CONTINUE MEDICATION

Children and adolescents are immature, developing organisms. Because of concerns about long-term untoward effects such as tardive and withdrawal dyskinesias and growth retardation as well as our inadequate knowledge of other long-term untoward effects of psychopharmacological agents on their biological and psychological maturation, there is virtually unanimous agreement that medication should be given for as short a period as possible.

The vicissitudes of the natural courses of psychiatric illnesses in children and adolescents are often not predictable for specific individuals. It is to be hoped, especially when there is a significant psychosocial etiological factor, that medication will augment the child's response to other therapeutic interventions and enhance his or her social and academic functioning, maturation, and development. Once real gains are made and internalized, the cycle of failures broken, and the maladaptive patterns replaced with more appropriate ones, it may be possible to discontinue the drug and maintain therapeutic gains. Even in chronic conditions with strong biological underpinnings, such as pervasive developmental disorder, schizophrenia, and depression, the clinical course may spontaneously vary so that in some patients psychoactive medication may be reduced or even discontinued.

Periodic Withdrawal/Tapering of Medication

It is usually considered mandatory to discontinue psychotropic medications (or to attempt to do so) in child and adolescent patients on a regular basis, certainly no less frequently than every 6 months to 1 year. There may be occasional exceptions to this—for example, the long-term prophylactic use of lithium carbonate or an antidepressant to prevent recurrences of mood disorders, or not withdrawing an antipsychotic in a child or adolescent being treated for a schizophrenia who has experienced serious relapses during prior withdrawal attempts. Whenever medication is continued beyond 6 to 12 months, it is important to document the clinical reasons for doing so in the medical record.

Withdrawal Syndromes/Untoward Effects

Rapidly metabolized drugs such as methylphenidate and amphetamines may be discontinued abruptly. However, with these drugs, which have short half-lives, there may be some rebound effect during routine daily administration of the drug as serum levels decline in late afternoon or evening.

It is recommended that most medications, especially those with longer serum half-lives, be gradually reduced rather than stopped abruptly in order to minimize the likelihood of developing withdrawal syndromes. The clinician should continue to complete the AIMS in patients who had preexisting abnormal movements prior to initiation of medication that may have been masked or ameliorated, or who are otherwise at risk for developing abnormal movements following withdrawal. If a withdrawal dyskinesia emerges upon discontinuing an antipsychotic drug, every effort should be made to keep the patient off antipsychotics. Any abnormal movements should continue to be recorded on the AIMS.

Gualtieri and his colleagues (1984b) reported both physical withdrawal symptoms, such as decreased appetite, nausea and vomiting, diarrhea and sweating, and acute behavioral deterioration, in about 10% of children and adolescents after their withdrawal from long-term treatment with antipsychotics. Both types of withdrawal symptoms ceased spontaneously within 8 weeks. It is extremely important that the clinician recognize that such symptoms may be expected withdrawal effects and that they are not necessarily a return of premedication symptoms. The symptoms must be monitored qualitatively and quantitatively over a sufficient period to see if they diminish, as would be expected with a withdrawal syndrome, or if they are an indication that the underlying psychiatric disorder still requires medication for symptom amelioration.

When tricyclics are withdrawn abruptly or too rapidly, some children experience a flu-like withdrawal syndrome resulting from cholinergic rebound. This characteristically includes gastrointestinal symptoms such as nausea, abdominal discomfort and pain, vomiting, and fatigue. Tapering the medication down over a 10-day period rather than abruptly withdrawing it will usually avoid this effect or significantly diminish the withdrawal syndrome. The clinician is cautioned that in patients with poor compliance, who in essence may undergo periodic self-induced acute withdrawals, the withdrawal syndrome may be confused with untoward effects, inadequate dose levels, or worsening of the underlying psychiatric disorder.

In significant numbers of cases, after an initial treatment period of varying duration, medication may no longer be required or adequate symptom control can be maintained on a lower maintenance dose. For example, Sleator et al. (1974) administered a 1-month-long period of placebo to 28 of 42 hyperactive children who had been treated with methylphenidate for between 1 and 2 years. Eleven of the 28 were able to continue performing adequately behaviorally and academically without medication. Seventeen of the 28 showed worsening during the placebo period; of the 17, 10 functioned well when their initial dose was resumed, whereas 7 needed an increase in dose to maintain their original gains.

In contrast, over time, occasionally higher doses may be required to maintain gains. This may reflect a worsening of the psychiatric disorder per se or a developmental/maturational effect, as in a child with autistic disorder who becomes both stronger and more aggressive as he or she enters adolescence. In other cases, the need for increased medication may be a consequence of an individual's normal physiological maturation's altering the drug's pharmacokinetics and/or normal or excessive weight gain.

•••••••••••••••••••••••••••••••

Specific
Drug
Treatments

Introduction

Child psychopharmacology is a relatively new field. The 1937 publication by Charles Bradley reporting the effects of administering racemic amphetamine sulfate (Benzedrine) to 30 children aged 5 to 14 years with various behavioral disturbances is usually considered to mark the beginning of the modern era of child psychopharmacology.

More than 20 years later, the first book concerned exclusively with psychopharmacological research in child psychiatry, *Child Research in Psychopharmacology,* evolved out of the 1958 Conference on Child Research in Psychopharmacology sponsored by the National Institute of Mental Health (Fisher, 1959). The book contains an annotated list of 159 references of studies of the effects of psychopharmacological agents administered to children with psychiatric problems, beginning with Bradley's 1937 publication. Interestingly, M. Molitch and coworkers also published, in 1937, three papers concerning the use of amphetamine sulfate in children, including two placebo-controlled studies (Molitch & Eccles, 1937; Molitch & Poliakoff, 1937; Molitch & Sullivan, 1937). Two of the studies found that amphetamine sulfate improved scores of children on intelligence tests, and one reported that 86% of 14 enuretic boys who had not responded to placebo were dry when given increasing doses of amphetamine sulfate and reverted to bedwetting within 2 weeks after the drug was discontinued.

In the 1950s the classes of drugs currently most important in general psychiatry were introduced: the antipsychotics (chlorpromazine and other compounds), the antidepressants, and lithium carbonate. The benzodiazepines, in particular diazepam and chlordiazepoxide, were introduced into clinical psychiatric practice in the early 1960s. Because of increased difficulties in conducting psychopharmacological research and of obtaining FDA approval of the safety and efficacy of psychoactive drugs in children and younger adolescents, the investigation and introduction into clinical practice of psychoactive drugs in children has always lagged somewhat behind that for adults. Weiner and Jaffe (1985) have written a brief but interesting overview of the history of child and adolescent psychopharmacology.

The reader who wishes an in-depth review of major issues of the past decade, spanning the entire field of psychopharmacology, is referred to *Psychopharmacology: The Third Generation of Progress* (Meltzer, 1987). Texts focusing entirely or significantly on child and adolescent psychopharmacology include those by Aman and Singh (1988), Campbell, Green, and Deutsch (1985), Gadow (1986a, 1986b), Klein, Gittelman, Quitkin, and Rifkin (1980), Weiner (1977, 1985), Rosenberg, Holttum, and Gershon (1994), Werry (1978), and Werry and Aman (1993).

In most instances, reviews of the literature establishing the clinical efficacy and safety of standard FDA-approved treatments for the psychiatric disorders of children and adolescents are not included in this book. Readers who wish to review the research data establishing these standard treatments will find such information to be readily accessible in the texts cited above.

Section II of this book summarizes the standard treatments but additionally focuses in greater detail on research into new and not yet approved uses of drugs in child and adolescent psychiatry and reviews these studies. Some knowledge of psychopharmacological research principles and techniques is essential to critically evaluate the data that appear in the psychiatric literature and to make informed clinical decisions about whether a trial of a particular drug is warranted for a particular patient.

Most important psychopharmacological research designs include comparison of the drug being investigated with either placebo or a drug approved as a standard treatment for the psychiatric disorder in question. Hence it is important to have a basic understanding of placebos.

Placebos

According to the *Oxford English Dictionary* (OED) (1933), the English word "placebo" was directly adopted from the Latin word meaning "I shall be pleasing or acceptable." By 1811 it was defined in *Hooper's Medical Dictionary* (OED, 1933) as "any medicine adapted more to please than benefit the patient." In 1982 the supplement to the OED added the following definition of placebo, which fairly accurately described its current use in psychopharmacological research: "A substance or procedure which a patient accepts as a medicine or therapy but which actually has no specific therapeutic activity for his condition or is prescribed in the belief that it has no such activity." Although placebos are often comprised of substances thought to be inert, in psychopharmacological research, placebos may also contain active ingredients chosen to simulate untoward effects of the drug to which the placebo is being compared. The purpose of this is to keep all participants "blind" by making it more difficult for patients and observers to distinguish between drug and placebo based solely on the drug's untoward effects.

Placebos play a crucial role in clinical psychopharmacological research by providing nonspecific treatment effects for comparison with the drug under investigation. These nonspecific psychological and physiological changes are not drug specific and may be measured by rating scales (Prien, 1988). These changes include both beneficial and untoward reactions produced by the expectations the patient or observers have about the drug, natural fluctuations in the clinical course of the disease as well as spontaneous alterations in the patient's condition that may have nothing to do with the illness under consideration, effects of the relationship between the patient and therapist and other medical staff, and other unknown effects.

Because of these nonspecific effects, even "inert" placebos have side effects. These commonly may include such symptoms as fatigue, tiredness, anxiety, muscle aches, nausea, diarrhea, constipation, dry mouth, dysmenorrhea, and behavioral changes such as increased or decreased aggressiveness, impulsiveness, attention span, or irritability. These are often symptoms that might appear periodically in the general population. It is the difference in incidence and severity of these unwanted effects between placebo and drug that is important.

The most methodologically sound use of a placebo for testing a new medication is a double-blind, randomized, parallel-groups design (Prien, 1988). Stanley (1988) has written an interesting article concerning ethical and clinical considerations in the use of placebos that considered such factors as withholding medication during a placebo period and whether treatment may be ethically withheld in a placebo-controlled trial when a known treatment is available. Prien (1988) offered six alternative study designs for use when it is not possible to use a double-blind, randomized, parallel-groups design and discussed some of their limitations. White et al. (1985) edited a fascinating book concerning the theory, ethics, use in research and clinical practice, and mediating mechanisms of placebos.

Evaluating Research Studies

Efficacy and safety are determined by a statistically significant benefit with acceptable untoward effects of the new medication compared with placebo. Statistics, however, inform us about groups of patients, not individuals. Hence if etiologically dissimilar groups are subsumed under the same diagnosis, a few patients may truly benefit, but their improvement could be so diluted by the larger majority who did not benefit that the drug may show no statistically significant benefit. Some researchers now note whether there are strong individual responders in a drug study even when there is no statistical difference between experimental and control groups. Thus individual case reports, studies of relatively small numbers, and open studies should not be summarily dismissed.

In evaluating the literature on child and adolescent psychopharmacology, it is important to remember that whether a drug is statistically significantly better than another drug or placebo does not necessarily mean that the drug is an optimal treatment for a given condition or for a specific child or adolescent. The drug may be effective only in certain environments (e.g., a laboratory) and cannot be generalized to more ordinary circumstances, or it may improve only certain symptoms but not affect other major target symptoms to a clinically meaningful degree, or the overall improvement may be relatively modest with significant symptoms or deficits remaining. For example, Sprague and Sleator (1977) found that 0.3 mg/kg of methylphenidate produced optimal enhancement of learning short-term memory tasks in hyperkinetic children in the laboratory, but 1 mg/kg of methylphenidate produced the maximum improvement of social behavior in the classroom as shown by ratings on the Abbreviated Conners Rating Scale. Another example is that although children with autistic disorder have shown statistically significant improvements with several drugs, the degree of their improvement is typically modest, with marked residual deficits remaining, and at present no drug is satisfactory for treatment of this condition (Green, 1988).

In evaluating research, diagnostic criteria and the diagnostic heterogeneity/homogeneity of the sample, and both the severity of the patients included and the clinical setting in which the drug was given, must be evaluated. Thus until the formalization by DSM-III (1980) of diagnostic distinctions between schizophrenia with childhood onset and autistic disorder (or their equivalents), both were subsumed under the diagnosis of schizophrenia, childhood type; many studies included diagnostically heterogeneous samples or the composition of the sample cannot be determined, rendering interpretation of the studies difficult or impossible (Green, 1989).

Gadow and Poling (1988) provide another relevant example. They noted that stimulant medication is not commonly prescribed for the mentally retarded in residential facilities where most of the residents are usually severely or profoundly retarded. They pointed out that some reviews of the use of stimulants in the mentally retarded falling into these diagnostic categories suggested that stimulants might not be useful in treating behavior disorders in the retarded and could even exacerbate attention deficit in these patients. Gadow and Poling (1988) noted that the large majority of mentally retarded individuals are not in institutions and that they are prescribed stimulants for management of disturbed behavior, particularly hyperactivity, much more frequently and with more favorable results than one might expect from reading the literature. In fact, these authors concluded that stimulants were highly effective in diminishing conduct problems and hyperactivity for some mentally retarded individuals, whatever their IQs.

As psychiatric nosology and diagnosis become more refined and the etiopathogeneses of more homogeneous subgroups are delineated, increasingly more focused research may be undertaken, and more specific and rational psychopharmacology will inevitably follow.

Specific Drug Treatments

In Section II of this book, psychopharmacological agents are organized and discussed by class rather than according to the psychiatric diagnoses for which they are treatments. The rationale for this organization is related to several of the issues discussed in the first part of the book. At the present time most diagnoses are based on phenomenology, that is, constellations of clinical symptoms, rather than on any basic understanding of the etiopathogenesis of the condition; thus a given drug may be used to treat several psychiatric diagnoses. Hence repetition of facts under each diagnostic category and extensive cross-referencing are avoided.

Each class of drugs is introduced with some general comments, including indications for use, contraindications, interactions with other drugs, and the most common untoward effects. The basic pharmacokinetics, including approximations of time of peak serum levels and the drug's serum half-life, major metabolites, and excretion, are discussed. Unless otherwise noted, all dosage recommendations are for oral administration.

Specific drugs of each class are reviewed individually; standard, FDA-approved treatments are discussed first. Some treatments not approved for advertising by the FDA but reported to be efficacious in the literature and used clinically by some practitioners are discussed as well. It is recommended that these drugs be used conservatively—that is, by experienced physicians and primarily after standard treatment regimens have proven unsuccessful. Likewise, a few drugs that have been investigated or are currently under investigation under research protocols and that seem to have potential therapeutic efficacy are also reviewed; they should be used even more cautiously, if at all, in clinical practice.

Most of the studies cited in this book either illustrate a particular point or provide the reader with some of the evidence, not readily accessible elsewhere, for using nonstandard treatments. This evidence ranges from reasonably convincing to merely suggestive of a possible alternative for a seriously disturbed patient who has not responded satisfactorily to any standard, approved treatment. Excellent and extensive literature reviews of the standard psychopharmacological treatments discussed below are readily accessible in the additional readings given above.

Although always important, informed consent, preferably written, is particularly important if FDA-approved drugs are used for nonapproved indications. If standard approved treatments for a seriously disabling disorder have been tried with little or no success, a clinical trial of a nonapproved or even an investigational medication is much more easily justified. The physician has the responsibility to become thoroughly familiar with the official package labeling information provided by the manufacturer of the drug or the relevant entry in the latest edition and supplements of the PDR (1995) prior to prescribing any drug.

The following table lists the most common psychiatric diagnoses in children and younger adolescents for which psychopharmacotherapy may be therapeutically indicated and the medication used in treating that disorder. Whenever a specific drug or class of drugs is generally preferred for a particular condition, an attempt has been made to rank them in order of usual preference, with FDA-approved uses preceding off-label indications.

Diagnoses in Childhood and Adolescence for Which Psychopharmacotherapy May Be Therapeutically Indicated

DSM-IV Diagnosis	Medication	
Attention-deficit/hyperactivity disorder	Stimulants	(pp. 56–77)
	Tricyclic antidepressants	(pp. 121–186)
	Antipsychotics	(pp. 79–80, 93)
	Clonidine	(pp. 240, 242–245)
	Guanfacine	(pp. 249–251)
	Fluoxetine	(pp. 172–173)
	Clomipramine	(pp. 161–162)
	MAOIs	(p. 186)
	Bupropion	(p. 183)
Conduct disorder (severe, aggressive)	Antipsychotics	(pp. 78–120)
	Haloperidol	(p. 104)
	Lithium	(pp. 79, 199–200)
	Propranolol	(p. 237)
	Carbamazepine	(pp. 227–228)
	Trazodone	(pp. 178–180)
	Clonidine	(pp. 245–246)
Encopresis	Lithium	(p. 200)
Enuresis	DDAVP	(p. 132)
	Imipramine	(pp. 8, 122, 132, 133)
	Benzodiazepines	(pp. 210–211)
	Carbamazepine	(p. 227)
	Amphetamines	(p. 47)
	Clomipramine	(pp. 159, 163)
	Desipramine	(p. 151)
Intermittent explosive disorder	Propranolol	(pp. 237–239)
Major depressive disorder	Antidepressants	(pp. 121–186)
	Lithium augmentation	(pp. 138–139)
	Lithium for Prophylaxis	(p. 122)

(continued)

continued
Diagnoses in Childhood and Adolescence for Which Psychopharmacotherapy May Be Therapeutically Indicated

DSM-IV Diagnosis	Medication	
Manic episode (acute and maintenance)	Lithium	(pp. 195–199)
	Antipsychotics	(p. 79)
	Valproic acid	(pp. 230–231)
Mental retardation (with severe behavioral disorder and/or self-injurious behavior)	Thioridazine	(pp. 79, 100–101)
	Chlorpromazine	(pp. 79, 98)
	Haloperidol	(pp. 79, 101–104)
	Lithium	(pp. 187–200)
	Propranolol	(pp. 237–239)
	Naltrexone	(pp. 234–235)
Obsessive-compulsive disorder	Clomipramine	(pp. 159–161)
	Fluoxetine	(pp. 170–171)
	Fluvoxamine	(pp. 175–177)
	Clonazepam	(pp. 214–215)
Overanxious disorder of childhood (subsumed under generalized anxiety disorder in DSM-IV)	Benzodiazepines	(pp. 201–214)
	Diphenhydramine	(pp. 221–222)
	Fluoxetine	(pp. 171–172)
	Buspirone	(pp. 215–218)
	Hydroxyzine	(pp. 222–223)
Panic disorder	Tricyclic antidepressants	(p. 142)
	Alprazolam	(p. 142)
	Clonazepam	(p. 213)
Pervasive developmental disorders	Haloperidol	(pp. 103–104)
	Fluphenazine	(p. 108)
	Naltrexone	(pp. 233–235)
	Fenfluramine	(p. 76)
	Clomipramine	(pp. 162–163)
	Buspirone	(p. 219)
	Clonidine	(p. 246)
Posttraumatic stress disorder (acute)	Propranolol	(p. 238)
Schizophrenia	Antipsychotics	(pp. 78–120)

continued
Diagnoses in Childhood and Adolescence for Which
Psychopharmacotherapy May Be Therapeutically Indicated

DSM-IV Diagnosis	Medication	
Selective mutism	Fluoxetine	(pp. 173–174)
Separation anxiety disorder	Imipramine	(p. 122, 140–142)
	Chlordiazepoxide	(p. 209)
	Fluoxetine	(pp. 170–171)
	Alprazolam	(pp. 142, 213)
	Buspirone	(pp. 217–218)
	Clomipramine	(pp. 163–164)
	Clonazepam	(p. 214)
Sleep disorders		
Primary insomnia	Benzodiazepines	(pp. 202–203, 207t)
	Diphenhydramine	(pp. 221–222)
	Hydroxyzine	(p. 223)
Circadian Rhythm Sleep disorder	Benzodiazepines	(pp. 201–204)
	Diphenhydramine	(pp. 221–222)
	Hydroxyzine	(pp. 222–223)
Sleep terror disorder	Benzodiazepines	(p. 211)
	Imipramine	(p. 142)
	Carbamazepine	(p. 227)
Sleepwalking disorder	Benzodiazepines	(p. 211)
	Imipramine	(p. 142)
Tourette's disorder	Haloperidol	(p. 79)
	Pimozide	(pp. 109–110)
	Clonidine	(pp. 246–249)
	Desipramine	(pp. 156–157)
	Guanfacine	(pp. 250–251)
	Nortriptyline	(pp. 146–147)
	Fluoxetine	(pp. 170–171)

3

Sympathomimetic Amines and Central Nervous System Stimulants

Introduction

These agents, commonly referred to as stimulants, are the drugs of choice for treating attention-deficit/hyperactivity disorder (ADHD).

Bradley's 1937 report on the use of racemic amphetamine sulfate (Benzedrine) in behaviorally disordered children is usually cited as the beginning of child psychopharmacology as a discipline. Since this initial report, more research has been published on the stimulants and ADHD than on any other childhood disorder. Double-blind, placebo-controlled studies have found consistently that stimulants are significantly superior to placebo in improving attention span and in decreasing hyperactivity and impulsivity. Although most of these studies have been done in children, two double-blind studies confirm the clinical efficacy of methylphenidate in treating adolescents diagnosed with attention deficit disorder (ADD) who also had ADD as children (Klorman et al., 1988a; 1988b).

Several investigators have reported that methylphenidate also improved academic performance and/or peer interactions (e.g., Pelham et al., 1985, 1987; Rapport et al., 1994). Whalen and her colleagues (1987) reported on 24 children between 6 and 11 years of age who were diagnosed with ADD or ADDH and who received either placebo, 0.3 mg/kg methylphenidate daily, or 0.6 mg/kg methylphenidate daily, in a random order so that all children received each dosage level for a total of 4 days. The authors reported that all children showed decrements in negative social behaviors when rated during relatively unstructured outdoor activities at the 0.3 mg/kg level, compared with placebo. The youngest 12 children showed further improvement in social behavior at the higher dose level, but the older children showed no further improvement.

Rapport et al. (1994) evaluated the acute effects of four dose levels (5, 10, 15 and 20 mg) of methylphenidate on classroom behavior and academic performance of 76 children diagnosed with ADHD in a double-blind, placebo-controlled, within-subject (crossover) protocol. Compared with baseline, the subjects showed a nearly linear increase in normalization of behavior as the dose of methylphenidate increased. On the Abbreviated Conners Teacher Rating Scale, scores improved in 16% and normalized in 78% of the subjects. Attention, measured by on-task behavior, improved in 4% and normalized in 72% of subjects. Academic efficiency, measured by the percentage of academic assignments completed correctly, improved in 3% and normalized in 50% of the subjects. Hence there are several different clinically significant subsets of children: those who improve in all domains; those who improve in the behavioral and attention domains but do not improve in the academic domain and require additional interventions, e.g., tutoring; those who show behavioral improvement but no significant improvement in attention or academic ratings; and a fourth subset who do not benefit from methylphenidate in any of the three domains.

In a double-blind, placebo-controlled study of 40 children (age range, 6 to 12 years; mean, 8.6 ± 1.3 years) who were diagnosed with ADHD, DuPaul et al. (1994) found that subjects (N = 12) who had additional internalizing symptoms such as anxiety or depression and who had high scores on the Internalizing scale of the Child Behavior Checklist (CBCL) were significantly less likely to benefit from methylphenidate at three different doses (5, 10, and 15 mg) in school, as evidenced by teachers' ratings, and in the clinic setting compared with subjects with borderline (N = 17) or low (N = 11) scores on the CBCL. There was a significant deterioration in functioning on methylphenidate among some children. In particular, 25% of the subjects in the high internalizing group were rated on the Teacher Self-Control Rating Scale as showing a worsening in classroom behavior compared with 9.1% in the low and none in the borderline internalizing groups. On the same scale, however, 50% of the high, 93.75% of the borderline, and 72.7% of the low internalizing groups were rated as improved or normalized.

ADHD and conduct disorder may frequently coexist; in fact, DSM-IV (APA, 1994) notes that if either diagnosis is present, the other diagnosis is commonly found as well. Psychostimulants also reduce some forms of aggression present in children diagnosed with ADDH (Allen et al., 1975; Klorman et al., 1988b). Amery et al. (1984) compared dextroamphetamine and placebo in 10 boys diagnosed with ADDH with a mean age of 9.6 ± 1.6 years. Dextroamphetamine was administered in doses of 15 to 30 mg/day. The authors reported that scores on the Thematic Apperception Test Hostility Scale and Holtzman Inkblot Test Hostility Scale, and observations for overt aggression in a laboratory free play situation, were reduced significantly ($P < .05$) during a 2-week period on dextroamphetamine, compared with a similar period on placebo. These data are important, as ADHD and conduct disorder frequently coexist, and stimulants are often not considered in treating children whose conduct disorders are the primary consideration.

About 75% of ADHD children treated with stimulants will show favorable responses (Green, 1995). Among these favorable responses, there will be a spectrum; some children will respond extremely well, and others will benefit but to a lesser degree. Also, some children with ADHD (or an earlier equivalent diagnosis) will respond favorably to one stimulant drug but less favorably, not at all, or unfavorably to another stimulant. For example, Arnold et al. (1976) conducted a double-blind crossover study of D-amphetamine, L-amphetamine, and placebo in 31 children with minimal brain dysfunction (MBD). Both isomers were statistically superior to placebo and did not differ significantly from each other. Interestingly, of the 25 children with positive responses, 17 responded well to both isomers, 5 responded favorably only to the D-isomer, and 3 responded favorably only to the L-isomer (Arnold et al., 1976).

In a double-blind crossover study, Elia et al. (1991) compared methylphenidate, dextroamphetamine, and placebo in treating 48 males (age range, 6 to 12 years; mean, 8.6 ± 1.7 years) with a history of hyperactive, inattentive, and impulsive behaviors that interfered with functioning in both home and school. Following a 2-week baseline period, subjects were assigned randomly for 3-week periods during each week in which the dosage was increased, unless untoward effects prevented it, to one of three regimens: (*1*) Methylphenidate doses were given at 9 AM and 1 PM: subjects weighing less than 30 kg received during week 1, 12.5 mg; week 2, 20 mg; and week 3, 35 mg. Subjects weighing 30 kg or more received during week 1, 15 mg; week 2, 25 mg; and week 3, 45 mg. The actual mean dosage for all subjects for week 1 was 0.9 mg/kg; week 2, 1.5 mg/kg; and week 3, 2.5 mg/kg. (*2*) Dextroamphetamine doses were given at 9 AM and 1 PM: subjects weighing less than 30 kg received during week 1, 5 mg; week 2, 12.5 mg; and week 3, 20 mg. Those weighing 30 kg or more received during week 1, 7.5 mg; week 2, 15 mg; and week 3, 22.5 mg. The actual mean dosage for all subjects during week 1 was 0.4 mg/kg; week 2, 0.9 mg/kg; and week 3, 1.3 mg/kg. (3) Placebo dosage was held at the preceding week's level, increased to a lower dosage than mandated by the next level, or decreased because of untoward effects in 19 subjects (40%), including 7 on methylphenidate, 7 on dextroamphetamine, and 5 on both drugs. The authors reported that 38 (79%) of subjects responded to methylphenidate and that 42 (88%) responded to dextroamphetamine; overall, 46 (96%) of the 48 subjects had a positive clinical response to one or both stimulants as rated on the Clinical Global Impression Scale (CGI) and, in particular, for restless and inattentive behaviors. Eight subjects did not respond to methylphenidate, 4 did not respond to dextroamphetamine, and 2 did not respond to either drug. Elia and colleagues (1991) distinguished between behavioral nonresponse and untoward effects, which few investigators have done. They noted that, although behavioral nonresponse to stimulants is rare when a wide range of doses is given, most subjects had some untoward effects. During week 2 or 3 of treatment, untoward effects required that for 19 (40%) of the subjects, the dose be only partially increased in 15 (6 on methylphenidate, 4 on dextroamphetamine, and 5 on both), held constant in 2 (1 on each medication), and decreased in 2 subjects receiving dextroamphetamine. When behavioral nonresponders were combined with subjects having untoward effects, the rate of nonresponse was similar to that reported in the literature. The authors noted that making a definitive clinical decision regarding improvement was often difficult because behavioral improvements had to be balanced against untoward effects, and different symptoms responded independently to dosage, setting, and subject (Elia et al., 1991).

Wender (1988) notes that the development of tolerance to the therapeutic effects of stimulant medication is unusual and that when it occurs, it progresses gradually over a period of 1 or 2 years. If this occurs, a trial of another stimulant is suggested, because complete cross-tolerance among the stimulants does not occur (Wender, 1988). There is a suggestion that the efficacy of stimulants typically decreases with age (Taylor et al., 1987).

Gadow and Poling (1988) reviewed the literature on the use of stimulants in the mentally retarded and concluded that stimulants are highly effective in reducing symptoms of hyperactivity and conduct disorder in some individuals, regardless of the degree of their retardation.

Normal prepubertal boys and college-aged men reacted similarly to patients diagnosed with ADHD when given single doses of dextroamphetamine; they exhibited decreased motor activity and generally improved attentional performance (Rapoport et al., 1978a, 1980a). Hence earlier teachings that stimulants have a paradoxical effect in hyperactive children are incorrect, and a positive response to stimulant medication cannot be used to validate the diagnosis of ADHD.

Pharmacokinetics of Stimulants

The stimulants undergo some metabolism in the liver and are primarily excreted by the kidneys. Table 3.1 gives the site of metabolism, main metabolic products, time of peak plasma levels, serum half-lives, and routes of excretion for the stimulants commonly used in child and adolescent psychiatry.

STANDARD STIMULANT PREPARATIONS COMPARED WITH LONG-ACTING OR SUSTAINED-RELEASE FORMS

Sustained-release tablets make once-daily dosage possible. One early report found the clinical efficacy of sustained-release methylphenidate to occur about 1 hour later and to be less than the standard release form of methylphenidate on several important measures of disruptive behavior in two studies of 22 boys with ADHD (Pelham et al., 1987). These authors thought that if once-daily dosage was necessary, then slow-release dextroamphetamine or magnesium pemoline would often be preferable to sustained-release methylphenidate. Birmaher et al. (1989) noted that the maximum serum level takes longer to develop when sustained-release tablets are administered and that peak serum levels are lower than for an equivalent dose of standard methylphenidate. These authors suggested that the relative inefficacy of sustained-release methylphenidate could result from differences in pharmacokinetics or absorption, or from tachyphylaxis.

Some subsequent studies, however, have reported significantly different results. Pelham et al. (1990) administered standard methylphenidate 10 mg every morning and noon, sustained-release methylphenidate 20 mg every morning; dextroamphetamine spansule (long acting), 10 mg every morning; pemoline, 56.25 mg every morning; and placebo in random order for from 3 to 6 days. Each double-blind, placebo-controlled, crossover study involved 22 boys, ages 8.08 to 13.17 years, diagnosed with ADHD. Midday placebos were given during the periods when long-acting drugs were administered. Subjects were rated on measures of social behavior and classroom per-

Table 3.1.
Some Pharmacokinetic Properties of Stimulant Drugs

Drug	Principal Metabolite(s)	Peak Serum Levels	Serum Half-Life	Principal Route(s) of Execution
Methylphenidate (Ritalin)	Liver → 75% ritalinic acid, which is pharmacologically inactive	1.9 hr (range, 0.3–4.4 hr); Ritalin S-R, 4.7 hr (range, 1.3–8.2 hr)	2–2½ hr	Kidney excretes 70%–80%, primarily as ritalinic acid, in 24 hr
Dextroamphetamine sulfate (Dexedrine)	Liver P-hydroxylation, N-demethyl- ation, deamination, and conju- gation	2 hours for tablet; 8–10 hr for spansule	6–8 hr in chil- dren, 10– 12 hr in adults	May be excreted unchanged by kidney. Amount varies according to urinary pH— from 2% to 3% in very alka- line urine to 80% in acidic urine.
Magnesium pemoline (Cylert)	Liver → pemoline conjugates: pemoline dione, mandelic acid, and other products	2–4 hr	8–12 hr	Kidney excretes about 40%– 50% unchanged, plus about 25%–40% as products of liver metabolism

formance, and on a continuous performance task. All four medication conditions had similar time courses, with effects evident between 1 and 9 hours after ingestion, and they were significantly, and approximately equally, better than placebo. The effects of the 3 long-acting preparations were as great, or almost as great, at 9 hours as at 2 hours after ingestion. Only 15 (68%) of the 22 patients improved sufficiently for the authors to recommend that they continue to receive stimulant medication. For these 15 patients dextroamphetamine spansules were recommended for 6, pemoline for 4, sustained-release methylphenidate for 4, and standard methylphenidate for 1. The clinical implications of this study are potentially very important because it suggests that the great majority (i.e., 14 [93.3%] of 15 children with ADHD) derive more overall benefit from long-acting than from standard release forms of stimulants. At the time of the study, it was estimated that about 90% of children receiving medication for ADHD were prescribed methylphenidate, and, of these, only about 10% received the sustained-release form.

Fitzpatrick et al. (1992) compared the efficacy of standard and sustained-release methylphenidate, and a combination of the two forms, in a double-blind placebo-controlled study of 19 children (17 males and 2 females; age range, 6.9 to 11.5 years) diagnosed with ADD. Dosage of sustained-release methylphenidate was 20 mg/day for all patients. Patients weighing less than and more than 30 kg received 7.5 mg and 10 mg, respectively, in the morning and at noon when on standard methylphenidate only, and 5 mg and 7.5 mg, respectively, in the morning and at noon when receiving standard methylphenidate in combination with sustained-release methylphenidate. Patients were rated on several scales by parents, teachers, and clinicians. All three active drug conditions were significantly better than placebo and were approximately equivalent in efficacy.

These studies, in which the medications were administered for relatively short periods, have relatively small numbers of subjects and need to be replicated with larger populations. They do, however, alert the clinician to the likelihood that sustained-release preparations are more efficacious than initially thought and they may be the preferred dosage forms for the majority of children with ADHD.

Contraindications for Stimulant Administration

Known hypersensitivity to the medication is a significant contraindication.

Stimulants may cause stereotypies, tics, and psychosis de novo in sensitive individuals or if given in high enough doses. Stimulants are relatively contraindicated in children and adolescents with a history of schizophrenia or other psychosis, pervasive developmental disorders, or borderline personality organization, because they appear to worsen these conditions in many cases. There is considerable controversy over whether they should be given to children and adolescents with Tourette's disorder, a tic disorder, or a family history of such disorders. Their use in pervasive developmental disorders and in Tourette's disorder or with tic disorders is discussed in greater detail below.

Stimulants may aggravate symptoms of marked anxiety, tension, and agitation, and are contraindicated when these symptoms are prominent (manufacturer's package insert).

Stimulants have a potential to be abused. They should not be prescribed to patients who have a history of drug abuse or when there is a likelihood that family members or friends would abuse the medication. In some cases in which the family is unreliable but stimulants are the drug of choice, it is worthwhile to attempt to work out a way to dispense and store all the stimulant medication at school, because, for most children, coverage during the time in school is the foremost consideration.

Magnesium pemoline should not be administered to patients with impaired liver function or to those with known hypersensitivity to it.

Interactions of Stimulants with other Drugs

Stimulants should not be administered with monoamine oxidase inhibitors (MAOIs) or until at least 14 days after MAOIs were last ingested, to avoid possible hypertensive crises.

In combination with tricyclic antidepressants, the actions of both may be enhanced.

Stimulants potentiate sympathomimetic drugs (including street amphetamines and cocaine) and may counteract the sedative effect of antihistamines and benzodiazepines.

Lithium may inhibit the stimulatory effects of amphetamines.

Amphetamines may act synergistically with phenytoin or phenobarbital to increase anticonvulsant activity.

Many other drug interactions, which are less likely to be encountered in child and adolescent psychiatry, may occur.

Untoward Effects of Stimulants

There is some evidence that, overall, the untoward effects of methylphenidate occur less frequently and with less severity than those from dextroamphetamine (Conners, 1971; Gross & Wilson, 1974). Gross and Wilson (1974) noted that side effects were infrequently severe enough to make immediate discontinuation of medication necessary—1.1% of 377 patients for methylphenidate and 4.3% of 371 patients for dextroamphetamine.

The most frequent and troublesome immediate untoward effects include insomnia, anorexia, nausea, abdominal pain or cramps, headache, thirst, vomiting, lability of mood, irritability, sadness, weepiness, tachycardia, and blood pressure changes. Many of these symptoms diminish over a period of up to a few weeks, although the cardiovascular changes may persist.

Since 1972 disturbances in growth—decrements in both height and weight percentiles—have been reported for both methylphenidate and dextroamphetamine, and the long-term untoward consequences of these effects have been of particular concern (Safer et al., 1972). There has been controversy about the significance of these changes. Mattes and Gittelman (1983) reported significant decreases in height and weight percentiles over a 4-year period. A subsequent controlled study found a significant reduction in growth velocity during the period when stimulants are actively administered (Klein et al., 1988). Despite this adverse effect on growth during the active treatment phase, it appears that an accelerated rate of growth or growth rebound occurs once the stimulant is discontinued and that there is usually no significant compromise of ultimate height attained (Klein & Mannuzza, 1988). It seems likely, however, that some children are at greater risk for growth suppression than others, and serial heights and weights of any child receiving stimulant medication should be plotted carefully on a growth chart (e.g., the National Center for Health Statistics Growth Chart) (Hamill et al., 1976).

Vincent et al. (1990) reported no significant deviations from expected height and weight growth velocities in 31 adolescents diagnosed with ADHD who had received methylphenidate continuously for a minimum of 6 months to a maximum of 6 years after their 12th birthdays. Mean age at beginning the study was 12.9 ± 0.8 years. The mean daily dose was 34 ± 14 mg or 0.75 ± 0.29 mg/kg and did not differ significantly with age or sex. The results suggested that early adolescent growth is not significantly adversely affected by methylphenidate.

A few children treated with stimulants may develop a clinical picture resembling schizophrenia. This condition occurs most frequently when untoward effects such as disorganization are misinterpreted as a worsening of presenting symptoms and the dosage is further increased until prominent psychotomimetic effects occur. It may also occur when stimulants are administered to children with borderline personality disorders or schizophrenia, conditions in which stimulants are usually contraindicated. In most such cases, the psychotic symptomatology improves rapidly after discontinuation of the drug (Green, 1989).

Some parents express concern that treatment with stimulants will predispose their child to later drug abuse or addiction. Most available evidence indicates that this is not the case. Although drug abuse itself is of major concern in our culture, children diagnosed with ADHD who have been treated with stimulants appear to be at no greater risk than controls for drug or alcohol abuse as teenagers and adults (Weiss & Hechtman, 1986).

REBOUND EFFECTS OF STIMULANTS

Rebound effects may occur beginning about 5 hours after the last dose of methylphenidate. Behavioral symptoms of rebound are often identical to those of the ADHD being treated and, in some cases, may even exceed baseline levels prior to administration of stimulants.

Rapoport and her colleagues (1978a) reported that normal children who received dextroamphetamine experienced behavioral rebound about 5 hours after a single acute dose. Symptoms included excitability, talkativeness, overactivity, insomnia, stomachaches, and mild nausea.

Stimulants' Relationship to Tics and Tourette's Disorder

Stimulants can exacerbate existing tics and precipitate tics and stereotypies de novo. There is disagreement among experts regarding whether stimulants should be given to persons with tics, Tourette's disorder, or a family history of either condition.

In a study of 1520 children diagnosed with ADDH and treated with methylphenidate, Denckla et al. (1976) reported that existing tics were exacerbated in 6 cases (0.39%), and tics developed de novo in 14 cases (0.92%). After the discontinuation of methylphenidate, all 6 of the tics that had worsened returned to their premedication intensity, and 13 of the 14 new tics completely remitted.

Shapiro and Shapiro (1981) reviewed the relationship between treating ADDH with stimulants and the precipitation or exacerbation of tics and Tourette's syndrome (TS). They also noted that they had treated 42 patients for symptoms of both MBD and TS with a combination of methylphenidate and haloperidol. Dosage of methylphenidate ranged from 5 to 60 mg/day and was individually titrated for each patient. The authors also used methylphenidate (dose range, 5 to 40 mg/day) in 62 additional patients with TS to counteract untoward effects of haloperidol, such as sedation, amotivation, dysphoria, cognitive impairment, and dullness. Shapiro and Shapiro (1981) concluded that the evidence suggests that stimulants do not cause or provoke TS, although high doses of stimulants can cause or exacerbate tics in predisposed patients. Clinically they noted that tics seemed less likely to be exacerbated by stimulants in patients who were also taking haloperidol for TS; when tics did increase in intensity, they remitted within 3 to 6 hours, the approximate duration of the usual clinical effects of methylphenidate.

Lowe et al. (1982) reported on a series of 15 patients diagnosed with ADDH who were treated with stimulant medications, including methylphenidate, dextroamphetamine, and pemoline. These patients subsequently had tics develop de novo, or had existing tics worsen, sometimes into full-blown cases of Tourette's disorder. Nine subjects had existing tics; 8 had family histories of tics or Tourette's disorder. Twelve of the 15 cases eventually required medication for control of the tics. The authors considered the presence of Tourette's disorder or tics to be a contraindication to stimulant medication and that stimulants should be used with great caution in the presence of a family history of tics or Tourette's disorder. They also considered the development of tics after treatment with stimulants sufficient reason to discontinue use of stimulant medication.

Lowe et al. (1982) noted that the early clinical signs of Tourette's disorder may be difficult to differentiate from ADDH. Shapiro and Shapiro (1981) noted that about 57% of children with tic and Tourette's syndromes (TTS) had concomitant minimal brain dysfunction (MBD), although most children with MBD do not develop TTS. Comings and Comings (1984) investigated the relationship between TS and ADDH. They found ADDH was present in 62% of 140 males under age 21 years diagnosed with TS. A study of their family pedigrees suggested that the TS gene could be expressed as ADDH but without tics. The authors thought that their data implied that patients diagnosed ADDH and treated with stimulants who subsequently developed tics had ADDH as a result of the TS gene and probably would have developed tics or TS even if they had not received stimulants. It is unclear whether stimulant medication might hasten the expression of such symptoms.

Gadow, Nolan, and Sverd (1992) treated with methylphenidate 11 boys, aged 6.1 to 11.9 years (mean, 8.3 ± 1.96 years), diagnosed with comorbid tic disorder and ADHD. The drug was administered under double-blind conditions; each subject was assigned to random 2-week periods of placebo and methylphenidate in doses of 0.1, 0.3, and 0.5 mg/kg/day. The authors noted that methylphenidate significantly decreased hyperactive and disruptive behaviors in class and reduced physical aggression on the playground. Vocal tics were also significantly reduced in the lunchroom and classroom. Based on this and other studies cited in their report, the authors concluded that methylphenidate is a safe and effective treatment for some children with comorbid ADHD and tic disorder over a short-term period; however, they cautioned that a risk of protraction or irreversible worsening of tics may exist for some individuals and that the consequences of long-term treatment of such patients are unknown.

At the present time, a conservative approach would consider the stimulants relatively or absolutely contraindicated in treating children and adolescents with tics or Tourette's syndrome, and a reason for caution in the presence of family history of such. In fact, one manufacturer of methylphenidate states that it is contraindicated in patients with motor tics or with a family history or diagnosis of Tourette's syndrome.

Stimulant Drugs Approved for use in Child and Adolescent Psychiatry

The stimulants are the most frequently prescribed psychiatric drugs during childhood. In 1977 more that half a million children were being treated with methylphenidate in the United States alone (Sprague & Sleator, 1977). By 1987 it was conservatively estimated that in the United States, 750,000 youth were being treated with medication for hyperactivity or inattentiveness (Safer & Krager, 1988). In Baltimore County, 6% of all public elementary school students were receiving such medication; methylphenidate accounted for 93% of the drugs prescribed and other stimulants for another 6% (Safer & Krager, 1988). Because methylphenidate is the most commonly prescribed drug for ADHD, it will be used to illustrate the use of the stimulants, despite its having appeared on the scene considerably later than dextroamphetamine sulfate.

METHYLPHENIDATE (RITALIN)

Indications in Child and Adolescent Psychiatry
    FDA approved for treating attention deficit hyperactivity disorder (ADHD) and narcolepsy.

Dosage Schedule for Treating ADHD
• Children under 6 years old: Not approved for use.
• Persons 6 years of age and older: Start with 5 mg once or twice daily and raise dose gradually 5 to 10 mg/week. Maximum recommended daily dosage is 60 mg.
• The usual optimal dose falls between 0.3 and 0.7 mg/kg administered two to three times daily (total daily dose range of 0.6 to 2.1 mg/kg (Duncan, 1990).

Dose Forms Available
• Tablets: 5 mg, 10 mg, 20 mg
• Sustained-release tablets (Ritalin-SR): 20 mg

Pharmacokinetics of Methylphenidate

Administration of methylphenidate with meals does not appear to adversely affect its absorption or pharmacokinetics and may diminish problems with appetite suppression (Patrick et al., 1987).

An improvement of target symptoms can be seen in as few as 20 minutes after a therapeutically effective dose is given (Zametkin et al., 1985). Peak blood levels occur between 1 and 2½ hours after administration (Gualtieri et al., 1982), and the serum half-life is about 2½ hours (Winsberg et al., 1982). Patrick et al. (1987) have reviewed the pharmacokinetics of methylphenidate in detail. The major metabolite produced in the liver is ritalinic acid, which is pharmacologically inactive. Between 70% and 80% of the radioactivity of radiolabeled methylphenidate, more than 75% of which is ritalinic acid, is recovered in the urine within 24 hours.

Because of these pharmacokinetics, the most frequent times to administer methylphenidate to children and adolescents are before leaving for school and during the lunch hour. This dosage schedule usually ensures adequate serum levels during school hours, which is the foremost consideration for most students.

Untoward Effects and Adjustment of Methylphenidate Dose Schedule

Children who develop significant behavioral or attention difficulties in the late afternoon or early evening may do so because of a return to baseline behavior as serum levels decline into subtherapeutic levels and/or because of a rebound effect as the drug wears off (Rapoport et al., 1978a). A third dose of medication given in the afternoon may be helpful for some such children. Johnston et al. (1988), however, suggested that psychostimulant rebound effects are not clinically significant for the large majority of children. Insomnia may also occur. It is clinically important to distinguish those children whose insomnia is an untoward effect of the drug from those whose insomnia may be due to the recurrence of behavioral difficulties as the medication effect subsides and/or a rebound effect. For the first group of children, a reduction in milligram dosage of the last dose of the day may be necessary. For the latter group, an evening dose or a dose about 1 hour before bedtime may be helpful. Chatoor et al. (1983) prescribed late afternoon or evening dextroamphetamine sustained-release capsules to seven children who had strong rebound effects as their medication wore off and who developed marked behavioral problems and difficulty settling down and sleeping at bedtime. Parents reported significant behavioral improvement and markedly less bedtime oppositional behavior and increased ease in falling asleep. The authors compared sleep EEGs in seven children recorded during periods on dextroamphetamine sustained-release capsules and on placebo. Compared with placebo, dextroamphetamine tended to delay onset of sleep slightly, significantly increased rapid eye movement (REM) latency (time to first REM period), and significantly decreased REM time (by about 14%) and the number of REM periods. Length of stage 1 and stage 2 sleep was significantly increased, and sleep efficiency (amount of time asleep during recording) decreased. Reduction in sleep efficiency was only 5%, which seemed minor compared with the significant behavioral improvement that occurred (Chatoor et al., 1983).

There is some evidence that methylphenidate may lower the convulsive threshold (manufacturer's package insert). McBride et al. (1986), however, found only a single case report in the literature in which a child who was previously seizure free had a seizure soon after treatment with methylphenidate was begun. The authors treated 23 children and adolescents, aged 4 to 15 years and diagnosed with ADD who had seizure disorders of various types (N = 20) or epileptiform EEG abnormalities (N = 3), with methylphenidate. Fifteen of the children with documented seizure disorder received concomitant antiepileptic drugs. Individual doses of 0.33 mg/kg ($\pm$0.13 mg/kg) were administered with total daily doses of 0.63 mg/kg ($\pm$0.25 mg/kg) for from

3 months' to 4 years' duration. The authors found no evidence of increased frequency of seizures following methylphenidate treatment in 16 children with active seizure disorders or 4 children who had had active seizure disorders but who had been seizure free and off antiepileptic drugs for from 2 months to 2 years. The three children with epileptiform abnormalities also developed no seizures during the period they received methylphenidate. This evidence suggests that methylphenidate may not lower the seizure threshold to a clinically significant degree at usual therapeutic doses and that the presence of a seizure disorder in a child or adolescent with ADHD is not an absolute contraindication for a trial of methylphenidate (McBride et al., 1986). Crumrine et al. (1987) also reported that they had administered methylphenidate 0.3 mg/kg twice daily to 9 males 6.1 years to 10.1 years of age who had diagnoses of ADHD and seizure disorder. The boys had been previously stabilized on anticonvulsant medication and experienced no seizures or changes in EEG background patterns or epileptiform activity during 4-week, randomized, double-blind crossover trials of methylphenidate or placebo. Subjects improved significantly on the hyperactivity, inattention, and hyperactivity index factors on the Conners Teacher Questionnaire (Crumrine et al., 1987).

These reports suggest that when clinically indicated, it is not unreasonable to undertake a trial of methylphenidate in children and adolescents with coexisting seizure disorders and ADHD. Clearly, frequency of seizures should be carefully monitored, and if their frequency increases or seizures develop de novo, the clinician may discontinue methylphenidate.

Swanson et al. (1986) reported on six children who developed behavioral and cognitive tolerance to their usual doses of methylphenidate during long-term treatment. To maintain satisfactory clinical response, their pediatricians had to titrate their total daily doses to levels of 120 mg to 300 mg administered in as many as five individual doses of 40 mg to 60 mg. These children performed a cognitive task better at their usual high dose (average, 60 mg three times daily) than at a lower dose (average, 30 mg three times daily), confirming cognitive tolerance. Overall, these children had high serum levels compatible with the high doses, suggesting that neither metabolic tolerance nor differential absorption was responsible for the behavioral tolerance.

Garfinkel et al. (1983) compared efficacy of methylphenidate with placebo, desipramine, and clomipramine in a double-blind crossover study of 12 males (mean age, 7.3 years; range, 5.9 to 11.6 years) diagnosed with ADD who required day hospital or inpatient hospitalization for the severity of their impulsivity, inattention, and aggressiveness. Methylphenidate was significantly better in improving symptoms on the Conners Scale as rated by teachers ($P < .005$) and program child care workers ($P < .001$).

REPORTS OF INTEREST

Methylphenidate in the Treatment of Hyperactivity in Children Diagnosed with Autistic Disorder. Methylphenidate has been investigated in the treatment of hyperactive children with autistic disorder. Although most of the earlier literature states that stimulants are contraindicated for autistic children and cause a worsening in behavior and/or stereotypies, several recent studies have reported that methylphenidate is effective in treating some children with autistic disorder who also exhibit such symptoms as hyperactivity, impulsivity, short attention spans, and aggression. Strayhorn et al. (1988) reported on two autistic children, a 6-year-old autistic boy given methylphenidate in a randomized trial with either placebo or methylphenidate given each day, and a preschool child treated openly with methylphenidate. The former child was reported to show improvement in attention and activity levels, less destructive behavior, and a decrease in stereotyped movements, but sadness and temper tantrums significantly worsened. The preschooler was said to have had similar results.

Birmaher et al. (1988) treated nine hyperactive autistic children aged 4 years to 16 years with 10 to 50 mg/day of methylphenidate. Eight of the children improved on all rating scales; the oldest child improved on all scales except the one measuring behavior in school.

In contrast, Realmuto et al. (1989), who treated two 9-year-old autistic boys with 10 mg of methylphenidate administered twice daily, found that one became fearful and unable to separate from significant adults, had a worsening of his hyperactivity, and developed a rapid pulse. The second youngster's baseline behaviors did not significantly change although he developed mild anorexia.

Until additional research with larger samples of autistic children clarifies these studies, the use of methylphenidate in treating autistic children or hyperactive subgroups of them must be regarded as investigational.

DEXTROAMPHETAMINE SULFATE (DEXEDRINE)

Indications in Child and Adolescent Psychiatry
FDA approved for treating attention deficit disorder with hyperactivity (ADDH), narcolepsy, and exogenous obesity. (ADDH is a DSM-III [APA, 1980a] diagnosis that, in large part, corresponds to the DSM-IV [APA, 1994] diagnosis ADHD; technically, as late as 1995, the FDA approval for advertising is still for treatment of ADDH; however, for purposes of medication and dosage, these diagnoses are essentially equivalent.)
The serum half-life for standard preparation detroamphetamine sulfate is approximately 6 to 8 hours in children. This half-life makes it possible for some children to take the medication before leaving for school and maintain clinical effectiveness for the duration of the school day without taking a noontime dose, which is required when the standard preparation methylphenidate is used.
Recently, a pill (Adderall, manufactured by Richwood) combining equal parts of dextroamphetamine saccharate, amphetamine aspartate, dextroamphetamine sulfate, and amphetamine sulfate has been introduced for the treatment of attention deficit disorder with hyperactivity and narcolepsy. The manufacturer states that its plasma half-life is 7 to 8 hours based on the amphetamine component. Whether this combination has clinically significant benefits compared with standard dextroamphetamine sulfate is uncertain at the present time.

Dosage Schedule for Treating ADDH/ADHD
• Children under 3 years of age: Not approved for use.
• Children 3 through 5 years: Begin with 2.5 mg daily; raise by 2.5-mg increments once or twice weekly; titrate for optimal dose.
• Patients 6 years and older: Begin with 5 mg daily; raise by 5-mg increments once or twice weekly; usual maximum dose is less than 40 mg/day.
• The usual optimal individual dose falls between 0.15 and 0.5 mg/kg for each dose (Duncan, 1990), administered two to three times daily (total daily dose range, 0.30 to 1.5 mg/kg/day).

Dose Forms Available
• Tablets: 5 mg
• Sustained-release capsules (Spansules): 5 mg, 10 mg, 15 mg.

Dextroamphetamine in the Treatment of ADDH/ADHD

Dextroamphetamine sulfate is the only amphetamine currently used with any frequency to treat ADHD and is the only stimulant currently in use that is approved by the FDA for administration to children as young as 3 years of age. Hence, it is officially the standard treatment for children up to age 6 years; however, many clinicians do prescribe methylphenidate for some patients under 6 years old. In addition, if methylphenidate does not provide satisfactory benefit in controlling symptoms of ADHD, it is recommended that dextroamphetamine and/or pemoline be tried before moving on to another class of drugs.

Amphetamines may obtund the maximal electroshock seizure discharge and have been reported to prevent typical 3-per-second spike-and-dome petit mal seizures and to abolish the abnormal EEG pattern in some children (Weiner, 1980). Dextroamphetamine may thus be the stimulant of choice for individuals who have seizures or who are at risk for developing them, although, as noted above, methylphenidate does not appear to increase the frequency of seizures or their development de novo when used in usual therapeutic doses.

REPORT OF INTEREST

Geller et al. (1981) reported that dextroamphetamine administered to two children with pervasive developmental disorder and ADDH improved their attention spans with no significant worsening of behavior.

MAGNESIUM PEMOLINE (CYLERT)

Indications in Child and Adolescent Psychiatry
  FDA approved for the treatment of attention deficit disorder with hyperactivity (ADDH). (ADDH is a DSM-III [APA, 1980a] diagnosis that, in large part, corresponds to the DSM-IV [APA, 1994] diagnosis ADHD; technically, as late as 1995, the FDA approval for advertising is still for treatment of ADDH; however, for purposes of medication and dosage, these diagnoses are essentially equivalent.)

Dosage Schedule for Treating ADDH/ADHD
• Children under age 6 years: Not recommended for use.
• Persons 6 years of age and older: The initial recommended daily dose of pemoline is 37.5 mg. This may be increased weekly by 18.75 mg until satisfactory clinical benefit occurs, untoward effects prevent further increase, or the maximum daily dose of 112.5 mg is reached.

Dose Forms Available
• Tablets: 18.75 mg, 37.5 mg, 75 mg.

Magnesium Pemoline in the Treatment of ADHD

Magnesium pemoline elicits central nervous system changes that are similar to those of methylphenidate and amphetamines, but it is structurally dissimilar to those drugs and has minimal sympathomimetic effects. Its serum half-life is approximately 12 hours. About 90% of an oral dose of magnesium pemoline is excreted by the kidneys; this excretion consists of unmetabolized magnesium pemoline (between 40% and 50%) and a remainder comprised of metabolic products of magnesium pemoline that were formed in the liver.

Sallee et al. (1985) reported a 200% variability in pemoline's bioavailability, a 300% variation in total body clearance of pemoline, and a 600% variation in elimination half-time among seven prepubescent hyperactive boys. They also suggested there may be a relatively narrow therapeutic margin and noted that choreiform movements occur frequently after an acute dose of 2 mg/kg/day of magnesium pemoline.

Advantages of pemoline over the sympathomimetic amines include minimal untoward cardiovascular effects; a longer serum half-life, permitting a single morning dose daily (if sustained release forms of the other stimulants are not available to the patient); and probably a less intense rebound effect than methylphenidate and dextroamphetamine. The disadvantages of pemoline are that its clinical effect is not as great as that of dextroamphetamine and methylphenidate, and improvement occurs gradually rather than promptly (Conners et al., 1972). If the manufacturer's recommended titration regimen is followed, significant clinical benefit from pemoline is often apparent only after 3 to 4 weeks. Another concern is hepatotoxicity. Elevated liver enzymes occur in a small percentage of children, perhaps 1% to 3%, treated with magnesium pemoline; these abnormalities appear to be reversible following drug withdrawal, but it is essential to monitor liver function regularly with liver function tests throughout the duration of therapy (PDR, 1995).

Sallee et al. (1985, 1989) reported that acute exposure to a single 2 mg/kg dose of pemoline resulted in abnormal involuntary movements including buccal-lingual chewing and choreoathetoid movements of the face, extremities, and trunk in 25% (5) of 20 severely hyperactive 6- to 12-year-old boys. The movements occurred at peak plasma pemoline concentration or immediately thereafter and lasted for up to 8 hours but persisted with repeated doses in only one subject. This subject and three additional patients also developed choreiform movements after receiving pemoline for a minimum of 3 weeks (3 patients received 2 mg/kg/day of pemoline, and 1 patient received 1.5 mg/kg/day of pemoline and 10 mg/day of imipramine). The authors noted that the low frequency of choreiform movements reported during the clinical use of pemoline may result from its gradual titration. These data would suggest that the clinician should not increase the dosage of pemoline more rapidly than recommended. Another important observation was that improvement in focusing attention occurred within 2 to 3 hours after the dose of pemoline in the acute trial, as opposed to the typically much longer lag period for significant clinical improvement when pemoline is prescribed as recommended (Sallee et al., 1989). Sallee et al. (1992) treated, with pemoline, 25 prepubescent boys diagnosed with ADHD. Pemoline was administered openly beginning with an initial dose of 2 mg/kg adjusted to the nearest 9.375-mg dose, which is equal to one half of an 18.75-mg tablet, the smallest available. This initial dose was chosen with the purpose of reaching therapeutic plasma levels of greater than 2 μg/ml. Mean peak plasma pemoline levels of 3.2 ± 1.2 μg/ml occurred a mean of 2.3 ± 0.8 hours after ingestion. Serum half-life of pemoline was 6.2 hours after 3 weeks of treatment and was not statistically different from that after an acute dose. In a subgroup of 13 subjects, a positive effect on neuroprocessing was evident on ratings for a memory scanning task for task efficiency that contained a motor component, but not on ratings for attention per se. In another subgroup of 12 subjects, positive effects were rated on Paired-Associates Learning tasks. These positive effects were noted within 2 hours after administration of pemoline in both subgroups, and they were sustained over at least the 6-hour period during which pemoline plasma levels remained at therapeutic levels. The authors noted that these features of pemoline's therapeutic response are different from the therapeutic response to methylphenidate or amphetamine. For the methylphenidate and amphetamine, the main therapeutic effects are thought to occur during the period of initial increasing serum levels as the drug is absorbed and to decline significantly once peak serum levels are maintained. Untoward effects of pemoline were not specifically addressed in this report.

Pelham et al. (1990) administered pemoline to 22 children in doses of 56.25 mg every morning over random 3-day periods in a study comparing its efficacy with that of standard methylphenidate and long-acting preparations of methylphenidate and dextroamphetamine. They reported that pemoline's effects on the second and third days of administration were essentially equivalent to the efficacy of standard dosage methylphenidate (10 mg in the morning and at noon) and long-acting dosage forms of both methylphenidate (20 mg/day) and dextroamphetamine (10 mg/day). Although this is higher than the initial dose of pemoline recommended by the manufacturer, the results supported some prior studies that found that pemoline yielded significant therapeutic benefits in much less than the 3 to 6 weeks often reported.

FENFLURAMINE (PONDIMIN)

Indications for Use in Child and Adolescent Psychiatry
Fenfluramine, a sympathomimetic amine with antiserotonergic properties, is approved by the FDA only as a short-term adjunct to the treatment of exogenous obesity in persons 12 years of age or older.

REPORTS OF INTEREST

Fenfluramine has been investigated in the treatment of ADDH and autistic disorder. Clinically fenfluramine was not efficacious, and it had no beneficial effects on motor activity or behavioral ratings in the treatment of ADDH (Donnelly et al., 1989). The rationale for fenfluramine's investigational use in the treatment of autistic disorder was based on the fact that it decreases serotonin levels, which have been found to be elevated in about 30% of mentally retarded and autistic children. Ritvo and his colleagues (1983) reported favorable results in a study of 14 autistic children, which stimulated several other investigators to study this drug.

A 1988 review of published studies of fenfluramine use with autistic children suggested that a subgroup of autistic children with the highest IQ levels and the lowest serotonin values and who had hyperactivity and motor stereotypies improved somewhat with the drug (Verglas et al., 1988). In contrast, a double-blind placebo-controlled study of 28 autistic children found that fenfluramine was not statistically superior to placebo and that it had a retarding effect on discrimination learning; the investigators noted that no individual children had a strong, positive response to the drug (Campbell et al., 1988).

Aman and Kern (1989) reviewed 25 published studies of fenfluramine used in treating subjects with autistic disorder. They concluded that fenfluramine may improve social relatedness and attention span and decrease stereotypies and excessive motor activity in some autistic children. However, broader areas of functioning, as measured by IQ tests and assessment of communicative abilities, did not appear to be affected. Untoward effects reported included lethargy, weight loss, irritability, restlessness, night awakenings, aggressiveness to self or others, diarrhea, and increased stereotypies.

Thus, the initial encouraging data have not been replicated, although a few individuals diagnosed with autistic disorders have shown symptomatic improvements.

CAFFEINE

Caffeine is included among the stimulants because there have been some suggestions that it may be useful in treating ADHD. Two reviews of the relevant literature concluded that caffeine is not a therapeutically useful drug in the treatment of ADHD (Klein, 1987; Klein et al., 1980). Bernstein et al. (1994) investigated the effects of caffeine on learning, performance, and anxiety in 21 prepubescent normal children, 12 males and 9 females, 8 through 12 years old (mean age, 10.6 ± 1.3 years) who ingested a minimum of 20 mg/day of caffeine in their usual diets (average daily caffeine consumption by subjects was 50.9 ± 52.2 mg/day or 1.3 mg/kg/day). Children with significant medical conditions or those ever diagnosed with ADHD were excluded. Subjects were enrolled in a double-blind, placebo-controlled, crossover study in which they were seen for four 2-hour sessions spaced about 1 week apart. The four rated conditions were baseline, placebo, low-dose (2.5 mg/kg) caffeine, and high-dose (5.0 mg/kg) caffeine. Caffeine intake was restricted for 12 to 15 hours before the sessions. Children reported feeling less "sluggish" after receiving caffeine and their performances improved significantly on 2 of 4 measures of attention and a test of manual dexterity for the dominant hand. Self-reported anxiety level showed a trend to increase after ingestion of caffeine.

4

Antipsychotic Drugs

Introduction

Although in adults antipsychotic drugs, also commonly known as neuroleptics or major tranquilizers, are used primarily to treat psychoses, in children they have additionally been used to treat other common nonpsychotic psychiatric disorders. One reason seems to be that the antipsychotic agents won by default; they were among the earliest psychoactive drugs used in child psychiatry, and the competition had not yet arrived. In addition, the risk of untoward effects such as cognitive dulling and irreversible tardive dyskinesia had not been fully appreciated. As clinical and research experience in child psychopharmacology progresses and other drugs become available, however, the use of these drugs in children is becoming more circumscribed. Indications for their use in children now are more closely approaching those for which they are prescribed in older adolescents and adults.

At the present time, antipsychotics are the drugs of first choice in childhood for schizophrenia and autistic disorder. There is, however, some evidence that antipsychotics are not as effective clinically in schizophrenia with childhood onset as in schizophrenia occurring in later adolescence and adulthood (Green et al., 1984). Meyers et al. (1980) noted that serum neuroleptic levels of 50 ng/ml of chlorpromazine equivalents correspond to the threshold for clinical response in adult schizophrenics and suggest that similar therapeutic serum levels are necessary in children. Because children may metabolize and excrete antipsychotics more efficiently than adults, determination of serum neuroleptic levels, if they are available, is recommended before a trial of an antipsychotic is deemed a failure.

Shapiro and Shapiro (1989) concluded that antipsychotics were also the drugs of choice for treating chronic motor or vocal tic disorder and Tourette's disorder when psychosocial, educational, or occupational functioning was so impaired that medication was required. Although antipsychotics are probably indicated in acute mania, paranoia, and schizoaffective disorder, these disorders are rarely diagnosed in childhood, and there is little information available on the use of antipsychotics to treat children with these diagnoses.

Antipsychotic drugs are also clinically effective in severely aggressive, conduct-disordered children, and some are approved for use in such children. Lithium is also effective in such children, however, perhaps more so when there is explosive affect present, and lithium has fewer clinically significant untoward effects than neuroleptics. Because lithium is still not approved for use either for children under 12 years of age or for this indication, and because of the necessity of monitoring serum lithium levels, many clinicians continue to use antipsychotic drugs.

The use of antipsychotics in the mentally retarded continues to be controversial, but they are prescribed frequently, especially for institutionalized patients. Only three neuroleptic drugs are recognized by the FDA as effective for the treatment of psychiatric disorders in the mentally retarded: thioridazine, chlorpromazine, and haloperidol (Gadow & Poling, 1988). In optimal doses antipsychotics are effective in decreasing irritability, sleep disturbances, hostility, agitation, and combativeness and may improve concentration and social behavior in agitated, severely retarded individuals (American Medical Association, 1986). Aman and Singh (1988) cautioned that the influential studies of the mentally retarded by Breuning, which showed significant detrimental effects on cognition resulting from antipsychotic use, appear to have been fabricated.

Antipsychotic Drugs in the Treatment of Attention-Deficit/Hyperactivity Disorders

Some antipsychotic agents (e.g., thioridazine) have been approved for treating children with symptoms such as excessive motor activity, impulsivity, difficulty sustaining attention, and poor frustration tolerance, which would be found in most children diagnosed with ADHD. Double-blind, controlled studies have shown antipsychotic drugs to be effective in treating children who would meet criteria for ADHD. However, studies comparing antipsychotic drugs with stimulants almost always show that stimulants are overall statistically more effective clinically than the antipsychotics (Green, 1995; Gittelman-Klein et al., 1976). In addition, many clinicians are reluctant to use antipsychotics to treat patients with ADHD because of the risk that an irreversible tardive dyskinesia might develop and the worry that the sedative effects of antipsychotics may interfere significantly with cognition and learning. Because of such factors, antipsychotics should be thought of as third-rank drugs to be used primarily in the treatment of ADHD, which is severely disabling and which has not responded to stimulants and other drugs with untoward effects of more acceptable risk.

Although these caveats in using antipsychotics are not to be dismissed, some recent data moderating these dictums should be cited. (*1*) The influential studies of Breuning and his colleagues, which showed significant detrimental effects on cognition in mentally retarded patients treated with antipsychotic drugs, appear to have been fabricated (Aman & Singh, 1988). (*2*) New studies have reported minimal impairment of cognition in subjects diagnosed with ADHD who were treated with appropriate doses of antipsychotics (Klein, 1990/1991). (*3*) There is a suggestion that thioridazine may be superior to stimulants in treating subgroups of mentally deficient patients diagnosed with equivalents of ADHD (Alexandris & Lundell, 1968; Aman et al., 1991a, 1991b).

In a randomized, crossover, double-blind study, Weizman et al. (1984) reported that the combination of propericiazine, a neuroleptic agent prescribed by child psychiatrists in Israel, and a stimulant was statistically superior to placebo-stimulant treatment of 14 children diagnosed with ADDH who had experienced some, but not satisfactory, improvement with stimulant medication only. The authors noted that the combination of a stimulant and neuroleptics may be useful in some children who do not respond adequately to stimulants alone. Clinically this may be a potentially useful option for a small subgroup of children who do not respond adequately to stimulants or to other drugs alone. The combination of stimulant and neuroleptic would presumably achieve a satisfactory result that either would not be achieved by the neuroleptic alone or would require higher doses of neuroleptics, which would carry an increased risk of untoward effects such as tardive dyskinesia and cognitive dulling.

Pharmacokinetics of Antipsychotic Drugs

Rivera-Calimlim et al. (1979) reported plasma chlorpromazine levels in a total of 24 children aged 8 to 16 years who were treated with chlorpromazine for psychiatric disorders, including various psychoses, mental retardation with aggression, hyperactivity, self-injurious behavior, and mood disorders with anxiety. The authors reported wide interpatient variations in chlorpromazine plasma levels for a given dose; for example, 9 children receiving 0.8 to 2.9 mg/kg/day achieved mean plasma levels of 6.6 ng/ml, with a range from undetectable to 18 ng/ml. One child receiving 9.8 mg/kg/day showed only trace levels of plasma chlorpromazine. Children and adolescents had chlorpromazine plasma levels that were from 2 times to 3.5 times lower than those for adults, for a given dose per kilogram of body weight. Clinical improvement in these children usually began when plasma chlorpromazine concentration was at least 30 ng/ml, and optimal levels ranged between 40 ng/ml and 80 ng/ml, compared with adults treated with chlorpromazine, in whom suggested optimal plasma levels were higher, i.e., between 50 ng/ml and 300 ng/ml. A final clinically important observation was that plasma chlorpromazine levels declined over time in most patients who were on fixed doses (Rivera-Calimlim et al., 1979). It was suggested that one possible reason might be autoinduction of enzymes that metabolize chlorpromazine.

Contraindications for the Administration of Antipsychotic Drugs

Known hypersensitivity to the drug and toxic central nervous system depression or comatose states are absolute contraindications. If a severe untoward effect develops (e.g., agranulocytosis, neuroleptic malignant syndrome, tardive dyskinesia, or a withdrawal dyskinesia), children and adolescents should be managed without antipsychotics if at all possible.

Neuroleptics may lower the seizure threshold; they should be used cautiously in patients with seizure disorders, and chlorpromazine probably should not be used in such patients.

Interactions of Antipsychotic Drugs with other Medications

The most frequent clinically important reactions are with other central nervous system depressants such as alcohol, sedatives and hypnotics, benzodiazepines, antihistamines, opiates, and barbiturates, in which an additive central nervous system depressive effect occurs.

Antipsychotic drugs also have varying degrees of anticholinergic effects. When combined with another anticholinergic (antiparkinsonian) agent, such as when one is used prophylactically to prevent acute dyskinesia, pseudoparkinsonism, or akathisia, central nervous system symptoms of cholinergic blockade may result. These symptoms may include confusion, disorientation, delirium, hallucinations, and worsening of preexisting psychotic symptoms. Of clinical importance, this picture may be mistaken for inadequate treatment or worsening of the psychosis, rather than an untoward effect.

The combination of antipsychotic drugs and lithium carbonate, particularly if high doses are used, may possibly lead to an increased incidence of central nervous system toxicity, including neuroleptic malignant syndrome.

Combined use with tricyclic antidepressants or monoamine oxidase inhibitors may increase plasma levels of antidepressants.

Neuroleptics may also have noteworthy interactions with many other medications.

Untoward Effects of Antipsychotic Drugs

Although antipsychotic drugs may have numerous serious untoward effects, those of greatest concern in children and adolescents are the effects of sedation on cognition and the extrapyramidal syndromes, in particular the possible development of irreversible tardive dyskinesia.

AGRANULOCYTOSIS

Agranulocytosis is a major concern in patients treated with clozapine; it is discussed in more detail below under that drug. Agranulocytosis has also been reported with other antipsychotics. It usually occurs relatively early in treatment (e.g., for chlorpromazine usually between the 4th and 10th weeks). Parents and older patients should be warned to report indications of sudden infections, such as fever and sore throat, to the physician. White blood cell count should be determined immediately, and if it is significantly depressed, medication should be stopped and therapy instituted.

UNTOWARD COGNITIVE EFFECTS

Both high-potency and low-potency antipsychotic agents are effective when given in equivalent doses, but they differ in the frequency and severity of their untoward effects. Usually, the higher-potency antipsychotic drugs cause less sedation, fewer autonomic side effects, and more extrapyramidal untoward effects; the lower-potency antipsychotic drugs cause greater sedation, more autonomic side effects, and fewer extrapyramidal effects (Baldessarini, 1990). Because of the great importance of minimizing any cognitive dulling in school children and in the mentally retarded, whose cognition is already compromised, high-potency, less-sedative antipsychotic drugs are often preferred. Over a period of days to weeks, however, considerable tolerance often develops to the sedative effects of high-dose, low-potency antipsychotic drugs, and thus they are still useful when untoward effects are carefully monitored (Green, 1989).

EXTRAPYRAMIDAL SYNDROMES

Significant numbers of children and adolescents receiving antipsychotic medication develop extrapyramidal syndromes. Baldessarini (1990) has enumerated six types of extrapyramidal syndromes associated with the use of antipsychotic drugs.

Effects Usually Appearing during Drug Administration

Acute Dystonic Reactions.   The period of maximum risk is within hours to 5 days after initiation of neuroleptic therapy. There may also be increased risk following increments in dose. High-potency, low-dose antipsychotic drugs are more likely to precipitate an acute dystonic reaction than are low-potency, high-dose antipsychotic drugs, and young males, both children and adolescents, may be at increased risk (APA, 1980b). Untreated acute dystonic reactions may last from a few minutes to several hours, and they may recur. Symptoms, which may be painful and frightening, particularly if the patient does not understand what is happening, include muscular hypertonicity; tonic contractions (spasms) of the neck (torticollis), mouth, and tongue, which may make speaking difficult; oculogyric crisis (eyes rolling upward and remaining in that position); and opisthotonos (spasm in which the spine and extremities are bent with a forward convexity). Acute dystonic reactions respond rapidly to anticholinergic and antiparkinsonian drugs, such as diphenhydramine (Benadryl), 25 to 50 mg orally or intramuscularly, or benztropine (Cogentin), 1 to 2 mg intramuscularly. (The manufacturer of benztropine cautions that, because of its atropine-like untoward effects, its use is contraindicated in children under 3 years of age and that it should be used with caution in older children [PDR, 1995].) If the dystonia is very severe, administering either 25 mg of diphenhydramine intramuscularly or 1 to 2 mg of benztropine intramuscularly will reverse the dystonia within a few minutes. The prophylactic use of anticholinergic and antiparkinsonian agents to prevent acute dystonic reactions is discussed below following the section on akasthisia.

Parkinsonism (Pseudoparkinsonism). Symptoms of parkinsonism include tremor, cogwheel rigidity, drooling, and decrease in facial expressive movements (mask-like or expressionless facies) and akinesia (slowness in initiating movements). These symptoms respond to antiparkinsonian medications; for example, benztropine (Cogentin), 1 to 2 mg given two or three times daily, usually provides relief within a day or two. Antiparkinsonian medication may be withdrawn gradually after 1 or 2 weeks to see if it is still necessary for symptomatic relief.

The period of maximum risk for developing parkinsonism is 5 to 30 days after initiation of neuroleptic therapy. The risk for development of parkinsonism appears to be greater for females and to increase with age. It is rarely seen in preschool children treated with therapeutic doses of neuroleptics; it occurs commonly in school-aged children and adolescents (Campbell et al., 1985). Richardson et al. (1991) reported that 21 (34%) of 61 hospitalized children and adolescents, of whom only 7 were diagnosed with psychotic or affective disorders, who were taking neuroleptics at the time of evaluation exhibited symptoms of parkinsonism when rated on several movement disorder scales. Three (14.3%) of the 21 children were rated as having parkinsonism despite the fact they were concurrently receiving antiparkinsonian drugs. Development of parkinsonism was significantly ($P = .05$) associated with a longer duration on medication at the time of evaluation (mean of 117 days for patients with parkinsonism and mean of 34 days for patients without parkinsonism).

Akinesia, perhaps the most severe form of parkinsonism, is defined by Rifkin et al. (1975) as a "behavioral state of diminished spontaneity characterized by few gestures, unspontaneous speech and, particularly, apathy and difficulty with initiating usual activities" (p. 672). It may be particularly difficult to differentiate from the negative symptoms of schizophrenia, such as apathy and blunting. Van Putten and Marder (1987) suggested that akinesia might be the most toxic behavioral side effect of antipsychotic drugs. The authors noted that a subjective sense of sedation or drowsiness, excessive sleeping, and a lack of any leg-crossing during an interview of about 20 minutes correlated with the presence of akinesia. Akinesia also interferes with social adjustment, and the patient may appear to have a "postpsychotic depression." Patients with akinesia often are less concerned with any psychotic symptoms and report that everything is fine; they may experience an absence of emotion and appear emotionally dead (Van Putten & Marder, 1987). Although antiparkinsonian drugs may be helpful, in some cases they do not adequately control symptoms of akinesia. There is some evidence that antiparkinsonian drugs become less effective at higher daily dosages of antipsychotics (Van Putten & Marder, 1987).

The prophylactic use of anticholinergic and antiparkinsonian agents to prevent pseudoparkinsonism is discussed below, following the section on akathisia.

Akathisia (Motor Restlessness). The period of maximum risk for developing this condition is 5 to 60 days after initiation of neuroleptic therapy, but it has been reported to occur in as few as 6 hours after an oral dose of a neuroleptic (Van Putten et al., 1984). Symptoms include constant uncomfortable restlessness, a feeling of tension in the lower extremities often accompanied by a strong or irresistible urge to move them, inability to sit still, and foot-tapping or pacing. Clinically, blunted affect, emotional withdrawal, and motor retardation may also be observed (Van Putten & Marder, 1987).

Akathisia may or may not respond to antiparkinsonian drugs such as trihexyphenidyl (Artane). Van Putten and Marder (1987) noted the dual nature of akathisia: a subjective experience of restlessness and observable motor restlessness. In their clinical experience, all patients with moderate or severe akathisia exhibited either rocking from foot to foot or walking on the spot. Akathisia was also strongly associated with depression, dysphoria, and, at times in severe and treatment-resistant cases, with exacerbation of psychotic symptoms and homicidal and suicidal ideation and behavior (Van Putten & Marder, 1987). Of particular clinical importance, patients who have unpleasant untoward effects, especially akathisia, with antipsychotics are more likely to be noncompliant and to unilaterally discontinue medication early in treatment (Van Putten & Marder, 1987).

Fleischhacker et al. (1989) have published a rating scale for akathisia that includes two subjective items: "a sensation of inner restlessness" and "the urge to move" and three items that characterize the frequency and magnitude of observed akathisia phenomena.

Propranolol may be helpful in ameliorating akathisia (Adler et al., 1986); benzodiazepines and clonidine have also been reported to be effective in some cases.

Clonazepam was administered to 10 first-onset psychotic adolescents (8 of whom were diagnosed with schizophrenia, paranoid subtype) between 16 and 19 years of age who experienced distressing akathisia following treatment with antipsychotics (Kutcher et al., 1987). Nine of the patients also had been receiving benztropine concomitantly with their antipsychotic medication. All patients reported subjective improvement, and scores on an akathisia subscale decreased significantly after 1 week's treatment with 0.5 mg/day of clonazepam.

In some cases, reduction in dose of the antipsychotic may be necessary. Neppe and Ward (1989) recommend that if only akathisia develops (i.e., without accompanying parkinsonism) that a β-blocker be used rather than an anticholinergic agent.

Prophylactic Use of Antiparkinsonian Agents for Acute Dystonic Reaction, Parkinsonism, and Akathisia. The use of antiparkinsonian (anticholinergic) agents prophylactically to minimize the likelihood of the patient's developing an acute dystonic reaction, parkinsonism, or akathisia from antipsychotic drug use is controversial. Some of the reasons relate to the effects caused by the anticholinergic agents themselves. Anticholinergic agents may affect cognition adversely and may aggravate psychotic symptomatology. In addition, there is some suggestion that at least part of the effectiveness of these agents is that they may lower the serum concentration of the antipsychotic drug (Rivera-Calimlim et al., 1976). Because of their reluctance to give an additional medication that itself may have untoward effects, many clinicians choose to minimize the risk of these extrapyramidal effects by beginning with a low dose and titrating the medication slowly. If an acute dystonic reaction should occur, it may be treated with diphenhydramine and the dosage of antipsychotic lowered temporarily if necessary. Conversely, some clinicians routinely prescribe an agent such as benztropine for approximately 1 month to 6 weeks covering the period of maximal risk for the development of both acute dystonic reactions and parkinsonian untoward effects. Another option for outpatients is to prescribe a small amount of an anticholinergic (e.g., diphenhydramine) with an explanation of how it is to be administered should a dystonic reaction occur (e.g., to take one capsule should such a reaction begin, to take another dose in 20 to 30 minutes if there is no improvement, and to go to an emergency room if the reaction is severe and alert the physician to the medication being taken).

In their review of the management of acute extrapyramidal syndromes induced by neuroleptics, Neppe and Ward (1989) note that anticholinergics can significantly reduce the rate of acute dystonias, especially in the highest-risk group, males under 30 years of age treated with high-potency antipsychotic agents. However, as acute dystonic reactions tend to be transient, prophylactic treatment for more than 2 weeks is not usually indicated. These authors recommend no prophylaxis for parkinsonism and akathisia, because they rarely present as dramatically emergent a picture as acute dystonia. The parents and/or patient as appropriate may be carefully informed about the possibility of these conditions arising, to aid in their early detection. The clinician can then decide how best to treat the particular symptom in the particular patient (Neppe & Ward, 1989).

Van Putten and Marder (1987) point out that prophylactic use of antiparkinsonian drugs may not fully prevent symptoms of akinesia from developing and that some schizophrenic patients who have been stabilized using antiparkinsonian medication may experience increased anxiety, depression, general dysphoria, and suffering when the anticholinergics are withdrawn.

The clinician should decide on a case-by-case basis which of the above possibilities is best for a given patient. This decision will be based on factors such as whether a high- or low-potency neuroleptic is given, how rapidly the dose is increased, previous experience of the patient, whether it is administered to an outpatient or an inpatient (who has ready access to clinical staff), how such a reaction might affect the relationship with the patient and/or the parents and subsequent compliance, and the patient's environment. For example, it can be particularly difficult for a patient and family if the patient develops an acute dystonic reaction while attending school. **Neuroleptic Malignant Syndrome.** This condition is life threatening and can occur after a single dose but most frequently within 2 weeks after initiation of neuroleptic therapy or an increase in dosage; males and younger individuals appear to be most often affected (for review see Kaufmann & Wyatt, 1987). Symptoms include severe muscular rigidity, altered consciousness, stupor, catatonia, hyperpyrexia, labile pulse and blood pressure, and occasionally myoglobinemia. Most patients have elevated creatine phosphokinase (CPK) levels. Neuroleptic malignant syndrome can persist for up to 2 weeks or longer after medication is discontinued and can be fatal. Treatment consists of immediate cessation of medication and hospitalization with supportive treatment. Dopaminergic agonists (e.g., bromocriptine and amantadine) and/or dantrolene have also been reported to reduce the mortality rate significantly (Sakkas et al., 1991). Antiparkinsonian drugs are not useful.

Latz and McCracken (1992) conducted an extensive literature search and reported a total of 49 cases of neuroleptic malignant syndrome (NMS) in patients 18 years old or younger. The youngest reported case was in an 11 month old. Five (83%) of the 6 preschoolers developed NMS after a single dose of neuroleptic that was either an accidental overdose or was prescribed for a nonpsychiatric illness. Overall lethality for all cases reviewed was 16.3% (8) of 49.

However, the death rate for patients 12 years of age or younger was 27% (3) of 11, more than twice the 13% (5) of 38 death rate for adolescents 13 to 18 years old.

Steingard et al. (1992) also published a review with detailed summaries of 35 cases of neuroleptic malignant syndrome in patients under 19 years of age. Fever, rigidity, altered mental status, and tachycardia were present in more than 70% of the cases. Five (14%) of the patients died; however, only one of these died within the past two decades and that was a 2 year old who had ingested chlorpromazine accidentally.

Late-Appearing Syndromes (after Months or Years of Treatment)

Tardive Dyskinesia.   Definitions and descriptions of tardive dyskinesia (TD) and related dyskinesias (withdrawal, masked dyskinesias) vary. Perhaps the most influential definition at the present time is the research diagnostic criteria proposed in 1982 by Schooler and Kane. They note that, if possible, the absence of abnormal involuntary movements prior to beginning pharmacotherapy should be documented. Schooler and Kane's (1982) research diagnostic criteria for tardive dyskinesia proposed three prerequisites for making the diagnosis:

1. Exposure to neuroleptic drugs for a minimum total cumulative exposure of 3 months
2. The presence of at least "moderate" abnormal involuntary movements in one or more body areas (face, lips, jaw, tongue, upper extremities, lower extremities, trunk) or at least "mild" movements in two or more body areas
3. Absence of other conditions that might produce abnormal movements

Once these prerequisites have been met by a patient, Schooler and Kane (1982) proposed six diagnostic categories of tardive dyskinesia:

1 (a) Probable tardive dyskinesia "concurrent neuroleptics" if the patient is currently receiving neuroleptic therapy, or (b) probable tardive dsykinesia "neuroleptic free" if no longer receiving neuroleptic medication. (Only one of these two diagnoses would be possible the first time the patient was examined.)

2. Masked probable tardive dyskinesia: Within 2 weeks after an increase in dose in a patient diagnosed with 1a (above) or resumption of neuroleptic drug treatment in a patient diagnosed with 1b (above), prerequisite 2 is no longer met.

3. Transient tardive dyskinesia: Within 3 months after a patient is diagnosed with 1a and with no increase in dose of neuroleptic (a dose reduction is permissible), prerequisite 2 is no longer met; or, within 3 months after a patient diagnosed with 1b, prerequisite 2 is no longer met, and the patient has remained neuroleptic free.

4. Withdrawal tardive dyskinesia: While receiving neuroleptics the patient does not meet prerequisite 2 but within 2 weeks following cessation of neuroleptics with usual serum half-lives or 5 weeks after stopping a long-acting neuroleptic (e.g., a depot dosage form), the patient develops abnormal movements consistent with prerequisite 2. If the movements cease or no longer satisfy prerequisite 2 within 3 months, this diagnosis stands.

5. (a) Persistent tardive dyskinesia "concurrent neuroleptics" if the patient was diagnosed with 1a and has continuously received neuroleptics over the subsequent 3 months and continues to satisfy prerequisite 2. (b) Persistent tardive dyskinesia "neuroleptic free" if the patient was diagnosed with 1a (and neuroleptic drug was immediately stopped), with 1b, or with 4 (withdrawal TD) and no neuroleptic was administered during the subsequent 3 months and the patient continues to fulfill prerequisite 2. (c) Persistent tardive dyskinesia "unspecified" if the patient was diagnosed 1a, 1b, or 4, and the patient received neuroleptics for part of the subsequent 3-month period and still meets prerequisite 2.

6. Masked persistent tardive dyskinesia if a patient diagnosed with 5a or 5c no longer meets prerequisite 2 within 3 weeks following an increase in dosage of the neuroleptic agent or if a patient diagnosed with 5b no longer meets prerequisite 2 within 3 weeks after resumption of a neuroleptic.

Four additional diagnostic criteria were suggested by the American Psychiatric Association Task Force on Tardive Dyskinesia (American Psychiatric Association, 1992):

1. The abnormal movements are exacerbated or may be provoked by a decrease or withdrawal of an antipsychotic drug. Increasing the dose of antipsychotic will suppress (or dampen) the movements at least temporarily.
2. Anticholinergic medication does not ameliorate and may worsen the movements.
3. Emotional stress may worsen the movements.
4. The movements decrease or disappear during sleep.

Tardive dyskinesia develops while actively receiving a neuroleptic drug, as opposed to a withdrawal dyskinesia that occurs when a neuroleptic is withdrawn or its dose is decreased. Tardive dyskinesia, which may be both severely disabling and irreversible, is the most clinically significant common long-term untoward effect of antipsychotic use. Baldessarini (1990) notes that in some cases, especially in younger patients, tardive dyskinesia will disappear over the course of weeks to as much as 3 years. It is believed that the risk of developing irreversible tardive dyskinesia increases with both total cumulative dose and duration of treatment. Older females appear to be at increased risk. It has been reported that fine worm-like (vermicular) movements of the tongue may be an early sign of tardive dyskinesia, and that discontinuation of the medication when this occurs may prevent further development of the syndrome (PDR, 1995). Symptoms of tardive dyskinesia most typically include involuntary choreoathetotic movements affecting the face; tongue; perioral, buccal, and masticatory musculature; and neck, but which may also involve the torso and extremities.

Atypical and less common forms of tardive dyskinesia, such as tardive akathisia, a persisting restlessness, and tardive dystonia, also occur. Burke et al. (1982) reported 42 cases of tardive dystonia that they diagnosed by the following criteria:

1. The presence of chronic dystonia
2. History of antipsychotic drug treatment preceding or concurrent with the onset of dystonia
3. Exclusion of known causes of secondary dystonia by appropriate clinical and laboratory evaluation
4. A negative family history for dystonia

Symptoms of tardive dystonia began after as few as 3 days and up to 11 years after initiation of antipsychotic medication. The incidence of tardive dystonia was more frequent in younger male patients than in older patients; was characterized by sustained abnormal postures accompanied by torticollis, torsion of the trunk and extremities, blepharospasm, and grimacing; and was incapacitating in severe cases. Spontaneous remission occurred in a few patients, but in most dystonia persisted for years. Of the many medications used to ameliorate the tardive dystonia, the most helpful were tetrabenzine, which improved symptoms in 68% of patients, and anticholinergics, which were helpful in 39% of patients (Burke et al., 1982).

In tardive dyskinesia and other choreoathetotic syndromes, emotional stress typically causes worsening of the movements, drowsiness or sedation causes them to diminish, and they disappear during sleep (APA, 1980b). There is no adequate treatment; antiparkinsonian drugs may worsen the condition (for review see APA, 1980b). There is evidence, however, that the atypical antipsychotic drug clozapine not only produces little or no tardive dyskinesia when it is the only neuroleptic ever used, but also significantly decreases or eliminates existing symptoms of tardive dyskinesia during the period it is prescribed (Small et al., 1987; Birmaher et al., 1992; Mozes et al., 1994). Upon its discontinuation, however, the dyskinetic movements that were suppressed by clozapine rapidly returned in 18 of 19 patients when it was discontinued (Small et al., 1987).

Vitamin E has also been reported to be helpful in treating tardive dyskinesia in adults. Adler et al. (1993) treated 28 adult patients diagnosed with tardive dyskinesia in a double-blind parallel-group comparison study of 8 to 12 weeks' duration. The 16 patients receiving 1600 IU of vitamin E daily showed significantly greater improvement on their scores on the AIMS than the 12 patients receiving placebo. The authors noted that their data also supported earlier findings that patients whose onset of tardive dyskinesia was within the preceding 5 years were more likely to respond to vitamin E therapy than patients with more longstanding tardive dyskinesia.

In addition, a withdrawal dyskinesia may emerge when neuroleptic medication is withdrawn or the dose is reduced. Withdrawal-emergent dyskinesias can occur for two different reasons: First, antidopaminergic drugs, including antipsychotics, can suppress tardive dyskinesia; thus decreasing their serum levels can "unmask" ongoing tardive dyskinesia. Second, Baldessarini (1990) points out that a "disuse supersensitivity" to dopamine agonists may also occur following withdrawal of antidopaminergic drugs; he suggests that this phenomenon may explain withdrawal dyskinesias that resolve within a few weeks.

The reported prevalence of neuroleptic-induced tardive dyskinesia and withdrawal tardive dyskinesia in children and adolescents has ranged from 0% to 51% (Wolf & Wagner, 1993). It is thought that the risk of developing tardive dyskinesia that will become irreversible increases with both total cumulative dose and duration of treatment. No cases of irreversible tardive dyskinesia developing in children or adolescents have been reported; the longest neuroleptic-free persistent tardive dyskinesia was reported to last was 4½ years. Usually withdrawal dyskinesias resolve within a few weeks to a few months after discontinuation of the neuroleptic (Wolf & Wagner, 1993).

Richardson et al. (1991) reported that 5 (12%) of 41 hospitalized children and adolescents (mean age, 15.5 years old), of whom only 10 were diagnosed with psychotic or affective disorders, who had taken neuroleptics for at least one period of 90 continuous days before the time of evaluation exhibited symptoms of treatment-emergent tardive dyskinesia (occurring while receiving neuroleptics) when rated on the Simpson Abbreviated Dyskinesia Scale. The 5 patients who developed tardive dyskinesia were significantly more likely to have had a history of assaultive behavior ($P = .003$) and a first-degree relative who had been hospitalized for a psychiatric disorder ($P = .009$) than patients who did not develop tardive dyskinesia. Using the more stringent research criteria of Schooler and Kane (1982), 3 (7%) were diagnosed with tardive dyskinesia.

If tardive dyskinesia develops, every effort should be made to discontinue or at least reduce the dose of antipsychotic drug as much as possible. The dyskinesia should be monitored with serial ratings on the AIMS. If the severity of the psychiatric disorder precludes discontinuation of antipsychotic medication (e.g., in a patient diagnosed with autistic disorder who exhibits severe self-injurious behavior and aggressiveness and who has not responded adequately to other medications such as lithium or propranolol), the clinician must carefully document the rationale for reinstituting antipsychotic medication and that the legal guardians (and patient when appropriate) have given their informed consent. Reinstating or increasing the dose of antipsychotic may suppress or mask tardive dyskinesia.

Because of such risks, antipsychotic agents should be given only to children and adolescents for whom no other potentially less harmful treatment is available; for example, although effective in some children diagnosed with ADHD, antipsychotic drugs should not be used unless stimulant medications and other nonstimulant drugs with safer untoward effect profiles have been treatment failures (Green, 1995).

Although antipsychotics are the only drugs that result in persistent tardive dyskinesia in a significant proportion of patients, a number of different drugs may cause dyskinesias after short- or long-term treatment. Jeste and Wyatt (1982) note that the dyskinesia produced by L-dopa most closely resembles the tardive dyskinesia resulting from antipsychotics and that, typically, the dyskinesias caused by most other drugs are usually acute, sometimes toxic, effects and almost always remit when the drug is discontinued. Among the drugs used in child and adolescent psychopharmacotherapy for which dyskinesias have been reported are amphetamines, methylphenidate, monoamine oxidase inhibitors, tricyclic antidepressants, lithium, antihistamines, benzodiazepines, and antiepileptic drugs (Jeste & Wyatt, 1982).

Rabbit Syndrome (Perioral Tremor). This condition, which may be a late-onset variant of parkinsonism, is uncommon. Its name derives from the fact that patients so afflicted make rapid chewing movements similar to those of rabbits (Villeneuve, 1972). It may respond to antiparkinsonian medication.

Other Untoward Effects of Antipsychotic Drugs

Table 4.1 is a compilation of most of the reported untoward effects of chlorpromazine, the prototype antipsychotic drug. Most of these untoward effects have also been reported to occur to a greater or lesser degree with other antipsychotic drugs.

Representative Antipsychotic Drugs Used in Child and Adolescent Psychiatry

Table 4.2 summarizes representative antipsychotic drugs commonly used in child and adolescent psychiatry. It compares their relative potencies and expectable potential sedative, autonomic, and extrapyramidal untoward effects with chlorpromazine, the prototype of the antipsychotics. FDA age limitations and recommended dosages for approved use in children and adolescents are also given when available.

Table 4.1.
Untoward Effects of Chlorpromazine

Allergic
  Mild urticaria
  Photosensitivity, exfoliative dermatitis
  Asthma
  Anaphylactoid reactions
  Laryngeal edema
  Angioneurotic edema
Autonomic nervous system
  Antiadrenergic effects
    Orthostatic hypotension
    Ejaculatory disturbances
  Anticholinergic effects
    Decreased secretion, resulting in dry mouth, dry eyes, nasal congestion
    Blurred vision, mydriasis
    Glaucoma attack in patients with narrow-angle closure
    Constipation, paralytic ileus
    Urinary retention
    Impotence
Cardiovascular
  Postural (orthostatic) hypotension
  Tachycardia
  ECG changes
  Sudden death due to cardiac arrest
Central nervous system
  Neuromuscular effects
    Dystonias
    Akasthisia (motor restlessness)
    Pseudoparkinsonism
    Tardive dyskinesia
  Seizures, lowering of seizure threshold
  Drowsiness, sedation
  Behavioral effects
    Increased psychotic symptoms
    Catatonic-like states

(continues)

CONSIDERATIONS ABOUT DOSAGE

The antipsychotic effects of neuroleptic agents evolve gradually. The depolarization inactivation of dopaminergic neurons, which is necessary for antipsychotic efficacy, takes about 3 to 6 weeks to develop. Hence, it is important to have a trial of adequate duration of an antipsychotic drug at usual therapeutic doses rather than rapidly increasing the dose, which can lead to the erroneous clinical impression that a much higher dose than necessary was responsible for the patient's clinical improvement. Studies have also sug-

Table 4.1. continued
Untoward Effects of Chlorpromazine

Dermatological
  Photosensitivity
    Skin pigmentation changes in exposed areas
    Rashes
Endocrinological
  Elevated prolactin levels
  Gynecomastia
  Amenorrhea
  Hyperglycemia, glycosuria, and hypoglycemia
Hematological
  Agranulocytosis
  Eosinophilia
  Leukopenia
  Hemolytic anemia
  Aplastic anemia
  Thrombocytopenic purpura
  Pancytopenia
Hepatological
  Jaundice
Metabolic
  Weight gain, increased appetite
Ophthalmologic
  Blurred vision
  Precipitation of acute glaucoma attack in persons with narrow-angle glaucoma
  Deposition of pigmented material and star-shaped opacities in lens
  Deposition of pigmented material in cornea
  Pigmentary retinopathy
  Epithelial keratopathy
Teratogenic effects possible (seen in animal studies)
Other
  Neuroleptic malignant syndrome
  Sudden death, which may be related to cardiac failure or suppression of cough
    reflex

gested that there is a therapeutic window of approximately 300 to 1000 mg of chlorpromazine or its equivalent for most psychotic adult patients. Patients receiving less than 300 mg tend to improve less, and those receiving more than 1000 mg of chlorpromazine or its equivalent show no increased benefit (for review see Levy, 1993). It is usually recommended that antipsychotic agents initially be administered in divided doses, most frequently three or four times daily. Once the optimal dose is established, however, their relatively long serum half-lives usually permit either once-daily dosage (e.g., before bedtime) or twice-daily dosage, in the morning and before bedtime.

Table 4.2.
Antipsychotic Drugs[a]

Antipsychotic Drug Tradename (Manufacturer)	Chemical Classification	Therapeutically Equivalent Oral Dose (mg)	Effects			Approved Age for Use	Usual Optimal Dose/ Maintenance Dose Range
			Sedation	Autonomic[b]	Extrapyramidal Reaction[c]		
Chlorpromazine[d] Thorazine (SmithKline Beecham)	Phenothiazine: aliphatic compound	100	+++	+++	++	Over 6 months	See text
Thioridazine[d] Mellaril (Sandoz)	Phenothiazine: piperidine compound	100	+++	+++	+	2 years	See text
Clozapine Clozaril (Sandoz)	Dibenzodiazepine	75	+++	+++	0?	16 years	As per adults See text
Mesoridazine Serentil (Boehringer Ingelheim)	Phenothiazine: piperidine compound	50	+++	++	+	12 years	No specific doses for children
Loxapine[d] Loxitane (Lederle)	Dibenzoxazepine	15	++	+/++	++/+++	16 years	As per adults
Molindone Moban (TEVA)	Dihydroindolone	10	++	+	+	12 years	No specific doses for children
Perphenazine[d] Trilafon (Schering)	Phenothiazine: piperazine compound	10	++	+	++/+++	12 years	No specific doses for children

Trifluoperazine[d] Stelazine (SmithKline Beecham)	Phenothiazine: piperazine compound	5	++	+	+++	6 years	See text
Thiothixene[d] Navane (Roerig)	Thioxanthene	5	+	+	+++	12 years	No specific doses for children
Fluphenazine[d] Permitil (Schering) Prolixin (Apothecon)	Phenothiazine: piperazine compound	2	+	+	+++	16 years	See text
Haloperidol[d] Haldol (McNeil)	Butyrophenone	2	+	+	+++	3 years	See text
Pimozide[e] Orap (TEVA)	Diphenylbutyl-piperidine	10	+	+	+++	Over 12 years	0.2 mg/kg/day or maximum, 10 mg/day

aAdapted from American Medical Association. Drug Evaluations Annual 1994. Chicago: American Medical Association, 1994.

bα-antiadrenergic and anticholinergic effects.

cExcluding tardive dyskinesia, which appears to be produced to the same degree and frequency by all agents except clozapine with equieffective antipsychotic doses. Clozapine has produced agranulocytosis; therefore, recommendations for its use are limited (see text).

dAvailable generically.

eOnly indicated for Tourette's disorder that has not responded to other standard treatments; not approved for use in psychoses.

Standard Antipsychotic Drugs

CHLORPROMAZINE (THORAZINE)

Indications in Child and Adolescent Psychiatry
In addition to being approved for uses similar to those for adults, including psychotic disorders, chlorpromazine is approved for the treatment of severe behavioral problems in children, marked by combativeness and/or explosive hyperexcitable behavior. It is also noted that dosages over 500 mg/day are unlikely to further enhance behavioral improvement in severely disturbed mentally retarded patients.
Chlorpromazine may lower the threshold to seizures; another antipsychotic should be chosen for seizure-prone individuals.

Dosage Schedule for Children and Adolescents
• Infants under 6 months of age: Not recommended.
• Children over 6 months to 12 years of age with severe behavioral problems or psychotic conditions:
Oral: 0.25 mg/kg every 4 to 6 hours as needed. Titrate upward gradually. In severe cases daily doses of 200 mg or higher may be required.
Rectal: 1 mg/kg every 6 to 8 hours as needed.
Intramuscular: 0.5 mg/kg every 6 to 8 hours as needed. Maximum daily intramuscular dose for a child under 5 years or under 22 kg is 40 mg; for a child 5 to 12 years of age or 22 kg to 45 kg, maximum daily dose is 75 mg.
• Adolescents: Depending on severity of symptoms, begin with 10 mg three times to 25 mg four times daily. Titrate upward with increases of 20 mg to 50 mg twice weekly. For severely agitated patients, 25 mg intramuscularly may be given and repeated if necessary in 1 hour. Any subsequent intramuscular medication should be at 4- to 6-hour intervals.

Dose Forms Available
• Tablets: 10 mg, 25 mg, 50 mg, 100 mg, 200 mg
• Syrup: 10 mg/5 ml
• Suppositories: 25 mg, 100 mg
• Concentrate: 30 mg/ml, 100 mg/ml
• Injectable: 25 mg/ml

REPORTS OF INTEREST

Chlorpromazine in the Treatment of Children and Adolescents Diagnosed with Attention Deficit Hyperactivity Disorder. Werry et al. (1966) reported that chlorpromazine was significantly superior to placebo (P =.005) in reducing hyperactivity in a double-blind, placebo-controlled, 8-week study of 39 hyperactive children (mean age, 8.5 years; IQ, 85 or greater), a large number of whom had additional symptoms of distractibility, irritability, and specific cognitive defects. Intellectual functioning and symptoms of distractibility, aggressivity, and excitability did not appear significantly affected by the drug. The authors concluded that chlorpromazine could be used for behavioral symptoms in therapeutic doses (mean dose was 106 mg/day with a maximum daily dose of 5 mg/kg or 150–200 mg) without fear of significantly impairing learning. The most frequent untoward effects were mild sedation and mild photosensitization of the skin (Werry et al., 1966).

Weiss and her colleagues (1975) reported that 5 years after initial diagnosis, there were no differences on measures of emotional adjustment, antisocial behavior, and academic performance among a group of hyperactive children treated with chlorpromazine for 1½ to 5 years, a similar group treated for 3 to 5 years with methylphenidate, and a group whose medication was discontinued after 4 months because of poor response.

THIORIDAZINE (MELLARIL)

Indications in Child and Adolescent Psychiatry
  In addition to psychotic disorders, thioridazine has FDA approval for treating severe behavioral problems marked by combativeness and/or explosive hyperexcitable behavior (out of proportion to immediate provocations). It is also approved in the short-term treatment of hyperactive children who show excessive motor activity with accompanying conduct disorders consisting of some or all of the following symptoms: impulsivity, difficulty sustaining attention, aggressivity, mood lability, and poor frustration tolerance.

Dosage Schedule for Children and Adolescents
• Children under 2 years of age: Not recommended.
• Children 2 to 12 years of age: Usual dosage ranges from 0.5 mg/kg/day to a maximum of 3 mg/kg/day. Start with a low dose and titrate upward for optimal therapeutic effect. More severely disturbed children may initially require 25 mg once or twice daily.
• Older adolescents: As in adults, a maximum of 800 mg/day is permitted to minimize the likelihood that pigmentary retinopathy will develop. The initial dose depends on the severity of the disorder; frequently 25 mg to 50 mg two or three times daily is an appropriate starting dosage.

Dose Forms Available
• Tablets: 10 mg, 15 mg, 25 mg, 50 mg, 100 mg, 150 mg, 200 mg
• Concentrate: 30 mg/ml, 100 mg/ml
• Suspension: 25 mg/5 ml, 100 mg/5 ml

REPORTS OF INTEREST

Thioridazine in the Treatment of Children and Adolescents Diagnosed with ADHD

  Klein (1990/1991) analyzed data collected in a 4-week, double-blind, placebo-controlled study of thioridazine in treating 77 children (ages, 6 to 12 years) who would meet DSM-III-R (APA, 1987) diagnostic criteria for ADHD. Subjects were administered a large number of tests measuring general and specific cognitive functions.

The mean daily doses of thioridazine at 4 and 12 weeks were 193 mg and 160 mg, respectively. At both 4 and 12 weeks, only a single psychometric test was significantly worse for patients on thioridazine than for those on placebo. Although significant decrements in cognitive test performance were expected on these relatively high doses of thioridazine, they did not occur. Klein concluded that thioridazine does not have a general deleterious effect of cognitive performance of children diagnosed with ADHD and treated for up to 12 weeks with therapeutic doses of thioridazine. It was suggested that thioridazine be administered in one nighttime dose to minimize the sedative effects, which are most acute following ingestion. Interestingly, Klein noted that over half of the subjects were rated as having at least mild-to-moderate daytime drowsiness, yet despite this, on testing, there was minimal effect on cognitive performance.

Thioridazine in Patients Diagnosed with ADHD and Mental Retardation

Aman et al. (1991b) studied effects on cognitive-motor performance in 27 children with a mean IQ of 54 (range, 30 to 90) who also had a DSM-III diagnosis of ADD and/or a conduct disorder in a double-blind, placebo-controlled, crossover study of methylphenidate (0.4 mg/kg/day) and thioridazine (1.75 mg/kg/day). Thioridazine had no adverse effect on performance of any of the cognitive motor performance tests and had no deleterious effect on IQ performance when subjects' correct answers were reinforced. Aman et al. (1991a) noted that more severely retarded children with IQs of 45 or less or a mental age below 4.5 years, whose functioning is characterized by a narrow attentional focus, tended to respond poorly to stimulants in contrast to less retarded individuals who responded more positively to stimulants. No such relationship was apparent between IQ and response to thioridazine. At the doses employed, thioridazine had relatively minor behavioral effects, although it was superior to placebo on teachers' ratings of conduct problems, hyperactivity, and overall improvement. The authors suggested that higher doses of thioridazine, up to 2.5 mg/kg, might be more effective in treating severe behavioral disorders and hyperactivity in more retarded individuals; they also noted that some such individuals might benefit from stimulants (Aman et al., 1991a, 1991b).

In an earlier study, Alexandris and Lundell (1968) compared the effects of thioridazine, amphetamine, and placebo in 21 mentally deficient (IQ range, 55 to 85) children (ages, 7 to 12 years) diagnosed with hyperkinetic syndrome. Thioridazine was significantly superior to amphetamine on scores related to concentration, aggressiveness, sociability, interpersonal relationship, comprehension, work interest, and work capacity. In no case was amphetamine or placebo significantly superior to thioridazine. The average dose of thioridazine after 6 months was 95 mg/day; dose range was 30 to 150 mg/day.

TRIFLUOPERAZINE (STELAZINE)

Indications in Child and Adolescent Psychiatry
One manufacturer has a specific disclaimer that trifluoperazine has not been proven effective in the management of behavioral complications in patients with mental retardation and recommends it only for the treatment of psychotic individuals and the short-term treatment of nonpsychotic anxiety in individuals with generalized anxiety disorder who have not responded to other medications.

Dosage Schedule for Children and Adolescents
• Children under 6 years of age: Not recommended.
• Children 6 to 12 years of age: A starting dose of 1 mg once or twice daily with gradual upward titration is recommended.
• Dosages in excess of 15 mg/day are usually required only by older children with severe symptoms.
• Adolescents: 1 to 5 mg twice daily. Usually the optimal dose will be 15 to 20 mg/day or less; occasionally up to 40 mg/day will be required. Titration to optimal dose can usually be accomplished within 2 to 3 weeks.

Dose Forms Available
• Tablets: 1 mg, 2 mg, 5 mg, 10 mg
• Concentrate: 10 mg/ml
• Injectable: 2 mg/ml. (One manufacturer notes there is little experience using intramuscular trifluoperazine with children and recommends 1 mg intramuscularly once, or maximally twice, daily if necessary for rapid control of severe symptoms.)

HALOPERIDOL (HALDOL)

Indications in Child and Adolescent Psychiatry
Haloperidol is approved for the treatment of psychotic disorders and Tourette's disorder. Only after the failure of treatment with psychotherapy and non–antipsychotic medications has haloperidol been approved for treating children with severe behavioral disorders—for example "combative, explosive hyperexcitability (which cannot be accounted for by immediate provocation)" (package insert) and the short-term treatment of hyperactive children with coexisting conduct disorders who exhibit such symptoms as "impulsivity, difficulty sustaining attention, aggressivity, mood liability and poor frustration tolerance" (package insert).

Shapiro and Shapiro (1989) concluded that the most effective neuroleptics in the treatment of tics and Tourette's disorder were haloperidol, pimozide (Orap), fluphenazine (Prolixin, Permitil), and penfluridol (Semap, an investigational drug).

Dosage Schedule for Children and Adolescents with Psychotic Disorders, Tourette's Disorder, or Severe Nonpsychotic Behavioral Disorders
• Children under 3 years of age: Not recommended.
• Children 3 to 12 years of age (weight, 15 to 40 kg): Begin with 0.5 mg daily; titrate upward by 0.5 mg increments at 5- to 7-day intervals.
   Therapeutic dose ranges are usually from 0.05 to 0.075 mg/kg/day for nonpsychotic behavioral disorders and Tourette's disorder; for psychotic children the upper range is usually 0.15 mg/kg/day but may be higher in severe cases. Morselli et al. (1983) reported good therapeutic results in children with tics and Tourette's disorder associated with haloperidol plasma levels in the range of 1 to 3 ng/ml. Higher haloperidol plasma levels, usually between 6 and 10 ng/ml, were necessary for significant improvement in psychotic conditions.
• Adolescents (over age 12): Depending on severity 0.5 to 5 mg two or three times daily. Higher doses may be necessary for more rapid control in some severe cases.

Dose Forms Available
• Tablets: 0.5 mg, 1 mg, 2 mg, 5 mg, 10 mg, 20 mg
• Concentrate solution: 2 mg/ml
• Injectable (haloperidol lactate): 5.0 mg/ml. Safety has not been established for children. If necessary, in acutely agitated adolescents an initial dose of 2 to 5 mg may be given intramuscularly. Additional medication may be given every 1 to 8 hours as determined by ongoing evaluation of the patient.

Pharmacokinetics of Haloperidol

Morselli et al. (1983) noted that steady-state haloperidol plasma levels in children may vary up to 15-fold at a given mg/kg daily dosage, but for a given individual the relationship between dosage and plasma level is fairly consistent. Most children had haloperidol plasma half-lives that were shorter than those of adolescents and adults. The authors also emphasized, however, that despite their more rapid metabolism of haloperidol, children did not require proportionally higher daily doses, because they also appear to be more sensitive to both the therapeutic and the untoward effects of haloperidol at lower plasma concentrations than were older adolescents and adults (Morselli et al., 1983).

REPORTS OF INTEREST

Haloperidol in the Treatment of Schizophrenia with Childhood Onset.   Green et al. (1992) administered haloperidol on an open basis to 15 hospitalized children under 12 years of age diagnosed with schizophrenia. They reported the optimal dose to range between 1 and 6 mg/day. Acute dystonic reactions occurred in about 25% of the children despite low initial doses and gradual increments of the drug.

Spencer et al. (1992) administered haloperidol to 12 patients (9 males, 3 females; ages, 5.5 to 11.75 years) in an ongoing, double-blind, placebo-controlled study of hospitalized children diagnosed with schizophrenia. Optimal haloperidol dose ranged from 0.5 to 3.5 mg/day (range, 0.02–0.12 mg/kg/day; mean, 2.02 mg/day). Haloperidol was significantly better than placebo on staff Global Clinical Judgments ($P = .003$) and on 4 of 8 Children's Psychiatric Rating Scale items selected for their pertinence to schizophrenia: ideas of reference ($P = .04$); persecutory ($P = .01$), other thinking disorders ($P = .04$), and hallucinations ($P = .04$). Two children (16.7%) experienced acute dystonic reactions. All 12 improved on haloperidol and were discharged on that medication.

Haloperidol in the Treatment of Autistic Disorder and Atypical Pervasive Developmental Disorders

At the present time, haloperidol is the most well-studied drug used in the treatment of autistic disorder and is recommended as the drug of first choice. In a study of 40 autistic children aged 2.33 to 6.92 years, haloperidol in optimal doses of 0.5 to 3 mg/day yielded global clinical improvement and decreased significantly the symptoms of withdrawal, stereotypies, abnormal object relationships, hyperactivity, fidgetiness, negativism, and angry and labile affect (Anderson et al., 1984). A high rate of dyskinesias remains a problem, however. Significant numbers of autistic children (22% or 8 of 36) developed tardive dyskinesia or withdrawal dyskinesia in a prospective study in which 0.5 to 3 mg/day of haloperidol was administered for from 3½ to 42½ months, thus close monitoring is necessary (Perry et al., 1985).

In autistic disorder, stereotypies existing at baseline may be suppressed by administration of haloperidol. When the drug is withdrawn, there is potential for confusion between the reappearance of stereotypies and a withdrawal dyskinesia; this is of special concern if a physician unfamiliar with the child at baseline assumes treatment responsibilities for the child while he or she is on maintenance medication.

Joshi et al. (1988) administered fluphenazine or haloperidol to 12 children aged 7 to 11 years who were hospitalized and diagnosed with childhood-onset or atypical pervasive developmental disorders (PDDs) (i.e., approximately equivalent to the DSM-III-R [APA, 1987] diagnoses of autistic disorder with childhood onset and PDD not otherwise specified [PDDNOS]). The children responded with remarkable improvement in peer interactions and reality testing and decreases in autistic-like behavior, aggressiveness, impulsivity, and hyperactivity. Seven of the 12 children were able to return home rather than be admitted to residential treatment as had been planned. Haloperidol was begun at a dose of 0.02 mg/kg/day and titrated based on behavioral response with increases at 3- to 5-day intervals. Mean optimal dose of haloperidol was 0.04 ± 0.01 mg/kg/day. Untoward effects were remarkably infrequent. Drowsiness occurred initially in some children, but it was transient and did not interfere with their later cognitive performance. Two children receiving haloperidol developed some rigidity and cogwheeling that responded to oral diphenhydramine during the first few days of treatment; the extrapyramidal symptoms did not recur when the diphenhydramine was discontinued.

Haloperidol in the Treatment of Aggressive Conduct Disorder

In a double-blind placebo-controlled study of 61 treatment-resistant hospitalized children, aged 5.2 to 12.9 years, with undersocialized aggressive conduct disorder, both haloperidol and lithium were found to be superior to placebo in ameliorating behavioral symptoms (Campbell et al., 1984b). Optimal doses of haloperidol ranged from 1 to 6 mg/day. The authors reported that, at optimal doses, the untoward effects of haloperidol appeared to interfere more significantly with the children's daily routines than did those of lithium.

Haloperidol in the Treatment of ADHD

Werry and Aman (1975) investigated the effects of methylphenidate and haloperidol on attention, memory, and activity in 24 children (ages, 4.11 to 12.4 years), over half of whom were diagnosed with hyperkinetic reaction and the remainder with unsocialized aggressive reaction. Each child received each of 4 drug conditions, placebo, methylphenidate (0.3 mg/kg), low-dose haloperidol (0.025 mg/kg), or high-dose haloperidol (0.05 mg/kg) in a double-blind, placebo-controlled, crossover (within subject) design. For all statistically significant measures of cognitive functions of vigilance and short-term memory, the rank order of the means was methylphenidate, haloperidol (low dose), placebo, and haloperidol (high dose). The data suggested that methylphenidate and low-dose haloperidol, although to a lesser degree, improved these cognitive functions whereas high-dose haloperidol appeared to cause them to deteriorate (Werry & Aman, 1975). The clinical importance of observing this biphasic effect is that it is the dose of haloperidol, not the drug itself, that may cause cognitive impairment. Based on this study, most children and adolescents treated for ADHD with haloperidol should receive doses between 0.5 and 2.0 mg/day (i.e., 0.025 mg/kg for a weight range of 20 to 80 kg).

THIOTHIXENE (NAVANE)

Indications in Child and Adolescent Psychiatry
Thiothixene is an antipsychotic drug of the thioxanthene series. It is indicated in the management of symptoms of psychotic disorders. It has not been evaluated in the management of behavioral disturbances in the mentally retarded nor is its use recommended in children under age 12 years, because safe conditions for its use in that age group have not been established (PDR, 1995).

Dosage Schedule for Children and Adolescents at Least 12 Years Old
• Milder conditions: Initial dose of 2 mg three times daily with titration to 5 mg three times daily if needed is usually effective.
• More severe conditions: Initial dose of 5 mg twice daily.
• The usual optimal dose is 20 to 30 mg/day; occasionally up to 60 mg/day are required. Daily doses of more than 60 mg rarely increase the beneficial response (PDR, 1995).

Dose Forms Available
• Capsules: 1 mg, 2 mg, 5 mg, 10 mg, 20 mg
• Concentrate: 5 mg/ml
• Intramuscular: 2 mg/ml, 5 mg/ml

REPORT OF INTEREST

Realmuto and his colleagues (1984) assigned 21 adolescent inpatients (mean age, 15.1 years; range, 11.75 to 18.33 years) diagnosed with chronic schizophrenia either thiothixene or thioridazine. Optimal dose was individually titrated over a period of about 2 weeks. For the 13 patients who received thiothixene, the mean optimal dose was 16.2 mg/day (range, 4.8 to 42.6 mg/day) or 0.30 mg/kg/day for 4 to 6 weeks. Hallucinations, anxiety, tension, and excitement decreased the most during the first week. Cognitive disorganization improved more slowly. There were no significant differences between the two drugs and rapidity of symptom improvement or extent of improvement at the end of the study. About 50% of patients improved, regardless of the medication. There was a suggestion, however, that untoward effects, particularly drowsiness, were less severe with thiothixene than with thioridazine and that because of this, high-potency antipsychotics may be preferable to the more sedating low-potency antipsychotics in treating adolescent schizophrenics (Realmuto et al., 1984).

LOXAPINE SUCCINATE (LOXITANE)

Indications in Child and Adolescent Psychiatry
Loxapine is a dibenzoxazepine compound with antipsychotic properties used in treating psychotic disorders. The manufacturer does not recommend its use in persons under 16 years of age.

Dosage Schedule for Children and Adolescents
• Children and adolescents under 16 years old: Not recommended.
• Adolescents at least 16 years old and adults: An initial dose of 10 mg twice daily is recommended and is titrated according to clinical response. The usual therapeutic and maintenance dose ranges from 60 to 100 mg daily. A maximum of 250 mg/day is recommended.

Dose Forms Available
• Capsules: 5 mg, 10 mg, 25 mg, 50 mg
• Oral concentrate: 25 mg/ml
• Injection (intramuscular): 50 mg/ml

REPORT OF INTEREST

Pool and colleagues (1976) conducted a 4-week double-blind study comparing the efficacies of loxapine, haloperidol, and placebo in 75 adolescents, 13 to 18 years of age, diagnosed with acute schizophrenia or chronic schizophrenia with an acute exacerbation. Loxapine was begun at a dose of 10 mg daily and titrated to a maximum of 200 mg daily (average daily dose, 87.5 mg). Extrapyramidal reactions, most commonly parkinsonian muscular rigidity, were the most frequent untoward effects of loxapine and occurred in 19 of 26 subjects. The second most frequent untoward effect, sedation, occurred in 21 of the 26 subjects. Both loxapine and haloperidol were significantly superior to placebo in diminishing schizophrenic symptoms. The authors concluded that loxapine was relatively safe and efficacious in the treatment of adolescent schizophrenia.

MOLINDONE HYDROCHLORIDE (MOBAN)

Molindone hydrochloride is a dihydroindolone compound with antipsychotic properties; it is structurally unrelated to the phenothiazine, butyrophenone, and thioxanthene antipsychotics. Its clinical action resembles that of the piperazine phenothiazines, e.g., perphenazine (Trilafon) (Drug Facts & Comparisons, 1995). Moban is rapidly absorbed from the gastrointestinal tract, and peak blood levels of unmetabolized drug are achieved about 1.5 hours after ingestion. Moban has many metabolites, and pharmacological effects from a single dose may last up to 36 hours (PDR, 1995).

Indications in Child and Adolescent Psychiatry
    Moban hydrochloride is not recommended for use in children under age 12 years, because safe conditions for its use in that age group have not been established (PDR, 1995).

Dosage Schedule for Children and Adolescents at Least 12 Years Old
    The usual starting dose for treatment of psychotic symptoms is 50 to 75 mg/day with an increase to 100 mg/day in 3 to 4 days. The medication should be titrated according to symptom response; up to 225 mg/day may be required in severely disturbed patients.

Dose Forms Available
• Tablets: 5 mg, 10 mg, 25 mg, 50 mg, 100 mg
• Concentrate: 20 mg/ml

REPORT OF INTEREST

Greenhill et al. (1985) compared molindone and thioridazine in treating 31 hospitalized boys, ages 6 to 11 years, who were diagnosed with undersocialized conduct disorder, aggressive type. Children were assigned randomly to either medication in an 8-week, double-blind, parallel-design study. Subjects were drug-free for the baseline week and were on placebo the second week of the study. During week 3, medication was raised until it produced sedation; this was followed by a fixed dose of drug during weeks 4 through 6. The final 2 weeks of the study were again placebo. The mean dose of thioridazine over the 4-week treatment period was 169.9 mg/day (4.64 mg/kg/day), and the mean dose of molindone was 26.8 mg/day (1.3 mg/kg/day).

The groups were similar on baseline ratings, which showed them to be severely aggressive. In fact, the initial or terminal placebo periods had to be shortened for 11 subjects and drug begun because of their severe symptomatology. Symptoms improved significantly during the 4 weeks on either drug compared with the placebo periods. On Clinical Global Impressions (CGI), nurses rated the severity of illness at the end of the study as less in the molindone group ($P < .08$) and the degree of improvement as significantly greater in the molindone group ($P < .035$). Untoward effects differed although not significantly between the drugs; acute dystonic reactions occurred more frequently in the molindone group (23.5% versus 6.1%), whereas sedation and gastrointestinal symptoms were more frequent among subjects treated with thioridazine. The authors concluded that molindone is relatively safe for inpatient children and adolescents and thought its efficacy in this population was similar to the more commonly used neuroleptics.

FLUPHENAZINE HYDROCHLORIDE (PROLIXIN, PERMITIL)

Indications in Child and Adolescent Psychiatry
Fluphenazine hydrochloride is approved for the treatment of psychotic disorders. It is not approved for administration to children under age 12 years, however, because of a lack of studies proving its efficacy and safety in this age group. A manufacturer notes that it has not been shown to be effective in treating behaviorally disturbed patients who are mentally retarded.

Dose Schedule for Children and Adolescents
• Children under 12 years of age: Not recommended.
• Children at least 12 years of age and adolescents: Manufacturer recommends an initial total daily dose of 2.5 to 10 mg divided and administered every 6 to 8 hours for adults. One should be at least this conservative in adolescents (see also Joshi et al. [1988] below).

Dose Forms Available
• Tablets: 1 mg, 2.5 mg, 5 mg, 10 mg
• Elixir: 0.5 mg/ml (2.5 mg/5 ml)
• Oral concentrate: 5 mg/ml
• Injectable (fluphenazine hydrochloride): 2.5 mg/ml
• Long-acting preparations for parenteral administration: Fluphenazine enanthate, 25 mg/ml, and fluphenazine decanoate, 25 mg/ml, are available. (They are used primarily in treating adults diagnosed with chronic schizophrenia.)

REPORT OF INTEREST

As discussed above for haloperidol, Joshi et al. (1988) found fluphenazine to be efficacious in treating children diagnosed with childhood onset PDD or atypical PDD. Fluphenazine was begun at 0.02 mg/kg/day and increased at 3- to 5-day intervals based on behavioral responses. Mean optimal dose of fluphenazine was 1.3 ± 0.7 mg/day. Untoward effects of fluphenazine were remarkably infrequent. Some initial drowsiness occurred in some children but it was transient.

PIMOZIDE (ORAP)

Indications in Child and Adolescent Psychiatry
Pimozide is an antipsychotic drug of the diphenylbutylpiperidine series.
It is indicated only in the treatment of patients with Tourette's disorder whose development and/or daily life function is severely compromised by the presence of motor and phonic tics and who have not responded satisfactorily to or cannot tolerate standard treatments, such as haloperidol. There is limited experience with its use in children under 12 years of age.

Pimozide Dosage Schedule for Children and Adolescents
Because there is very limited information available on the use of pimozide in children, it should be introduced at a very low dose and gradually adjusted upward. It is

(continues)

(continued)

suggested that treatment should be initiated with 0.5 mg/day and gradually increased by increments of 0.5 mg once or twice weekly. Most patients are maintained at less than 0.2 mg/kg/day or 10 mg/day, whichever is less. Doses greater than 0.2 mg/kg/day or 10 mg/day are not recommended. Unexplained deaths, perhaps cardiac related, and grand mal seizures have occurred in patients taking high doses of pimozide (more than 20 mg/day) (PDR, 1995).

Dose Forms Available
• Scored tablets: 2 mg

Pharmacokinetics of Pimozide

Peak serum levels usually occur 6 to 8 hours after ingestion of pimozide. Pimozide is metabolized primarily in the liver; the drug and its metabolites are excreted primarily through the kidneys. There are wide interindividual variations in half-life and in peak serum levels for equivalent doses. Mean serum half-life in schizophrenics is about 55 hours. There are few correlations between plasma levels and clinical findings (package insert).

Untoward Effects of Pimozide

Pimozide prolongs the Q-T interval of the ECG. An ECG should be done at baseline and monthly during the period of dose titration. Increase of the Q-T interval beyond an absolute limit of 0.47 second in children or 0.52 second in adults or more than 25% above the patient's original baseline should be considered a mandate for no further increase in dose and for possibly lowering the dose. Because hypokalemia is associated with ventricular arrhythmias, potassium levels should be monitored during therapy.

Contraindications for Pimozide Administration

In addition to considerations for antipsychotics in general, pimozide is contraindicated in the treatment of simple tics or tics other than those associated with Tourette's disorder. Pimozide also should not be given to patients with congenital long Q-T intervals or a history of cardiac arrhythmias.

REPORTS OF INTEREST

Use of Pimozide in Children and Adolescents with Treatment-Resistant Tourette's Disorder

Shapiro, Shapiro, and Eisenkraft (1983) treated 31 patients aged 10 to 50 years (mean age, 19.6 ± 9.2 years) diagnosed with Tourette's syndrome with pimozide in an open study. All had previously received haloperidol and either had unsatisfactory symptom control, an unacceptable level of untoward effects, or a desire to try pimozide. Pimozide was titrated in 1-mg increments every 4 to 7 days until optimal dose was achieved. The mean optimal dose of pimozide was 12.9 ± 12.5 mg/day (median dose, 8 mg/day; range, 1 to 64 mg/day). In this subgroup of patients, the therapeutic efficacy of pimozide was superior to that of haloperidol. Significantly more patients treated with pimozide (74.4%) achieved more than 70% symptomatic improvement than with haloperidol (45.4%). The mean score for untoward effects was significantly less for pimozide than for haloperidol. The authors hypothesized that the superiority of pimozide was related to its relative lack of norepinephrine antagonism compared with haloperidol, which decreases norepinephrine levels and more readily induces untoward effects such as sedation, depression, impaired motivation, cognitive dulling, irritability, phobias, and dysphoria, limiting the use of higher doses of haloperidol (Shapiro et al., 1983).

Shapiro and Shapiro (1984) performed a double-blind placebo-controlled study of pimozide in 20 patients (mean age, 24.65 ± 2.71 years; range, 11 to 53 years) diagnosed with Tourette's syndrome. Six patients had a concomitant diagnosis of ADDH. The study was 14 weeks long—2 drug-free weeks followed by 6 weeks of one condition and then 6 weeks of the other. Initial dose of pimozide was 1 mg/day at bedtime, and dosage was flexibly adjusted every 2 to 3 days over 6 weeks to a maximum of 10 mg/day (approximately 0.2 mg/kg/day) for children and 20 mg/day for adults. Average optimal dose for pimozide was 6.88 ± 1.26 mg/day. The authors noted that effective dosage was relatively independent of age and that younger patients often required higher dosages than adults. Benztropine was used in 18 patients at some time during treatment to counteract extrapyramidal and akinesic effects. Pimozide was significantly more clinically effective (most measures at the $P = .0001$ level) than placebo on multiple dependent measures. The untoward effects of pimozide were similar to those of other high-potency antipsychotic drugs but were mostly of only slight to moderate intensity, an advantage over haloperidol (Shapiro & Shapiro, 1984).

Use of Pimozide in Children and Adolescents with Other Psychiatric Disorders

Pangalila-Ratulangi (1973) reported a pilot study in which eight boys and two girls aged 9 to 14 years, eight of whom were diagnosed with schizophrenia or schizophrenia-like symptoms and two of whom had symptoms suggestive of epilepsy and blunted affect, improved clinically on doses of 1 to 2 mg/day of pimozide.

Naruse and colleagues (1982) assigned 87 children and adolescents, aged 3 to 16 years, randomly to haloperidol, pimozide, or placebo in a crossover double-blind study. The subjects were diagnosed with various behavioral disorders, and 34 were autistic. Global ratings found pimozide to be clinically as effective as haloperidol and both to be superior to placebo. Pimozide, however, was more clinically efficacious than haloperidol on behavioral rating scales. Sleepiness was the most common untoward effect and occurred in 24% (20) of the subjects receiving pimozide and 23% (19) receiving haloperidol versus only 4% (3) receiving placebo. Insomnia was the next most common side effect occurring in 4% (3) of subjects on pimozide, 5% (4) of subjects on haloperidol, and 11% (9) of subjects on placebo.

"Atypical" Antipsychotic Drugs

Atypical antipsychotic drugs, such as risperidone and clozapine, differ from the traditional antipsychotic drugs in that in addition to being dopamine receptor (D_2) blockers, they are significant serotonin receptor (S_2) blockers. The simultaneous blocking of D_2 and S_2 receptors in the brain is thought to account for the increased efficacy of these drugs in improving "negative" symptoms of schizophrenia as well as the decreased incidence of extrapyramidal untoward effects that occur with the atypical antipsychotic drugs compared with standard antipsychotic drugs (Borison et al., 1992; PDR, 1995). These drugs also may have a positive therapeutic effect when administered to some patients with preexisting tardive dyskinesia (Chouinard et al., 1993; Birmaher et al., 1992; Mozes et al., 1994).

RISPERIDONE (RISPERDAL)

Risperidone belongs to the new chemical class of benzisoxazole derivatives. It was approved by the FDA for marketing in the United States in late 1993. The manufacturer suggests that its antipsychotic properties may be mediated through its antagonism of dopamine type 2 (D_2) and serotonin type 2 ($5HT_2$) receptors; it also has a high affinity for α-1 and α-2-adrenergic and H_1 histaminergic receptors (package insert).

Risperidone appears to have significantly greater efficacy in improving "negative" symptoms of schizophrenia than the traditional antipsychotics (Chouinard et al., 1993).

Risperidone has significantly fewer extrapyramidal symptoms than typical antipsychotics. At the usual recommended dose of 6 mg/day and at doses up to 10 mg/day, the incidence of extrapyramidal symptoms in patients treated with risperidone is not significantly different from the incidence of those symptoms in patients treated with placebo. However, the appearance of extrapyramidal symptoms is dose related and becomes increasingly greater than that for placebo with further increases in dosage.

Although the manufacturer notes that there have been isolated reports of tardive dyskinesia associated with risperidone, it is likely that the incidence of tardive dyskinesia occurring with risperidone only will be significantly less than with typical antipsychotic agents.

Indications in Child and Adolescent Psychiatry
The manufacturer notes that the safety and effectiveness of risperidone in the pediatric age group has not been established. The youngest subjects treated in any published clinical trial were 16 years of age; data, however, were not analyzed separately for adolescent patients.

Dosage Schedule for Children and Adolescents
• Children and adolescents under 16 years of age: Not recommended.
• Adolescents at least 16 years of age: An initial dose of 1 mg bid is recommended, with an increase to 2 mg twice daily on the second day and a further increase to 3 mg twice daily on the third day. It is recommended that any subsequent adjustments of dosage be made at weekly intervals to allow adequate time for steady-state serum levels to be achieved. If adjustments are necessary, small, e.g., 0.5 mg or 1 mg twice daily, increments or decrements are suggested. Doses above 6 mg/day have not been demonstrated to have any increased clinical efficacy.

Dose Forms Available
• Tablets: 1 mg, 2 mg, 3 mg, and 4 mg

Pharmacokinetics of Risperidone

Food does not affect the rate or extent of the absorption of risperidone. Peak serum levels of risperidone occur a mean of 1 hour after ingestion. Risperidone is metabolized in the liver by cytochrome $P_{450}IID_6$ to 9-hydroxyrisperidone, its major metabolite, which is similar to risperidone in its receptor binding activity. Because of genetic polymorphism about 7% of Caucasians and a very low percentage of Asians are slow metabolizers. Peak 9-hydroxyrisperidone levels occur at about 3 hours in extensive metabolizers and 17 hours in poor metabolizers. Half-life ($T_{1/2}$) of risperidone is about 3 hours in extensive metabolizers and 20 hours in poor metabolizers; $T_{1/2}$ of 9-hydroxyrisperidone is about 21 hours in extensive metabolizers and 30 hours in poor metabolizers.

Contraindications for Risperidone Administration

Risperidone is contraindicated in patients with a known hypersensitivity to it.

Risperidone should be administered with caution to patients with hepatic impairment, which may increase free risperidone by up to 35%, and/or renal impairment, which may decrease clearance of risperidone and its active metabolite by up to 60%.

Untoward Effects of Risperidone

Extrapyramidal Symptoms. The incidence of extrapyramidal symptoms in patients treated with risperidone appears to be dose related; however, it is not significantly different from placebo for patients receiving up to 10 mg daily.

Other Untoward Effects. Orthostatic hypotension, dizziness, tachycardia, increase of QT_c interval on ECG to greater than 450 msec, weight gain, insomnia or somnolence, constipation, rhinitis, and many other untoward effects have been reported.

REPORT OF INTEREST

Cozza and Edison (1994) treated two 15-year-old adolescents, one male and one female, with risperidone; they were diagnosed with schizophrenia and had not responded satisfactorily to usual antipsychotics. Risperidone was begun at 1 mg daily and rapidly titrated to 6 mg/day. Both adolescents developed significant extrapyramidal side effects suggesting that adolescents may be more sensitive to these effects than adults. Risperidone was decreased to 1 mg twice daily and untoward effects improved. Both patients showed significant improvement in positive and negative symptoms within 1 week. However, both patients also reported an upwelling of such uncomfortable emotions that they were ambivalent about continuing on risperidone, and the female eventually became noncompliant.

CLOZAPINE (CLOZARIL)

Clozapine, a dibenzodiazepine, was approved by the FDA for marketing in the United States in late 1989. It differs from typical antipsychotic drugs in its dopaminergic effects. It functions as a dopamine blocker at both D_1 and D_2 receptors but does not induce catalepsy or inhibit apomorphine-induced stereotypy. Clozapine also appears to block limbic dopamine receptors more than striatal dopamine receptors. This may account for the fact that no confirmed cases of tardive dyskinesia have been reported in more than 15 years of worldwide experience in patients who have received only clozapine (PDR, 1995).

Clozapine has significantly greater efficacy in treating the "negative" symptoms of schizophrenia and a lesser incidence of extrapyramidal symptoms than traditional antipsychotics. There also is evidence that clozapine has a positive therapeutic effect on some patients with preexisting tardive dyskinesia. Like traditional antipsychotic drugs, clozapine initially suppresses the involuntary movements, but, unlike with traditional antipsychotics, the abnormal movements do not worsen over time with clozapine, sometimes even with dose reduction. There is a suggestion that, although it may not be curative, clozapine may alleviate tardive dyskinesia over time in some patients (Jann, 1991).

Because of the increased risk for serious and potentially life-threatening untoward effects that has been reported in patients receiving clozapine, its administration is appropriate only for severely dysfunctional patients with schizophrenia who have not responded satisfactorily to adequate trials of at least two other standard antipsychotic drugs, or who cannot tolerate the untoward effects present at therapeutic dose levels.

Indications in Child and Adolescent Psychiatry
    The manufacturer noted that safety and efficacy of clozapine have not been established in children under 16 years of age.

Dosage Schedule for Children and Adolescents
• Children and adolescents under 16 years of age: Not recommended.
• Adolescents at least 16 years of age: Initially, a dose of 25 mg once or twice daily is recommended. The dose can be increased daily by 25 to 50 mg, if tolerated, to reach a target dose of 300 to 450 mg by 2 weeks' time. Subsequent dose increases of a maximum of 100 mg may be made once or twice weekly. Total daily dosage should not exceed 900 mg.

Dose Forms Available
• Tablets: 25 mg, 100 mg

Untoward Effects of Clozapine

Agranulocytosis is reported to occur in association with administration of clozapine in between 1% and 2% of patients. Because of this, weekly monitoring of white blood cell counts is mandatory with discontinuation of treatment if the white blood cell counts decrease significantly. Alvir et al. (1993) reported that 73 of 11,555 patients who received clozapine during a 15-month period developed agranulocytosis and, of these, 2 died from complications of infection. The cumulative incidence of agranulocytosis was 0.80% after 1 year and 0.91% after 18 months. Agranulocytosis occurred during the first 3 months of treatment in the large majority of cases (61 [83.6%] of 73). In general, older patients and females appear to be at higher risk for developing agranulocytosis. An exception, however, appeared to be that patients under 21 years of age were at somewhat higher risk than patients between 21 and 40 years of age. The authors also noted that subsequent to the time period of their study, an additional 5 patients between 40 and 72 years of age died from complications resulting from agranulocytosis within 3 months after they began taking clozapine (Alvir et al., 1993). The manufacturer reports that more than 68,000 patients in the United States had been prescribed clozapine as of January 1, 1994. Of these 317 developed agranulocytosis and despite weekly monitoring, 11 cases were fatal (PDR, 1995).

Administration of clozapine is also associated with an increased incidence of seizures that is apparently dose dependent. At doses below 300 mg/day, about 1% to 2% of patients develop seizures; at moderate doses of 300 to 599 mg/day, about 3% to 4% develop seizures; at high doses of 600 to 900 mg/day, about 5% of patients develop seizures. Baseline EEG and periodic monitoring should be mandatory for children and adolescents receiving clozapine.

Other untoward effects include adverse cardiovascular effects such as orthostatic hypotension, tachycardia, and ECG changes.

REPORTS OF INTEREST

Siefen and Remschmidt (1986) administered clozapine to 21 inpatients, 12 of whom were younger than 18 years old (average age, 18.1 years). Their patients had an average of 2.4 inpatient hospitalizations and had been tried on an average of 2.8 different antipsychotics without adequate therapeutic response or with severe extrapyramidal effects. In addition, the authors considered it a risk that their patients' psychotic symptoms would become chronic if clozapine was not administered.

Clozapine was administered over an average of 133 days. The average maximum dose was 415 mg/day (range, 225 to 800 mg/day) and the average maintenance dose was 363 mg/day (range, 150 to 800 mg/day). In addition, 11 of the 21 subjects were administered one or more other unidentified drugs during about half of the time they were receiving clozapine.

About 67% of symptoms that had been relatively resistant to previous treatment with antipsychotics disappeared or improved markedly in 11 (52%) of the patients, and an additional 6 (29%) patients showed at least slight improvement in the same number of symptoms. Four patients, however, had no changes or worsening of over half of their psychopathological symptoms during clozapine therapy. Positive symptoms of schizophrenia improved more than negative symptoms. Specifically, improvements in incoherent/dissociative thinking, aggressiveness, hallucinations, agitation, ideas of reference, anxiety, inability to make decisions, psychomotor agitation, motivation toward achievement, impoverished and restricted thinking, and ambivalent behavior were reported. Symptoms such as lack of self-confidence, fear of failure, psychomotor retardation, irritability, slowed thinking, blunted affect, and unhappiness showed no improvement or deteriorated during treatment with clozapine (Siefen & Remschmidt, 1986).

The most frequent untoward effects observed early in treatment with clozapine were daytime sedation, dizziness, tachycardia, orthostatic hypotension, sleepiness, and increased salivation. No patients developed agranulocytosis, and the hematological changes that occurred in about 25% of patients were clinically insignificant and normalized during continued maintenance on clozapine (Siefen & Remschmidt, 1986).

Schmidt et al. (1990) reported a total of 57 cases of children and adolescents (age range, 9.8 to 21.3 years; mean 16.8 years; 30 males and 27 females) who were treated with clozapine. Forty-eight patients were diagnosed with a schizophrenic disorder, 5 with schizoaffective disorder, 2 with monopolar manic disorder, and 2 with pervasive developmental disorders. These patients had a mean duration of illness of 19.4 months (range, 0 to 74 months) prior to this hospitalization, which was the first for 16 patients, the second for 16 patients, and the third or more for the remaining 25 patients. Clozapine was begun on average about 3 months after hospitalization following treatment failures with other antipsychotic drugs and concern about chronicity, intolerable untoward effects, or uncontrolled excitation. Average dose during the length of hospitalization was 318 mg/day (range, 50 to 800 mg/day); average dose at discharge was somewhat lower, 290 mg/day (range, 75 to 800 mg/day). Thirty-five patients received only clozapine. In 22 cases, one or more additional other neuroleptics, primarily phenothiazines, were administered simultaneously, but in about half of these cases the additional drugs were tapered off and discontinued so that eventually 80% of the patients were on clozapine only. Mean duration on clozapine during hospitalization was 78 days (range, 7 to 355 days), and 17 (31%) patients were discharged on clozapine.

Clozapine was discontinued in 15 (28%) of the patients between the 8th and 132nd day of treatment (average, 50th day) when they were taking a mean dose of 143 mg/day (range, 25 to 350 mg/day) for the following reasons: insufficient antipsychotic effect in seven cases; poor compliance and a change to depot medication in five cases; and severe untoward effects in three cases (cholinergic delirium, seizure, and questionably clinically significant decrease of erythrocytes to 2.3 million). The authors reported that two-thirds of the patients significantly improved in the whole range of symptoms. Paranoid-hallucinatory symptoms and excitation responded best followed by a reduction in aggressivity. Clozapine was less effective in decreasing agitation and improving negative symptoms, and these symptoms sometimes worsened. Untoward effects were noted in all subjects. These included increased heart rates (during the first 8 weeks only) of 94 to 109 beats per minute in 37 (65%) patients; daytime sedation in 29 (51%) patients; hypersalivation in 20 (35%) patients; orthostatic hypotension in 20 (35%) patients; and an unspecified rise in temperature in 15 (26%) patients. Abnormal movements were observed in 9 patients including tremor (6 cases), akathisia (1 case) and unspecified extrapyramidal symptoms in 2 cases. During the first 16 weeks of clozapine therapy, a significant decrease of various hematological parameters including number of erythrocytes was observed but did not reach pathological values; a relative shift from lymphocytes to neutrophils was seen in the differential during the first 2 weeks. There was a reversible increase of liver enzymes that peaked during the third and fourth weeks. On EEGs, there was evidence that clozapine induced increased neuronal disinhibition, e.g., spike discharges, and a shift of background activity to lower frequencies. Pathological EEG changes were present in 30 (55%) patients on clozapine compared with 17 (30%) patients before clozapine ($P <$ .01). One patient developed a seizure (Schmidt et al., 1990). The authors later noted that they considered EEG monitoring before and during treatment with clozapine to be mandatory (Blanz & Schmidt, 1993).

Birmaher et al. (1992) treated three inpatient adolescents (an 18-year-old female and two 17-year-old males) with clozapine; they were diagnosed with schizophrenia that was chronic and resistant to treatment with standard antipsychotics. Clozapine was titrated upward resulting in markedly better symptom control than was achieved in previous drug trials. Doses at discharge were 100 mg/day for the female and 300 mg/day for the two males. The female patient experienced a reexacerbation of symptoms after about 1 year despite good compliance, and rehospitalization was required. She was able to be discharged in 2 weeks, but it was necessary to increase clozapine to 400 mg/day; her functioning was described as satisfactory, but some auditory hallucinations remained. The only untoward effects that these three patients complained about were sedation and increased salivation, and these gradually remitted. The buccolingual dyskinesia, which one of the males had developed during treatment with standard antipsychotics, disappeared while on clozapine (Birmaher et al., 1992).

Mandoki (1993) administered clozapine to two hospitalized males, aged 14 and 16 years, diagnosed with schizophrenia who had unsatisfactory responses to trails of many medications including antipsychotics. The younger patient had predominantly severe negative symptoms and the older one predominantly severe positive symptoms. Clozapine in doses of 300 to 400 mg/day resulted in significant improvements. The 14 year old was discharged on 300 mg/day of clozapine 11 weeks after clozapine treatment began. At follow-up he was attending school. Clozapine had been increased to 200 mg every morning and 400 mg at bedtime. Untoward effects were significant weight gain, mild hypersalivation, and severe drowsiness. The 16 year old was discharged on 300 mg/day of clozapine 2 months after beginning clozapine. Dose was increased to 400 mg/day after 2 months because inappropriate touching behaviors recurred. No untoward effects were reported. At follow-up both adolescents were continuing to experience gradual clinical improvement.

Remschmidt et al. (1994) reported a retrospective study of 36 adolescent inpatients, age range of 14 to 22 years, diagnosed with schizophrenia who were treated on an open basis with clozapine following treatment failures with at least two other antipsychotic drugs. Doses ranged from 50 to 800 mg/day (mean, 330 mg/day) and the mean duration of clozapine administration was 154 ± 93 days. Twenty-seven patients (75%) had clinically significant improvement; of these, 4 (11%) had complete remissions. Three patients (8%) showed no improvement. Six (17%) developed untoward effects necessitating the discontinuation of clozapine: leukopenia without agranulocytosis (2 patients); hypertension, tachycardia, and ECG abnormalities (2); elevations in liver transaminases to 10 times normal values without other signs of hepatitis (1); and worsening of symptoms and development of stupor when given in combination with carbamazepine 400 mg/day (1). Overall, positive symptoms improved significantly more than negative symptoms. For example, delusions, hallucinations, and excitation improved in about 65% of patients. Negative symptoms such as anhedonia, flat affect, and autistic behavior showed little improvement, but other negative symptoms such as anergy, muteness, bizarre behavior, and thought blocking showed improvement in 11% to 22% of the patients. Nine (90%) of 10 patients who had predominantly negative symptoms did not improve clinically.

Levkovitch et al. (1994) treated 13 adolescents (7 males and 6 females; mean age, 16.6 years; range, 14 to 17 years) who were diagnosed with adolescent-onset schizophrenia with clozapine. All had experienced treatment failures with an average of 3 traditional antipsychotics. Patients received an average daily dose of 240 mg of clozapine for a mean of 245 days. After 2 months, 10 patients (76.9%) showed significant improvement of at least a 50% decrease in scores on the Brief Psychiatric Rating Scale; 2 patients showed more modest improvements. Clozapine was discontinued after 2 days in one patient because of significant orthostatic hypotension. Other untoward effects were tiredness in 4 (30.8%) patients, hypersalivation in 1 (7.7%), and temperature elevation in 1 (7.7%). No leukopenia occurred during weekly monitoring.

Frazier et al. (1994) treated 11 hospitalized adolescents (age range, 12 to 17 years; mean, 14.0 ± 1.5 years) diagnosed with childhood-onset schizophrenia with a 6-week open trial of clozapine. Subjects were chronically and severely ill and had received at least two previous neuroleptic medications without significant clinical benefit or experienced intolerable untoward effects. Following a 4-week washout/observation period, clozapine was begun at 12.5 mg/day or 25 mg/day. Dose was titrated individually based on symptom response versus untoward effects and increased by one to two times the initial dose every 4 days to a potential maximum of 900 mg/day. The main untoward effects responsible for limiting dose increases were tachycardia (3 patients) and sedation (7 patients). Other untoward effects reported included hypersalivation (8 patients), weight gain (7), enuresis (4), constipation (4), orthostatic hypotension (2), nausea (1), and dizziness (1)

Extrapyramidal untoward effects also occurred: 4 adolescents developed akathisia after several months and 1 developed a coarse tremor. The mean dose of clozapine at the end of the 6-week period was 370.5 mg/day (range, 125 to 825 mg/day). Six (55%) of the patients improved over 30% on the Brief Psychiatric Rating Scale (BPRS) on optimal dose of clozapine compared with admission ratings when 9 of the patients were receiving other drugs; 9 (82%) of the patients improved on clozapine over 30% on the BPRS compared with ratings during the washout period. Nine of the 11 patients also received 6-week courses of haloperidol following 4-week washout/observation periods during their hospitalizations; of these, five (56%) showed more than a 30% improvement on the BPRS while on clozapine, compared with earlier ratings while on haloperidol. Both positive and negative symptoms of schizophrenia improved (Frazier et al., 1994).

Mozes et al. (1994) treated four children with clozapine; the 3 males and 1 female, 10 to 12 years of age, were diagnosed with schizophrenia and had not responded satisfactorily to other neuroleptics,. Clozapine was begun in doses of 25 to 100 mg/day and titrated upward. Three patients had significantly reduced symptomatology in less that 2 weeks. Further decreases in both positive and negative symptoms occurred during the next 10 to 15 weeks of treatment. All four children improved significantly on the BPRS with a mean reduction of 41 within 15 weeks. At the time of the report, patients had been in treatment between 23 and 70 weeks, and maintenance dosage ranged from 150 to 300 mg/day. The most frequent untoward effect was drooling, which spontaneously decreased over time; drowsiness, experienced by 3 patients, peaked during the first week and then gradually faded away. Excitatory EEG changes occurred in 3 patients, and dosage was not increased to decrease the likelihood of seizures. Of note, two cases of tardive dyskinesia caused by previous neuroleptic drugs disappeared on clozapine.

Siefen and Remschmidt (1986) and Birmaher et al. (1992) concluded that clozapine was a particularly useful addition to the drug armamentarium in treating adolescents who do not respond satisfactorily to treatment with standard antipsychotics. Because prepubertal children diagnosed with schizophrenia differ from adolescents and adults diagnosed with schizophrenia on some significant parameters and frequently respond less satisfactorily to treatment with standard antipsychotics, specific investigations of clozapine will be necessary to determine its efficacy in this age group (Green & Deutsch, 1990).

5

Antidepressant Drugs

Introduction

The tricyclics are probably still the most frequently prescribed antidepressants used to treat psychiatric disorders of children and younger adolescents. However, selective serotonin reuptake inhibitor (SSRI) antidepressants are being prescribed with increasing frequency because of their significantly safer untoward effect profile, in particular the reduced risks of cardiotoxicity and lethality of overdose. For these reasons, Ambrosini et al. (1993) recommend prescribing SSRIs and not tricyclics to patients with suicidal and/or impulsive tendencies.

Tricyclic Antidepressants

INDICATIONS

The tricyclic antidepressants have FDA approval for the treatment of depression in persons with a minimum age of 12 years. A literature review of the use of tricyclic antidepressants in children and adolescents with major depression found them to be clinically effective in several open studies, but no double-blind placebo-controlled study has reported that tricyclics were superior to placebo (Ambrosini et al., 1993). However, the placebo-controlled double-blind study of Preskorn et al. (1987) found that desipramine was superior to placebo when plasma levels were controlled (reviewed below). Geller et al. (1993) caution that the use of tricyclic antidepressants in depressed 6 to 12 year olds may precipitate switching to mania and hasten the onset of bipolarity and perhaps increase later rapid cycling.

Imipramine is additionally approved for the treatment of enuresis in persons at least 6 years of age. There is, however, a considerable body of literature suggesting that imipramine is effective in the treatment of attention-deficit hyperactivity disorder (ADHD), school phobia (separation anxiety disorder), disorders of sleep (sleep terror disorder and sleepwalking disorder), and major depressive disorder (MDD) in some children treated on an open basis.

Clomipramine, another tricyclic antidepressant, has been shown to be effective in the treatment of childhood obsessive-compulsive disorder (Flament et al., 1985). It is well established that prepubertal children can be diagnosed with MDD using research diagnostic criteria (RDC) (Spitzer et al., 1978) or DSM-III (APA, 1980a) criteria (Puig-Antich, 1987).

Currently, there are no formal criteria for the prophylactic use of tricyclic antidepressants in children and adolescents. The risks versus benefits of long-term use for prevention of recurrences of mood disorders in this age group have not yet been established, and such use must be based on the physician's clinical judgment (National Institute of Mental Health/National Institutes of Health Consensus Development Panel, 1985).

Tricyclic Antidepressants in the Treatment of Children and Adolescents Diagnosed with ADHD

Although the treatment of ADHD is not an approved indication, tricyclic antidepressants are probably the second-line drugs most frequently prescribed in treating patients diagnosed with ADHD who have not responded to stimulant medication; they are used as the drug of first choice by some clinicians when comorbid diagnoses such as depression or anxiety disorder are present (Green, 1995). Imipramine hydrochloride and desipramine hydrochloride are the best studied and most frequently used, although nortriptyline hydrochloride, amitriptyline hydrochloride, and the antiobsessional drug, clomipramine hydrochloride, have also been found to be effective. Overall, desipramine hydrochloride appears to have a lower risk of untoward effects than imipramine, amitriptyline, and clomipramine (Biederman et al., 1989a); however, cardiotoxicity remains a major concern (see below). There are few studies of long-term safety and efficacy of the tricyclic antidepressants in treating ADHD (Green, 1995).

The mechanism of action of tricyclic antidepressants in ADHD is different from their action in depression; optimal doses are usually considerably lower, and the onset of clinical response is rapid (Don-nelly et al., 1986; Linnoila et al., 1979), although one study required 3 to 4 weeks for subjects treated with desipramine to show signifi-cant clinical improvement compared with subjects receiving placebo (Biederman et al., 1989b). When used to treat ADHD, tricyclics im-prove mood and decrease hyperactivity but usually are sedating and do not appear to improve concentration (Wender, 1988). Tricyclic an-tidepressants have also been reported to cause small but significant declines in motor performance, which are usually of limited clinical significance (Gualtieri et al., 1991).

The preponderance of published studies suggests strongly that tricyclic antidepressants are effective in the treatment of ADHD. In fact, in the early 1970s, some authors considered imipramine to be the drug of choice in treating ADHD (Huessy & Wright, 1970; Waizer et al., 1974). Most double-blind studies comparing tricyclic antidepressants with a stimulant, a placebo, or both have found that both drugs are superior to placebo; however, the stimulant drug is usually equal or superior to the tricyclic on the majority of clinically significant measures of improvement and, overall, the literature suggests that stimulants are superior (Campbell et al., 1985; Klein et al., 1980; Pliszka, 1987; Rapoport & Mikkelsen, 1978).

Paralleling the situation with stimulants, there is evidence that patients diagnosed with ADHD may not respond to one tricyclic an-tidepressant but may have a markedly positive response to another. For example, Wilens et al. (1993) found that 31 (70%) of 44 subjects who had had unsatisfactory responses to desipramine subsequently had positive responses to nortriptyline.

One difference noted in several studies relates to the longer serum half-lives of the tricyclic antidepressants compared with those of methylphenidate and dextroamphetamine; the therapeutic effects last longer with the tricyclics, and behavior after school and in the evenings of subjects receiving tricyclics is typically rated bet-ter by parents and others than behavior of subjects on the stimu-lants. The latter is true because when the last dose of the stimulant is given at lunchtime, it loses its clinical efficacy by late afternoon (Green, 1995; Yepes et al., 1977).

PHARMACOKINETICS OF TRICYCLIC ANTIDEPRESSANTS

About 7% of the general population has a genetic variation that results in decreased activity of the drug-metabolizing enzyme cytochrome $PA_{450}IID_6$ (PDR, 1995). Such individuals metabolize tricyclic antidepressants more slowly than usual and may develop toxic serum levels at therapeutic doses of less than 5 mg/kg. Individuals taking the same oral dose of desipramine have been reported to have up to a 36-fold variation in plasma levels (PDR, 1995, p 1417).

There may be large interindividual variations in steady-state plasma levels of tricyclics and their metabolites, although intraindividual levels are usually reproducible and correlate linearly with dose. Preskorn and his coworkers (1989a) reported that steady-state imipramine plus desipramine levels varied 22-fold (from 25 to 553 ng/ml) among 68 hospitalized children, aged 6 to 14 years, who were prescribed a fixed daily dose of 75 mg of imipramine to treat major depression (N = 48) or enuresis (N = 20); likewise, Biederman et al. (1989b) found that desipramine serum levels varied up to 16.5-fold when fixed doses of desipramine were administered.

Potter and his colleagues (1982) found that about 5% of 47 subjects, including 32 enuretic boys aged 7 to 13 years, were deficient desipramine hydroxylators and that such subjects had two to four times the steady-state concentrations of either imipramine or desipramine per unit dose as the general population. Preskorn and his colleagues (1989b) warned that persons who metabolize tricyclics slowly may develop central nervous system toxicity, which may be confused with worsening of depression, or severe cardiotoxicity when taking conventional doses of tricyclics, and that deaths have occurred. Because of these variables, it is necessary to obtain plasma levels to avoid treatment failures for subtherapeutic levels or possible toxic effects from excessive levels.

Dugas and his colleagues (1980) have recommended administering tricyclic antidepressants to children in two or three divided doses daily if more than 1 mg/kg/day is given to avoid or minimize untoward effects related to peak serum levels. Long-acting preparations (e.g., imipramine pamoate capsules) are designed for once-daily dosing; their use is not recommended in children and younger adolescents because of their high unit potency and greater sensitivity of the age group to cardiotoxic effects.

Table 5.1 summarizes the development of symptoms of central nervous system toxicity. Preskorn et al. (1989b) have urged that therapeutic drug monitoring of tricyclic antidepressants be considered a routine standard of care for patients receiving these drugs.

Table 5.1.
Evolution of Central Nervous System Tricyclic Antidepressant Toxicity[a]

Affective Symptoms	Motor Symptoms	Psychotic Symptoms	Organic Symptoms
Mood	Tremor	Thought disorder	Disorientation
↓Concentration	Ataxia	Hallucination	↓Memory
Lethargy	Seizures[b]	Delusions	Agitation
Social withdrawal			Confusion

[a]From Preskorn SH, Jerkovich GS, Beber JH, Widener P. Therapeutic drug monitoring of tricyclic antidepressants: A standard of care issue. Psychopharmacol Bull 1989;25:281–284.
[b]Seizures typically occur late but can occur earlier in the evolution.

WITHDRAWAL OF MEDICATION

Some children experience a flu-like withdrawal syndrome, with gastrointestinal symptoms including nausea, abdominal discomfort and pain, vomiting, headache, and fatigue. These symptoms result from cholinergic rebound and may be considered a cholinergic overdrive phenomenon. Ryan (1990) noted that because of their rapid metabolism of tricyclics, some prepubertal children and younger adolescents may show daily withdrawal effects if they receive their entire daily tricyclic medication in one dose; hence it may be necessary to divide the medication into two or three doses.

When maintenance medication is discontinued, tapering the medication down over 10 days to 2 weeks rather than abruptly withdrawing the medication will usually avoid the development of a clinically significant withdrawal syndrome. The clinician is cautioned that in patients with poor compliance, who in essence may undergo periodic self-induced acute withdrawals, the resulting withdrawal syndrome may be confused with untoward effects of the medication, inadequate treatment, or worsening of the underlying condition.

CONTRAINDICATIONS FOR TRICYCLIC ANTIDEPRESSANT ADMINISTRATION

Known hypersensitivity to tricyclic antidepressants is an absolute contraindication.

Tricyclic antidepressants are contraindicated for children and adolescents with cardiac conduction abnormalities.

Tricyclic antidepressants should not be administered concomitantly with an MAOI. At least a 14-day period must elapse after discontinuing an MAOI before administering a tricyclic antidepressant.

Tricyclics may lower the seizure threshold and should be used with caution in individuals with seizure disorder. Tricyclic antidepressants may activate psychotic processes in schizophrenic patients.

INTERACTIONS OF TRICYCLIC ANTIDEPRESSANTS WITH OTHER DRUGS

Hyperpyretic crises or severe convulsive seizures may occur in patients receiving MAOIs and tricyclic antidepressants simultaneously.

Anticholinergic effects of tricyclic antidepressants may be additive with those of antipsychotics and result in central nervous system anticholinergic toxicity.

The central nervous system depressive effects of tricyclic antidepressants may be additive with those of alcohol, benzodiazepines, barbiturates, and antipsychotics.

Tricyclic antidepressants may diminish or reverse the efficacy of antihypertensive agents.

Cigarette smoking may decrease the efficacy of tricyclic antidepressants.

Many other interactions with various drugs have also been reported.

UNTOWARD EFFECTS OF TRICYCLIC ANTIDEPRESSANTS

Tricyclic Antidepressants and Cardiotoxicity

At least six sudden deaths have been reported in children taking tricyclic antidepressants. Although these deaths have not been proven to be cardiac related, cardiac arrhythmias, particularly tachyarrhythmias, are particularly suspected. Five of the sudden deaths occurred in children taking desipramine, and three of these occurred after exercise. Four of the children who died were 9 years old or younger, one was 12 years old, and one was 16 years old.

A 6-year-old girl taking imipramine for chronic school phobia and separation anxiety died 3 days after the dose had been raised to 300 mg (14.7 mg/kg) at bedtime (Saraf et al., 1974).

Sudden deaths were reported in three boys treated with desipramine ("Sudden Death," June 1, 1990). These were two 8-year-old boys diagnosed with ADD (one received desipramine for 2 years at an unknown dose and one received the same drug for 6 months at 50 mg/day) and a 9-year-old boy whose diagnosis, dose, and duration of desipramine administration were not reported. All three of the boys had plasma levels in the therapeutic or subtherapeutic ranges

("Sudden Death," 1990). A fourth child, a 12-year-old girl who had been prescribed a single daily 125-mg dose of desipramine for the treatment of ADD died a few days after the dose was increased to 50 mg three times daily; she was found unconscious after playing tennis and retiring for a nap and was not successfully revived (Riddle et al., 1993). The fifth sudden death, reported by Zimnitzky (1994), was a 15-year-old male who was prescribed 300 mg/day of desipramine. His serum level on 225 mg/day was 132 ng/ml. He was in a residential treatment facility and collapsed and died a short time after swimming in the pool.

Several reports, editorials, and comments rapidly followed the report of these deaths. It became clear how little is known about the cardiac effects of tricyclics in prepubertal and even older subjects. Basically the response has been to be even more cautious when administering tricyclics to children but also to adolescents (Geller, 1991). In particular, it is recommended that a rhythm strip be obtained at baseline, during titration of medication, and at maintenance levels emphasizing measurement of the QT_c to aid in identifying potentially vulnerable children (Riddle et al., 1991). Elliot and Popper (1990/1991) recommended obtaining ECGs at baseline, at a dose of about 3 mg/kg/day, and at a final dose of not greater that 5 mg/kg/day; they also suggested using the following parameters as guidelines for cardiovascular monitoring in children and adolescents receiving tricyclic antidepressants.

PR interval: less than or equal to 210 milliseconds
QRS interval: widening to no more than 30% over baseline
QT_c interval: less than 450 milliseconds
Heart rate: maximum of 130 beats per minute
Systolic blood pressure: maximum of 130 mm Hg
Diastolic blood pressure: maximum of 85 mm Hg

Although a more conservative viewpoint would be to obtain an ECG after each dose increase, Elliot and Popper (1990/1991) have pointed out that simply increasing the frequency of ECG monitoring does not necessarily reduce the risk of sudden death.

Cardiovascular toxicity of tricyclic antidepressants is of concern in all age groups but especially in children and younger adolescents. Of particular concern is the slowing of cardiac conduction as reflected on the ECG by increases in P-R and QRS intervals, cardiac arrhythmias, tachycardia, and heart block.

Schroeder et al. (1989) reported that the cardiovascular effects of desipramine in 20 children, aged 7 years to 12 years, who were treated with an average dose of 4.25 mg/kg/day (maximum of 5 mg/kg/day) were a 21% increase in cardiac rate and a 2.5% increase in the Q-T interval. Arrhythmias and clinically meaningful blood pressure changes did not occur. The authors concluded, concerning potential cardiotoxicity, that desipramine was safe in children without heart disease, although ECG monitoring was essential (Schroeder et al., 1989). Baldessarini (1990) noted that children are more sensitive to cardiotoxic effects of tricyclic antidepressants than are adolescents and adults; he suggested that this increased vulnerability may be related to the relative efficiency with which they convert tricyclic antidepressants to potentially cardiotoxic 2-OH metabolites. However, Wilens and colleagues (1992) studied steady-state serum concentrations of desipramine (DMI) and 2-OH-desipramine (OHDMI) in 40 child, 36 adolescent, and 27 adult psychiatric patients. Serum levels of desipramine per weight-corrected (mg/kg) dose rose from 50 ng/ml in children (age range, 6 to 12 years), to 56 ng/ml in adolescents (age range, 13 to 18 years), and to 91 ng/mg in adults (age range, 19 to 67 years). Contrary to expectations, 2-OH-desipramine levels also increased with age from 17 ng/ml in children, to 20 ng/ml in adolescents, and to 26 ng/ml in adults. The results did not support the hypothesis that children would develop relatively higher levels of OHDMI than adolescents and adults because of more efficient hepatic oxidative metabolism of DMI. Children were either more efficient in clearing both DMI and OHDMI than adults or absorbed DMI relatively inefficiently. In fact, the data supported the clinical impression that children and adolescents usually require higher mg/kg doses of DMI than adults to reach similar serum DMI and OHDMI concentrations (Wilens et al., 1992).

In a subsequent study, Wilens et al. (1993a) analyzed the effects of serum levels of desipramine and 2-OH-desipramine on ECGs in 50 children, 39 adolescents, and 30 adult psychiatric patients treated with desipramine. With these expanded numbers of subjects, children and adolescents continued to have lower serum levels of DMI and OHDMI for weight-corrected doses than did adults. Children and adolescents showed no significant associations between serum drug and metabolite levels and heart rate or conduction (PR and QRS) intervals, although there was a weak relationship between sinus tachycardia and higher total DMI plus OHDMI levels. When data from all 119 subjects were combined, there was a modest correlation among DMI, OHDMI, and DMI plus OHDMI serum levels and PR and QRS intervals; however, the authors concluded that these were not likely to be clinically significant in any age group. About 10% of the subjects had combined DMI plus OHDMI serum levels of 250 ng/ml or greater, which may increase risk of cardiovascular toxicity. They recommended monitoring serum levels, and obtaining a baseline ECG and ECGs with increases in daily dose of more than 3 mg/kg (Wilens et al., 1993a).

Because routine ECGs may not record infrequent cardiac arrhythmias, Biederman et al. (1993) examined 24-hour ECG recordings and echocardiographic findings in 35 children and 36 adolescents receiving long-term (1.5 ± 1.2 years) desipramine therapy for psychiatric disorders. Compared with untreated healthy children, subjects' ECGs had significantly higher rates of single or paired premature atrial contractions and runs of supraventricular tachycardia and a decreased rate of sinus pauses and junctional rhythm. DMI levels correlated significantly only with paired premature atrial contractions. All echocardiographic findings but one were normal; the abnormal one was thought to be caused by a pericardial effusion of viral origin and not drug related. Overall, the data supported prior impressions that treatment with desipramine is associated with minor and benign cardiac effects (Biederman et al., 1993).

Walsh et al. (1994) reported on the effects of desipramine on the autonomic control of the heart in 13 children, adolescents, and young adults (age range, 7 to 29 years; mean, 17.5 ± 6.4 years). They noted that parasympathetic input to the heart decreases substantially with age and suggested that, because of the tricyclics' anticholinergic effects and their blockading the more active parasympathetic nervous systems of this age group, they increase supine blood pressure and pulse notably more in children and adolescents than in middle-aged and older adults. Their study documented that desipramine reduces parasympathetic input to the heart and suggested that desipramine may increase the ratio of sympathetic to parasympathetic cardiac input more in younger patients because of their relatively higher pretreatment levels of autonomic activity; this may explain the findings that desipramine increased the ratio of low-frequency to high-frequency variability in heart rate and overall substantial decrease in heart period variability found in their study. Because reductions in heart period variability are associated with increased vulnerability to serious arrhythmias, treatment with tricyclic antidepressants may increase the risk of arrhythmias in children and adolescents. The authors emphasize that their data are preliminary and that further studies are needed before clinical recommendations may be made.

The above studies appear to conclude that tricyclic antidepressants in the usual clinical dose range (under 5 mg/kg/day) and at the usual serum drug and metabolite levels (250 to 300 ng/ml or less of DMI plus OHDMI) are usually associated with minor and clinically benign effects on cardiac function in all age ranges. They further suggest that children and adolescents are not at significantly greater risk for developing such effects than are adults. The Ad Hoc Committee on Desipramine and Sudden Death of the American Academy of Child and Adolescent Psychiatry, established to investigate these concerns, reported at a members' forum at the 1992 Annual Convention that the risk of sudden death for children 5 to 14 years old who are treated with desipramine in therapeutic doses is approximately the same as the risk of sudden death for similarly aged children in the general population, between 1.5 and 4.2/million/year ($P > .23$) (AACAP, 1992, p. 8). The matter remains controversial, however. Werry (1994), in a letter to the editor of the *Journal of the American Academy of Child and Adolescent Psychiatry* proposed severe restrictions on the use of desipramine, whereas Riddle, Geller and Ryan (1994) rebutted his suggestion, noting

> based on the available data, there is as yet no established cause of the deaths nor any scientific evidence that they were related to the desipramine. As the number of sudden deaths is so small, the causal mechanism(s) are unknown and no specific cardiac finding has any known predictive value, clinically it should be considered mandatory to monitor both ECG changes and serum drug and metabolite levels and to keep them within recommended parameters whenever tricyclic antidepressants are prescribed.

Other Untoward Effects of Tricyclic Antidepressants

Central nervous system untoward effects may include drowsiness, EEG changes, seizures, incoordination, anxiety, insomnia and nightmares, confusion secondary to anticholinergic toxicity, delusions, and worsening of psychosis.

Tricyclic antidepressants may cause blood dyscrasias; if patients develop fever and sore throats during treatment with tricyclics, a complete blood count should be performed.

Anticholinergic untoward effects may include dry mouth, blurred vision, and constipation.

Changes in libido, both increases and decreases, have been reported; gynecomastia and impotence have also been reported.

Preskorn et al. (1988) reported that cognitive toxicity was associated with supratherapeutic plasma levels of tricyclics.

Tricyclic antidepressants, including clomipramine, may cause acute psychotic episodes if inadvertently administered to individuals with schizophrenia who have been incorrectly diagnosed.

Tricyclic Antidepressants in Child and Adolescent Psychiatry

IMIPRAMINE HYDROCHLORIDE (TOFRANIL), IMIPRAMINE PAMOATE (TOFRANIL-PM)

Because imipramine has been the most widely used clinically and has been more thoroughly studied in children and adolescents than the other tricyclics, it will serve as the prototype.

Indications in Child and Adolescent Psychiatry
Imipramine is approved for use in treating symptoms of depression in adolescents and adults. Its use in children is restricted to the treatment of enuresis in children who are at least 6 years old. Manufacturers state that a maximum dose of 2.5 mg/kg should not be exceeded in children (PDR, 1995).

Dosage Schedule for Children and Adolescents for Treating Depression
• Children under 12 years of age: Not recommended (however, see the reviews below of imipramine's use in this age group).
• Children at least 12 years of age and adolescents: An initial dosage of 30 to 40 mg with gradual titration upward is suggested. It is generally not necessary to exceed 100 mg/ day (manufacturer's package insert) (however, see the discussion below on treating adolescents and the importance of determining serum levels).
• For treating enuresis:
    Recommended dose differs from that for depression and is given below in the section "Imipramine in the Treatment of Enuresis."
• For treating ADHD:
    Recommended doses are given below in the section "Imipramine in the Treatment of ADHD."

Dose Forms Available
• Tablets (imipramine hydrochloride): 10 mg, 25 mg, 50 mg
• Capsules (imipramine pamoate): 75 mg, 100 mg, 125 mg, 150 mg. These capsules are designed for once-daily dosing. Because of their high unit potency and greater sensitivity of children to the cardiotoxic effects of imipramine, their use is not recommended in children and younger adolescents.

Untoward Effects of Imipramine

Imipramine has many untoward effects, some of which are potentially life threatening. Cardiovascular effects, including arrhythmias, tachycardia, blood pressure changes, impaired conduction and heart block, and a decreased seizure threshold, are particularly worrisome. See also the section "Untoward Effects of Tricyclic Antidepressants," above.

Imipramine in the Treatment of Enuresis

Although the pharmacological treatment of enuresis has been shown to be effective (Poussaint & Ditman, 1965; Rapoport, et al. 1980), it should not be employed until possible organic etiologies have been ruled out by appropriate physical examination and tests. It should be emphasized that behavioral therapies (e.g., conditioning with a bell and pad apparatus) are the treatments of choice for functional enuresis. There is a tendency for some children to become tolerant of imipramine's antienuretic effects, and many children relapse after medication withdrawal. Desmopressin acetate nasal spray (DDAVP), a synthetic analog of the natural hormone arginine vasopressin, may also be effective in some cases that do not respond satisfactorily to other treatments (package insert).

Imipramine's antienuretic effect occurs rapidly and appears to be unrelated to its antidepressant effects; it may directly inhibit bladder musculature and increase outlet resistance (American Medical Association, 1986). It also appears that the imipramine plus desipramine plasma level required for the effective treatment of enuresis is lower than that required for treating major depressive disorder. DeGatta et al. (1984) treated 90 enuretic patients, aged 5 to 14 years, with imipramine and reported that the minimum efficient serum concentration of imipramine plus desipramine in most cases was 80 ng/ml. However, about 20% of the subjects did not respond satisfactorily to imipramine even with adequate serum levels.

Fritz et al. (1994) reviewed prior studies of plasma levels of imipramine (IMI) and desipramine (DMI), its metabolite, in enuretic children treated with imipramine and reported on levels in 18 additional patients. The therapeutic efficacy of imipramine was moderately but significantly related to increasing levels of mg/kg dosage. Intersubject plasma combined IMI and DMI levels varied at least sevenfold at every dosage. The combined IMI and DMI levels at 2.5 mg/kg averaged 136.0 ng/ml (range, 35 to 170 ng/ml) for complete responders; 116 ng/ml (range, 37 to 236 ng/ml) for partial responders, and 96.0 ng/ml (range, 60 to 157 ng/ml) for nonresponders. The authors noted that despite the lack of a clear therapeutic window, serum level monitoring is useful in identifying subjects with low serum levels and suboptimal responses; in such cases, the dose of imipramine may be raised before concluding that the medication is ineffective. Knowledge of the serum level is essential, however, to avoid the danger of further dose increases resulting in toxic serum levels in nonresponsive subjects who have relatively high serum levels.

A trial of imipramine may occasionally be indicated when safer and more efficacious methods have failed and the symptom is psychologically handicapping or distressing to the patient, or, perhaps, when rapid control is essential to permit a child to go to summer camp or to travel.

The most frequent untoward effects reported in the treatment of enuretic children with imipramine are nervousness, sleep disorders, tiredness, and mild gastrointestinal disturbances (PDR, 1995). De-Gatta et al. (1984) reported that 40% of their 90 enuretic subjects had at least one side effect; 42% had loss of appetite, 16% had light sleep, 11% had abdominal pains, 8% had dry mouth, and 8% had headaches.

In clinical practice, initial ECGs often have not been done for the treatment of enuresis, because the final total daily dosage of imipramine usually remains below 2.5 mg/kg and the risk of cardiotoxicity is low. In light of the several sudden deaths reported in children receiving tricyclic antidepressants, even in usual doses, the author recommends a baseline ECG to screen for cardiac abnormalities that may increase the risk of conduction disorders secondary to tricyclic administration. It is suggested that bedwetters who void soon after falling asleep benefit if imipramine is given earlier and in divided doses (e.g., 25 mg in midafternoon and 25 mg before bed) (PDR, 1995). A maximum dose of 2.5 mg/kg should not be exceeded because of the possibility of developing ECG abnormalities. Doses over 75 mg/day do not increase efficacy and do increase untoward effects (PDR, 1995).

Dosage Schedule for Treating Enuresis
- Children under 6 years of age: Not recommended.
- Children at least 6 years of age through 11 years: Begin with 25 mg 1 hour before bedtime. If not effective within 1 week, increase to maximum dose of 50 mg.
- Persons at least 12 years of age: Proceed as above, with the option to increase the dose to a maximum of 75 mg.

REPORTS OF INTEREST

Imipramine in the Treatment of Childhood (Prepubertal) MDD. At the present time, imipramine and nortriptyline are the only tricyclics approved by the FDA for investigational use for depression in children aged 12 years and younger. Current FDA guidelines for ECG changes during treatment with either drug are as follows:

1. The P-R interval should not exceed 0.21 second.
2. Resting heart rate should be less than 130 beats per minute.
3. The QRS interval should not exceed 0.02 seconds more than the baseline interval.

The blood pressure of children receiving imipramine, which can both elevate the blood pressure and produce orthostatic hypotension, should not be permitted to exceed 145/95 mm Hg (Geller & Carr, 1988). Imipramine levels above 5 mg/kg are not usually permitted in investigational protocols (Hayes et al., 1975).

Baseline studies that should be completed before initiating treatment with a tricyclic antidepressant include sitting and supine blood pressure, complete blood count with differential, electrolytes, thyroid function tests, blood urea nitrogen (BUN), serum creatinine, urinalysis with osmolality, liver function tests, and an ECG.

Several investigators have noted that in clinical practice an absolute upper dose maximum for tricyclic antidepressants is not very useful because of the marked intersubject variability in pharmacokinetics (e.g., metabolism and elimination) and the fact that, although children as a group tend to metabolize and/or eliminate tricyclic antidepressants more rapidly than older adolescents and adults, some children, perhaps genetically slow hydroxylators, may reach very high serum levels on doses well below the recommended maximum (Biederman et al., 1989b). Hence careful clinical monitoring, including serum levels, is essential.

Puig-Antich and his colleagues (1987) investigated the use of imipramine in prepubescent children diagnosed with MDD. In a double-blind placebo-controlled study of 38 subjects, there was no significant difference between response to imipramine (56%; 9 of 16 subjects) and response to placebo (68%; 15 of 22 subjects).

These authors also studied total maintenance plasma level (imipramine plus desipramine) in 30 prepubescent children and found a positive correlation between plasma level and clinical response. Responders had significantly higher ($P < .007$) mean maintenance total plasma levels (284 ± 225 ng/ml) than did nonresponders (145 ± 80 ng/ml). The authors reported that a maintenance total plasma level of 150 ng/ml was the most important differentiating point between responders and nonresponders. Eighty-five percent (17) of 20 subjects whose values were above 150 ng/ml had positive responses, but only 30% (3) of 10 children with lower values responded positively. The authors also found nothing, including dosage, that predicted plasma levels (Puig-Antich et al., 1987). This is consonant with the finding that combined imipramine and desipramine steady-state plasma levels varied sixfold (from 56 to 324 ng/ml) in 11 boys receiving 75 mg/day of imipramine (Weller et al., 1982).

Other important findings of Puig-Antich and his colleagues (1987) were: (a) the more severe the pretreatment depressive symptoms on the Kiddie-Schedule for Affective Disorders and Schizophrenia (K-SADS) nine-item depressive score, the less likely was a favorable response to imipramine ($P < .008$); (b) prepubescent children with the RDC psychotic subtype of MDD were much less likely to have a favorable response to imipramine than nonpsychotic depressed children ($P < .05$); and (c) some children would require dosages over 5 mg/kg/day to reach plasma levels in the range associated with positive response.

These authors also reported that the following untoward effects were found in more than 30% of the children treated with imipramine: excitement, irritability, nightmares, insomnia, headache, muscle pain, increased appetite, abdominal cramps, constipation, vomiting, hiccups, dry mouth, bad taste in the mouth, sweating, flushed face, drowsiness, dizziness, tiredness, and restlessness. Similar untoward effects were present in the placebo group, although at lower frequencies. The untoward effects were severe enough in 17 of the 30 children to prevent upward titration to 5 mg/kg/day; cardiac side effects were responsible in 10 of these cases. Nine children had increases in the P-R interval to the maximum, and one child's resting heart rate reached 130 beats per minute. No child on placebo showed ECG changes from baseline, whereas nearly every child receiving imipramine had at least minor changes (Puig-Antich et al., 1987).

Preskorn et al. (1987) reported a double-blind, randomly assigned, placebo-controlled study of 22 hospitalized, prepubertal depressed children ages 6 to 12 years; it found imipramine to be statistically better than placebo ($P < .05$) by 3 weeks, when imipramine plus desipramine plasma levels were used by laboratory workers to adjust dosage of impramine to reach a therapeutic range of 125 to 250 ng/ml. Doses of imipramine could range between 25 and 150 mg/day. The authors also noted that dexamethasone suppression test (DST) nonsuppressors showed greater improvement than DST suppressors. Total plasma levels below 125 ng/ml yielded a response rate only somewhat better than placebo, and levels above 250 ng/ml

were associated with a lower response rate and an increased incidence of toxic untoward effects; the latter included prolongation of
intracardiac conduction, increased blood pressure and heart rate,
and mental confusion. The authors noted that, in a prior study in
which clinicians were unaware of plasma levels and further increased dosages resulting in some children developing total
imipramine plus desipramine plasma levels greater than 450 ng/ml,
the antidepressant response was poor and several children developed toxic confusion that was incorrectly interpreted as a worsening
of the depressive condition. This underscored the importance of
monitoring plasma drug levels because a reduction in dosage, not an
increase, would be indicated.

Based on their own data and that of Puig-Antich and his coworkers, Preskorn et al. (1989a) concluded that plasma imipramine plus
desipramine levels ranging from 125 to 250 ng/ml were both efficacious and safe in treating MDD in children. These authors suggested
using an initial oral dose of 75 mg imipramine daily and then determining the combined plasma concentration of imipramine plus
desipramine 7 to 10 days later when steady-state levels would be expected. Based on their experience, 78% of children initially had
plasma levels outside of the therapeutic range; 66% were below 125
ng/ml and 12% were above 250 ng/ml. Because intraindividual
plasma levels were reproducible and linearly correlated with dose,
the authors used a formula

$$\text{new dose} = (\text{initial dose/initial level}) \times \text{desired level}$$

to adjust the dosage. The desired level was 185 ng/ml, the midpoint
of the optimal range. Using this strategy, 84% of their patients
achieved levels within the therapeutic range. The remaining 16%
had subtherapeutic levels, possibly requiring additional adjustments (Preskorn et al., 1989a).

**Imipramine in the Treatment of Comorbid Prepubertal
MDD and Conduct Disorder.**   Puig-Antich (1982) reported that
16 of 43 prepubertal males accepted for treatment for major depressive disorder had a codiagnosis of conduct disorder. These subjects
did not differ on significant demographic and clinical variables from
subjects diagnosed with MDD only. Approximately one-third of each
group had auditory hallucinations consistent with RDC criteria for
psychotic subtype major depression. Major depression was found by
history to precede the onset of conduct disorder in 14 (87%) of the 16
cases. Thirteen of the 16 patients who completed the study had a full

antidepressant response between 5 and 18 weeks after beginning medication. Although this was a double-blind study, only 1 patient had a full response during the 5-week double-blind period; the others received either imipramine openly or were switched to desipramine and titrated upward. Dosage of 5 mg/kg/day was the desired dosage, but doses above and below this occurred; exact dosage was not reported for these patients. Of particular interest, however, was the fact that 11 of the 13 boys who definitely recovered from the major depression also experienced total remission of their conduct disorders. In a majority of cases, conduct disorders reappeared following recurrence of another major depressive episode. In 6 of these patients, who were treated with the same drug and dosage associated with remission, conduct disorders persisted in 2 (33%) following remission of the depressive symptoms. Puig-Antich (1982) emphasized the potential importance of treating these comorbid disorders and avoiding recurrence of the depression during childhood and adolescence in significantly improving the prognosis of this subgroup of conduct disorders, which appear to develop following the onset of major depression.

Imipramine in the Treatment of Adolescent MDD. Thirty-four adolescents with MDD treated with imipramine in an open study with monitoring of plasma imipramine levels showed some differences from prepubescent children (Ryan et al., 1986). Imipramine was titrated to a dose of 5 mg/kg/day; the adolescents had an overall positive response rate of 44% (15) of 34, but there was no relationship between positive response and higher plasma imipramine levels. Another difference between the adolescents and prepubertal children with MDD was that, as a group, nonpsychotic subjects did not respond more favorably than the psychotic subtype. The authors hypothesized that adolescents with MDD were less responsive to imipramine because of an antagonistic effect of sex hormones, levels of which increase during adolescence (Ryan et al., 1986).

Strober et al. (1990) treated 35 adolescents, aged 13 years to 18 years (mean, 15.4 years), openly with imipramine; they had been hospitalized and diagnosed by RDC criteria with MDD with at least probable certainty. Ten of the adolescents also met criteria for delusional subtype. After failing to improve after 1 week's hospitalization, subjects were treated for 6 weeks with imipramine. Six (17.7%) of the 34 subjects who completed the study were unable to achieve the target dose of 5 mg/kg/day, because of untoward effects. Average daily dose was 222 ± 49 mg/day, and steady-state imipramine plus desmethylimipramine levels varied 11-fold (mean, 237 ± 168 ng/ml;

range, 79 to 888 ng/ml). Eight (33%) of the 24 nondelusional subjects and 1 (10%) of the 10 delusional subjects were considered responders, suggesting greater refractoriness in patients with psychotic features. No responders had a plasma imipramine plus desmethylimipramine level below 180 ng/ml, but the difference between responders and nonresponders was not significant. Overall, only 10 (29.4%) patients were rated very much improved or much improved on the Clinical Global Impressions Improvement scale.

Lithium Augmentation in Adolescents Diagnosed with MDD Who Were Treatment Resistant to Imipramine. Ryan et al. (1988a) reported in a retrospective chart review their treatment of 14 adolescents, aged 14 to 19 years (mean, 16.9 years), who were diagnosed by RDC with nonbipolar MDD; these patients had not responded to treatment with various tricyclic antidepressants (for a period of at least 6 weeks in 12 cases and for 4 weeks in 2 cases) by lithium augmentation while continuing treatment with amitriptyline, desipramine, or nortriptyline. Lithium carbonate was titrated to achieve therapeutic serum levels. Six patients (43%) were responders and improved to the extent that they had, at most, mild symptoms of depression and were no longer being functionally impaired by their depression. Most responders improved gradually over the first month after the addition of lithium treatment. Their serum lithium level was 0.65 ± 0.06 mEq/l and was not significantly different from that of the nonresponders. The authors suggested that the addition of lithium carbonate may be a useful adjunct to the treatment of some adolescents with major depression who do not respond satisfactorily to treatment with tricyclic antidepressants (Ryan et al., 1988a).

Strober et al. (1992) treated 24 adolescents diagnosed with major depressive disorder who had not responded to 6 weeks of treatment with imipramine by augmentation with lithium. The dosage of imipramine at the end of the sixth week was held constant, and lithium was added on an open basis for a 3-week period beginning with doses of 300 mg three times a day that were then titrated upwards based on clinical response to a final mean serum lithium level of 0.89 mEq/l. As a comparison group, the authors used 10 patients diagnosed with MDD in an earlier study who did not respond to imipramine during the first 6 weeks and who continued receiving imipramine only for the subsequent 3 weeks. Both groups improved significantly during the final 3 weeks of treatment as measured on the Hamilton Rating Scale for Depression (HAM-D). Although the group receiving lithium showed greater improvement, the difference between the two groups was not significant. Two patients (8.3%) in the lithium-augmented group were rated as "marked responders," as evidenced by a decrease of at least 50% in the HAM-D and a final score of less than 10, between 2 and 7 days after addition of lithium. Eight additional patients (33.3%) showed partial improvement over a period of 14 to 21 days following lithium administration. The authors noted that lithium's efficacy as an adjunct in adolescents with tricyclic-resistant major depression appears to be much less than in adults, in whom up to 70% respond favorably. They also suggested that a small subgroup of adolescents may show an initial robust positive effect and that other adolescents may show gradual but less improvement over time. A trial of longer than 3 weeks may be necessary to determine if additional adolescents might benefit and whether further clinical gains would occur in adolescents who showed some improvement: the authors note that Thase et al. (1989) reported on a subgroup of adults who showed improvement only after 4 to 6 weeks of lithium augmentation.

Imipramine in the Treatment of ADHD. There is a considerable body of literature attesting to the clinical efficacy of imipramine in the treatment of attention-deficit hyperactivity disorder (ADHD), although most studies find stimulants superior (for review see Campbell et al., 1985; Rapoport & Mikkelsen, 1978; Rapoport et al., 1974). Although imipramine does not have FDA approval for use in ADHD, some clinicians consider imipramine or desipramine the next drug of choice if a patient does not respond to stimulants. Wender (1988), however, notes that when used to treat ADHD, tricyclics improve mood and decrease hyperactivity but usually are sedating and do not appear to improve concentration.

The mechanism of action of imipramine in ADHD is different from that in depression; it is rapidly effective, and often lower doses are required. Mean dosages reported in the literature have ranged from 20 to 173.7 mg/day. The development of tolerance by some children to the therapeutic effects of imipramine within about 6 weeks presents difficulties.

Rapoport et al. (1974) compared imipramine and methylphenidate in a double-blind placebo-controlled study of 76 hyperactive boys. Mean daily dose of imipramine was 80 ± 21 mg (maximum 150 mg), and mean daily dose of methylphenidate was 20 mg (maximum 30 mg). Although both drugs were significantly better than placebo, most measures favored the stimulant drug. Some tolerance to the therapeutic effects of imipramine appeared to develop after about 10 weeks of treatment.

In a double-blind, placebo-controlled, crossover-design study of 30 hyperactive children, Werry et al. (1980) found imipramine to be statistically more effective than methylphenidate in its overall therapeutic effect; untoward effects of imipramine, however, were greater and more troublesome than those of methylphenidate. Methylphenidate was given in doses of 0.40 mg/kg; imipramine was given in doses of 1 and 2 mg/kg/day. The authors found few significant differences between the two imipramine doses but thought that the lower dose resulted in a slightly better clinical response and milder side effects (Werry et al., 1980).

A 1-year follow-up study of 76 hyperactive boys treated with imipramine or methylphenidate found that significantly more subjects on imipramine discontinued the medication because of lack of benefit or untoward effects but that subjects in both treatment groups who continued on either drug were equally improved (Quinn & Rapoport, 1975). The large dropout rate is a considerable clinical disadvantage in using imipramine. It appears that tolerance to imipramine may develop, resulting in deterioration after an initial improvement (Gross, 1973; Klein et al., 1980; Quinn & Rapoport, 1975; Waizer et al., 1974).

Dosage Schedule for Treating ADHD
 No official recommendations for age or dose exist. Based on the literature and experimental protocols, the following is suggested for children over 6 years of age: Monitoring prerequisites for imipramine should be followed. Begin with a low dose, either 25 mg/day or 0.5 mg/kg/day, and slowly titrate upward with increases of 25 mg once or twice weekly.

Imipramine in the Treatment of Separation Anxiety Disorder (School Phobia). Gittelman-Klein and Klein (1971) reported a double-blind placebo-controlled study using imipramine to treat 35 children diagnosed with school phobia (separation anxiety). Of the 45 children between ages 6 and 14 years old who entered the study, 35 (19 females and 16 males; mean age, 10.8 years) completed the 6-week protocol. Dosage was administered in the morning and evening for a total of 75 mg/day for the first 2 weeks and then adjusted weekly. At the completion of the study, doses ranged from 100 mg/day to 200 mg/day (mean, 152 mg/day). All subjects also were treated simultaneously with a multidisciplinary treatment program.

Dry mouth was much more frequent in the active drug group, occurring in 50% of the subjects ($P < .003$). One child developed orthostatic hypotension requiring reduction of dosage, but all other side effects reportedly disappeared without dosage adjustment. The authors noted that doses of imipramine below 75 mg/day were indistinguishable from placebo in this study. Using return to school regularly within 6-weeks as the criterion, there was no statistical difference between imipramine and placebo at the 3-week mark, but by 6 weeks, imipramine was significantly ($P < .05$) better than placebo (Gittelman-Klein & Klein, 1971). Klein et al. (1980) emphasize that imipramine is effective in reducing separation anxiety but that anticipatory anxiety may continue to be problematic. Imipramine doses of between 75 and 200 mg/day were effective for school-phobic children between 6 and 14 years of age; however, children with severe separation anxiety without school phobia sometimes responded to doses as low as 25 to 50 mg/day. School-phobic children who responded to imipramine were found to show at least some improvement when doses reached 125 mg/day; once improvement began, further dose increases usually produced additional benefit. Response was usually maximal within 6 to 8 weeks. It was suggested that maintenance be continued for a minimum of 8 weeks following remission of symptoms and then tapered and discontinued (Klein et al., 1980).

Klein et al. (1992) compared the efficacy of imipramine and placebo in a double-blind randomized study of 21 children (14 males and 7 females; age range, 6 to 15 years; mean, 9.5 ± 0.8 years) diagnosed with separation anxiety disorder by DSM-III criteria. Nine subjects (43%) were diagnosed with comorbid DSM-III anxiety disorders, overanxious disorder being the most frequent. The 21 subjects comprised the nonresponders of a larger group (N = 45) who were treated for the month preceding entry into the study with vigorous behavioral therapy. Behavioral treatment continued throughout the 6-week treatment period, during which 11 patients received imipramine and 10 patients received placebo.

Imipramine was begun at 25 mg/day for 3 days, increased to 50 mg for the next 4 days, and then titrated to a maximum dose of 5 mg/kg/day. Baseline ECGs were obtained with subsequent ECGs recorded after every dose increase above 50 mg/day. Daily doses of imipramine ranged from 75 to 275 mg/day (mean, 153 mg/day or 4.67 mg/kg) at the completion of the study. Children treated with imipramine had significantly more untoward effects than those who received placebo. Irritability or angry outbursts occurred in 5 (45%), dry mouth in 5 (45%), and drowsiness in 2 (18%) of the children receiving imipramine. ECG changes occurred, but no dosage reductions were required because they did not exceed the recommended maximum values or changes from baseline (Klein et al., 1992). There were no significant differences between the imipramine and placebo groups on any measure; both groups showed about 50% overall improvement. These results are strikingly different from those in the earlier study (Gittelman-Klein & Klein, 1971). The authors note that although imipramine may still be useful in treating separation anxiety disorder, its efficacy appears to be considerably less than previously thought (Klein et al., 1992)

Recently, it was reported that three children with panic disorder who also had severe separation anxiety and agoraphobia responded well to a combination of imipramine and alprazolam, a benzodiazepine (Ballenger et al., 1989).

Imipramine in the Treatment of Somnambulism and Night Terrors. Four children with night terrors, two children with somnambulism, and one child with both disorders were treated with imipramine (10 to 50 mg at bedtime). The sleep disorders remitted completely in all children (Pesikoff & Davis, 1971).

NORTRIPTYLINE HYDROCHLORIDE (PAMELOR)

Indications in Child and Adolescent Psychiatry
Nortriptyline is approved by the FDA for the treatment of symptoms of depression in adolescents and adults. The drug is not recommended for use in the pediatric age group because its safety and effectiveness have not been established in children.

Dosage Schedule for Children and Adolescents
• Children: Not recommended.
• Adolescents: Manufacturer recommends giving a total of 30 to 50 mg/day. One should start at a low dose and titrate upward based on clinical response (however, see recommendations of Geller and her colleagues, below, on the usefulness of serum levels.)

Dose Forms Available
• Capsules: 10 mg, 25 mg, 50 mg, 75 mg
• Oral solution: 10 mg/5 ml

Untoward effects of the tricyclic antidepressants are discussed above as well as in the discussions of the individual tricyclic antidepressants, below.

REPORTS OF INTEREST

Nortriptyline in the Treatment of Major Depressive Disorder in Children and Adolescents.   Geller and her colleagues have studied pharmacokinetic parameters of nortriptyline and its use in treating children and adolescents diagnosed with major depressive disorder (MDD) (Geller et al., 1985, 1986, 1987a, 1987b, 1989, 1990, 1992). There are no double-blind placebo-controlled studies establishing nortriptyline's superiority over placebo in treating MDD in children or adolescents. In an open study, Geller et al. (1986) found that therapeutic efficacy correlated with nortriptyline plasma levels. Twenty-two children, aged 6 to 12 years, diagnosed with MDD were treated on an outpatient basis with fixed doses of either 10 mg twice daily or 25 mg twice daily for 8 weeks. Initial dose was based on individual subjects' rate of metabolism of nortriptyline, as determined by baseline single-dose kinetics, with the slower metabolizers receiving the lower fixed dose. Fourteen subjects (63.6%) responded favorably to nortriptyline. Responders were not significantly different from non-responders in terms of age, sex, weight, social class, duration of illness, or baseline or 2-week Children's Depression Rating Scale scores. Responders, however, had significantly higher mean milligram per kilogram daily doses (1.02 ± 0.21 mg/kg; range, 0.64 to 1.57 mg/kg) than nonresponders (0.82 ± 0.51 mg/kg; range, 0.40 to 2.01 mg/kg). The mean nortriptyline steady-state plasma level was also higher in responders (60.31 ± 20.90 ng/ml; range, 18.8 to 111.5 ng/ml) than in nonresponders (30.86 ± 17.64 ng/ml; range, 12 to 54.3 ng/ml). Twelve of the 13 subjects who received at least 0.89 mg/kg/day responded. All subjects with steady-state nortriptyline plasma levels of at least 60 ng/ml responded, as did 4 of 7 children with levels ranging from 40 to 59 ng/ml. At the end of the 8-week protocol, 7 of the 8 nonresponders recovered when the dose was increased to achieve steady-state nortriptyline plasma levels of 60 to 100 ng/ml. Overall, 21 of the 22 subjects had good clinical response with minimal and transient side effects, and all ECGs remained within recommended parameters for prepubertal children. These authors thought that because children's plasma nortriptyline levels are stable over time, ECGs need to be performed only at baseline and once at steady-state plasma levels if they remain within recommended parameters (Geller et al., 1986).

Geller and her colleagues (1989, 1992) enrolled 72 prepubescent children, aged 6 years to 12 years, who were diagnosed with MDD, nondelusional type, by Research Diagnostic Criteria (RDC) (Spitzer et al., 1978) and DSM-III (1980) criteria in a double-blind placebo-controlled study of the efficacy of nortriptyline. The study design was a 2-week, single-blind, placebo washout phase followed by an 8-week random assignment, double-blind, placebo-controlled phase.

All subjects were outpatients, and most had coexisting separation anxiety. The children were chronically depressed: 96% had been ill for at least 2 years, and 50% had had MDD for 5 or more years before entering the study. Of the 72 subjects entering the study, 12 (16.7%) responded during the placebo phase, 10 were discontinued for various reasons during the active treatment phase, and 50 (24 on placebo and 26 on nortriptyline) completed the study.

Using Table 5.2, below, the initial dose necessary to achieve a steady-state nortriptyline level of 80 ± 20 ng/ml was determined from 24-hour plasma levels. Any necessary adjustments to obtain mean steady-state plasma levels of nortriptyline and of total, trans-10-hydroxynortriptyline, and cis-10-hydroxynortriptyline (10-OH-NT) were made during the first 4 weeks of the double-blind phase.

Both the nortriptyline and the placebo groups had a low rate of positive response (30.8% on nortriptyline and 16.7% on placebo), and there was no significant difference between them. There was no significant correlation between mean nortriptyline plasma level and response, nor between mean nortriptyline plus mean total, cis-10-OH-NT, or trans-10-OH-NT plasma levels and response. Because of the poor response rate and the unlikelihood of finding a statistical difference between the placebo and active groups if the protocol were completed, Geller et al. (1989, 1992) stopped their study at this point.

Geller et al. (1990) enrolled 52 postpubertal adolescents, aged 12 to 17 years and diagnosed with MDD by RDC (Spitzer et al., 1978) and DSM-III (1980a) criteria, in a random assignment, double-blind, placebo-controlled study of nortriptyline. Adolescents with delusional symptoms were not enrolled. Subjects had scores on the Children's Depression Rating Scale (CDRS) and the Kiddie Global Assessment Scale (KGAS) placing them in the severe range of pathology. Of the 31 subjects completing the study, 27 (87.1%) had a duration of symptoms of at least 2 years (10 [32.3%] between 2 and 5 years and 17 [54.8%] more than 5 years). The study was comprised of a 2-week, single-blind, placebo washout phase and an 8-week, double-blind, placebo-controlled phase. Using Table 5.2, below, the initial dose necessary to achieve a steady-state nortriptyline level of 80 ± 20 ng/ml was determined from 24-hour plasma levels. Mean nortriptyline plasma level was 91.1 ± 18.3 ng/ml.

Of the 52 subjects enrolled, 17 (32.7%) responded to placebo by the end of week 2, and 4 additional subjects dropped out for other reasons. Of the 31 completing the study, 12 were assigned to nortriptyline and 19 to placebo. The results of the study showed such a

Table 5.2.
Suggested Nortriptyline Dose Schedules for Children and Adolescents[a]

Predicted doses from 24-hour plasma levels after a single dose of 25 mg administered to 5- to 9-year-olds.[b]

24-Hour Plasma Level (ng/ml)	Suggested Total Daily Dose (mg)
6–10	50–75
11–14	35–40
15–20	25–30
21–25	20

Predicted doses from 24-hour nortriptyline plasma levels after a single dose of 50 mg administered to 10- to 16-year-olds.[b]

24-Hour Plasma Level (ng/ml)	Suggested Total Daily Dose (mg)
10–14	75–100
15–19	50–75
20–24	40–50
25–29	35
30–34	30
35–40	25
>40	20

[a]Adapted from Geller B, Cooper TB, Chestnut EC, et al. Child and adolescent nortriptyline single dose kinetics predict steady state plasma levels and suggested dose: Preliminary data. J Clin Psychopharmacol 1985;5:154–158.
[b]Total daily dose should be divided and given twice daily because of relatively short half-life.

low rate of response to nortriptyline that the study was terminated early. Only 1 (8.3%) of 12 subjects receiving nortriptyline responded, whereas 4 (21.1%) of the 19 subjects on placebo responded. (The one responder to nortriptyline went on to have a bipolar course.) Subjects with higher nortriptyline levels achieved significantly worse scores on the CDRS (P =.002). There were, however, no significant differences between the two groups on final CDRS or KGAS scores.

It is most interesting that 17, or about one-third, of enrolled patients with chronic and severe depression responded to placebo within 2 weeks. However, 13 of the 17 placebo responders relapsed, 9 of them within 1 to 4 weeks (Geller et al., 1990).

Nortriptyline in the Treatment of Children and Adolescents Diagnosed with ADHD. Saul (1985) treated 60 patients diagnosed with ADD (age range, 9 to 20 years) with nortriptyline. The first group of 30 subjects was diagnosed with ADD and also scored more than 9 points on the Kovacs Children's Depression Inventory (KCDI). The second group of 30 subjects had ADD but scored

9 or less on the KCDI; they were initially prescribed stimulant medication but responded poorly and were switched to nortriptyline. Nortriptyline for both groups was begun at 10 mg nightly for 2 weeks. Because no patients experienced difficulty at this dose level, the dose was then increased to 25 mg twice daily. Fifty-four (90%) of the 60 subjects had positive responses. Satisfactory clinical response usually occurred at 50 mg daily; 75 mg/day was the maximum dose given. Within 5 to 6 weeks, typically there was a marked change in attitude followed by an increase in attention span and a decrease in impulsivity. The most clinically significant untoward effects at the initial dose were dizziness and sleepiness; their inconvenience was minimized by administering the drug near bedtime.

Wilens et al. (1993b) conducted a retrospective chart review of 58 patients (age range, 7 to 18 years; mean 12.1 ± 2.9 years) who were diagnosed with ADHD and received nortriptyline. All but 9 subjects had comorbid diagnoses including 34 with mood disorder, 18 with oppositional defiant disorder, and 5 with conduct disorder. These were treatment-resistant patients who had not responded satisfactorily to an average of 4 prior medication trials. About half of the subjects were also receiving one or two other medications concomitantly. Nortriptyline was administered for a mean of 11.9 ± 14.0 months (range, 0.4 to 57.9 months) in mean daily doses of 73.6 ± 33.1 mg (range, 20 to 200 mg/day) or a mean weight-corrected daily dose of 1.94 ± 0.99 mg/kg (range, 0.4 to 4.5 mg/kg). Overall, 28 patients (48%) were rated as marked responders and 16 (28%) as moderate responders. Subjects with and without comorbidity responded equally well; all five subjects with comorbid conduct disorder responded favorably.

There were no significant differences between responders and nonresponders in mean daily dose (74.8 ± 31.9 versus 70.0 ± 38.0 mg), in weight-corrected mean daily dose (1.9 ± 0.9 versus 2.1 ± 1.2 mg/kg), or serum nortriptyline levels (96.3 ± 51.6 versus 83.4 ± 43.1. ng/ml). Significantly more ($P < .03$) of the "markedly improved" subjects had serum nortriptyline levels between 50 and 150 ng/ml. Untoward effects were usually mild and necessitated stopping nortriptyline in only one child who became agitated. No clinically significant conduction abnormalities were noted on ECG follow-up assessment.

Nortriptyline in Comorbid ADHD and Chronic Motor Tic Disorder or Tourette's Syndrome.   In a retrospective study of 12 children and adolescents (age range, 5 to 16 years; mean, 10.9 ± 1.0 years) diagnosed with ADHD and comorbid chronic motor tic disorder (N = 2) or Tourette's syndrome (N = 10), Spencer et al. (1993c) reported that 8 (67%) of subjects were rated as being marked or very much improved (P = .01) in their movement disorders and 11 (92%) were rated much or very much improved (P = .0001) in their ADHD symptoms. The average dose of nortriptyline was 105 ± 11.7 mg/day or 2.8 ± 0.3 mg/kg/day. Mean serum nortriptyline level was 122.7 ± 12.1 ng/mg for the 10 patients for whom such values had been determined. There were few untoward effects. The only cardiac symptom was a mild tachycardia in one patient; no clinically significant changes occurred in EEGs.

Nortriptyline Dosage Schedule for Children and Adolescents. Pharmacokinetic studies of tricyclic antidepressants in adults have shown that their elimination half-lives are sufficiently long to permit the frequent practice of giving a single bedtime dose once titration is completed (Rudorfer & Potter, 1987). Geller et al. (1987b), however, noted that 41 children, aged 5 to 12 years, had a significantly shorter mean nortriptyline plasma half-life (20.8 ± 7.2 hours; range, 11.2 to 42.5 hours) than 32 adolescents 13 to 16 years old (31.1 ± 19.8 hours; range, 14.2 to 76.6 hours). Geller et al. (1985) also found that correlations between the milligram per kilogram dose of nortriptyline and steady-state plasma levels were not significant in 33 children and adolescents 5 to 16 years of age. The clinical significance of these data, including the interindividual variation of half-life by as much as six- or sevenfold, prompted Geller et al. (1987b) to advise that nortriptyline should be administered twice daily for all patients up through 16 years of age and that plasma level monitoring is essential to be sure of achieving therapeutic plasma nortriptyline levels.

Geller et al. (1985) have used a single test dose of nortriptyline to predict steady-state plasma levels and to determine the initial dose of nortriptyline and presented tables suggesting daily doses to reach therapeutic nortriptyline plasma levels (Table 5.2). To use this method, the clinician must have access to a laboratory that can reliably assay nortriptyline levels of less than 20 ng/ml.

To use this table clinically Geller et al. (1985) and Geller and Carr (1988) suggested the following:

1. At 9:00 AM administer a single dose of 25 mg to patients 5 to 9 years of age, or 50 mg to patients 10 to 16 years of age.
2. Twenty-four hours later (9:00 AM the next day) draw blood to determine the plasma nortriptyline level.

3. Use the table to determine the suggested medication dose for the patient's nortriptyline level and age.
4. Seven days later determine plasma nortriptyline level 9 to 11 hours after a dose. If the level is not in the therapeutic range (60 to 100 ng/ml), adjust the dosage using the following equation (Geller & Carr, 1988):

$$\frac{\text{Day 7 plasma levels}}{\text{Current dose}} = \frac{80 \text{ ng/ml}}{\text{Adjusted dose}}$$

Geller et al. (1987b) have recommended that nortriptyline be withdrawn gradually over approximately 10 days to 2 weeks to avoid withdrawal symptoms. Only 6 of 30 children and adolescents 6 to 16 years old developed withdrawal symptoms when this was done. In all cases symptoms were mild, and in 5 subjects they were limited to the gastrointestinal system and consisted of stomachache, nausea, and/or emesis.

AMITRIPTYLINE HYDROCHLORIDE (ELAVIL, ENDEP)

Indications in Child and Adolescent Psychiatry
    Amitriptyline is approved to treat symptoms of depression. It is noted that endogenous depression is more likely to be alleviated than are other depressive states. It is not recommended for patients under 12 years of age because of limited experience with treating this age group with amitriptyline.

Dosage Schedule in Children and Adolescents
• Children under 12 years of age: Not recommended.
• Children and adolescents at least 12 years old: An initial dose of 25 mg/day titrated upward in 25-mg increments is suggested. Ten milligrams three times daily and 20 mg at bedtime may be adequate for adolescents who do not tolerate higher doses. Usual maintenance is 50 to 100 mg/day. Adequate therapeutic response may take up to 30 days to develop.

Dose Forms Available
• Tablets: 10 mg, 25 mg, 50 mg, 75 mg, 100 mg, 150 mg
• Injectable: 10 mg/ml

Untoward effects of amitriptyline are discussed above in "Untoward Effects of Tricyclic Antidepressants."

REPORTS OF INTEREST

Amitriptyline in the Treatment of Children and Adolescents Diagnosed with ADHD.   Yepes et al. (1977) administered amitriptyline, methylphenidate, or placebo to 50 children diagnosed with hyperkinetic reaction of childhood for randomly determined 2-week periods during which each drug was titrated. The initial dose of amitriptyline was 25 mg three times daily; dose was titrated to achieve optimal clinical response. Dose range was 50 to 150 mg/day; the mean was 92.1 mg/day. Amitriptyline was, with few exceptions, comparable to methylphenidate in effectiveness in reducing hyperactivity and aggression in both the home and school environments. The authors noted, however, that amitriptyline was more sedating than imipramine and that, frequently, doses of amitriptyline sufficiently high to control symptoms could not be tolerated. Sedation remained a problem throughout the 2-week period on amitriptyline. In an earlier study (Krakowski, 1965), however, 50 children with various diagnoses with hyperkinesis received maintenance doses of 20 to 75 mg/day (i.e., about one-half that used in the above study) for up to 9 months with positive results, and only one instance of severe sedation occurred (the other subjects developed tolerance or the sedative effect disappeared with reduction of dosage).

Amitriptyline in Depressed Children. Kashani et al. (1984) performed a double-blind cross-over study comparing amitriptyline and placebo in nine prepubertal depressed children. Dosage ranged from 45 to 110 mg/day. Six (66.7%) of the subjects improved on amitriptyline, a finding that was not significant ($P < .09$).

Amitriptyline in Depressed Adolescents. Kramer and Feiguine (1981) compared the efficacy of amitriptyline and placebo in treating 20 adolescents diagnosed with depression. Age range was 13 to 17 years. Amitriptyline was initially given in 25-mg doses four times daily and increased within 3 days to a maximum of 200 mg/day in divided doses. The length of the study was 6 weeks. Both placebo and active medication groups improved over the 6-week period, and there was no significant difference between the two groups. Although this pilot study suggests that amitriptyli e is no more effective than placebo in treating adolescent depression, more studies and larger numbers are necessary before making this conclusion definitively.

DESIPRAMINE HYDROCHLORIDE (NORPRAMIN, PERTOFRANE)

Indications in Child and Adolescent Psychiatry
 Desipramine is indicated in the treatment of symptoms in various depressive syndromes, especially endogenous depression. Its efficacy and safety have not been established for children.

Dosage Schedule for Children and Adolescents
• Children: Not recommended.
• Adolescents: Usual dose is between 25 and 100 mg/day. One should start at a lower dose and titrate according to clinical response. A dose of 150 mg/day should not be exceeded. Adequate treatment response may take 2 to 3 weeks to develop.

Dose Forms Available
• Tablets: 10 mg, 25 mg, 50 mg, 75 mg, 100 mg, 150 mg

Untoward Effects of Desipramine

Untoward effects of the tricyclics, including sudden death with desipramine, are discussed above in "Untoward Effects of the Tricyclic Antidepressants."

REPORTS OF INTEREST

Desipramine in the Treatment of Adolescent Major Depressive Disorder. From 113 adolescents referred for depression, Boulos et al. (1991) identified a group of 52 adolescents who were diagnosed with nonpsychotic major depressive disorder by DSM-III criteria and who did not have an eating disorder, had not been treated with psychiatric medication, and had ratings of at least 17 on the Hamilton Rating Scale for Depression (HAM-D) and of at least 16 on the Beck Depression Inventory. These subjects were enrolled in single-blind placebo washout for 1 week. The 43 subjects whose rating scores continued to fulfill the above criteria then entered a 6-week double-blind protocol in which they received either placebo or desipramine in identical capsules. Desipramine was initiated at a dose of 100 mg at bedtime. Additional doses of 50 mg were added the next two mornings to achieve a daily dose of 200 mg (100 mg twice daily), which was maintained for the duration of the study. Thirty patients completed the study; 12 were receiving desipramine and 18 were receiving placebo. Seven patients dropped out for "personal reasons" and 6 because of untoward effects. A positive treatment response was reported if there was a reduction of at least 50% in the pretreatment score on the HAM-D. There was no significant difference ($P < .59$) between the placebo group (6 [33%] of 18) and the desipramine group (6 [50%] of 12). There were no significant differences between the groups in subjective untoward effects that were reported. However, major adverse effects that necessitated discontinuing medication in 6 patients occurred only in the desipramine group ($P < .05$) and included an allergic-type pruritic maculopapular rash (3 patients), vomiting and laryngospasm (1), and orthostatic hypotension (2). ECG abnormalities including tachycardia, sinus arrhythmia, and nonspecific T wave changes occurred only in the desipramine group but were clinically nonsymptomatic and did not require withdrawal from the study. Serum metabolite levels were not reported.

Kutcher et al. (1994) enrolled 70 adolescents who were diagnosed with major depressive disorder in a fixed-dose, placebo-controlled desipramine protocol. During the initial single-blind, one-week placebo period, 10 subjects were judged to be placebo responders and were dropped. The remaining 60 subjects (42 females, 18 males; age range, 15 to 20 years; mean age, 17.8 years) were assigned randomly to 6-weeks of placebo (N = 30) or desipramine (N = 30). Desipramine was begun with a 100 mg 8:00 PM dose, and 50 mg was added at 8:00 AM the second day and increased to 100 mg on the third day. Desipramine was continued at 100 mg twice daily throughout the remaining 6 weeks. Eighteen subjects dropped out. Significantly more of these were on active medication (13 [72%] of 18), and 10 of them did not complete the study because of untoward effects. Nine (90%) of the 10 were receiving desipramine; 5 subjects had allergic-type reactions (4 had maculopapular and 1 had mild laryngospasm), 2 patients had clinically significant orthostatic hypotension, and 2 had significant gastrointestinal complaints. The patient receiving placebo dropped out because of severe agitation. At the completion of the protocol, 2 of the 26 items on the Side Effect Scale were rated significantly higher among subjects in the DMI group: trouble sleeping ($P = .03$) and delay in urinating ($P = .007$). Although heart rate was significantly increased in the DMI group, there were no significant differences in systolic blood pressure while seated or standing, diastolic blood pressure while seated, or PR and QRS intervals on the ECG between the DMI and placebo groups.

Forty-two subjects completed the protocol; the ratings of 15 subjects (36%) decreased by at least 50% from baseline on the Hamilton Depression Rating Scale at the end of week 6. There was no significant difference ($P = .53$) between improved subjects receiving imipramine (N = 8 [47%] of 17) and placebo (N = 7 [28%] of 25).

Mean combined DMI level (205.06 ng/ml) plus 2-OH-DMI level (70.01 ng/ml) was 275.07 ng/ml. There was no significant correlation between DMI, 2-OH-DMI, or combined serum levels and treatment outcome; in fact the 17 subjects receiving DMI who did not improve had higher mean values of DMI, 2-OH-DMI, and combined serum levels than the 8 subjects who improved. The authors concluded that their data were consonant with other studies of tricyclic medication in depressed adolescents that did not show the significant treatment benefit seen in adults, but that did show a relatively high rate of significant and unpleasant untoward effects (Kutcher et al., 1994)

Desipramine in the Treatment of Enuresis. Rapoport et al. (1980b) found that 75 mg of desipramine at bedtime had a short-term antienuretic effect that was not statistically different from that of imipramine.

Desipramine in the Treatment of ADHD. Garfinkel et al. (1983) studied 12 males (mean age, 7.3 years; range, 5.9 to 11.6 years) who were diagnosed with attention deficit disorder and required day hospital or inpatient treatment for the severity of their symptoms of impulsiveness, inattention, and aggression. The subjects received placebo, methylphenidate, desipramine, and clomipramine in a double-blind crossover experiment. Mean dose of desipramine was 85 mg/day and did not exceed 100 mg/day or 3.5 mg/kg/day for any subject. Methylphenidate was significantly better than the other three conditions in improving overall classroom functioning as rated on the Conners Scale by teachers ($P < .005$) and program child care workers ($P < .001$).

In an open study, Gastfriend, Biederman, and Jellinek (1984) treated 12 adolescents, age range of 12 to 17 years, who were diagnosed with ADD with desipramine for 6 to 52 weeks. Eleven of them had previously responded poorly to stimulants or had intolerable untoward effects. Although these were outpatients, their symptoms were so severe that residential schooling or hospitalization had been considered for many of them. Desipramine was initiated with a dose of 10 or 25 mg/day and increased weekly to a maximum or 5 mg/kg or until an optimal clinical result was obtained or untoward effects prevented further increase. The mean daily dose after 4 weeks was 1.57 mg/kg (range, 0.58 to 2.63 mg/kg); 11 of the 12 patients improved, and 5 of them were rated "much" or "very much" improved on the Clinical Global Impressions scale. Ten patients were followed for 21 to 52 weeks; their optimal daily doses ranged from 0.93 mg/kg to 5.95 mg/kg. Nine of the 10 patients sustained their improvement for more than 6 months, and 8 of these were rated "much" or "very much" improved. Plasma levels for a given dose varied as much as 10-fold. Untoward effects were most troublesome during the first month; 6 patients (50%) experienced drowsiness, 3 (25%) postural dizziness, 3 (25%) weight loss and/or decreased appetite, 2 (16%) headache, 1 (8%) insomnia, and 1 (8%) racing thoughts. The untoward effects lessened in all cases following reduction in dosage.

Subsequently, in another open study, Biederman, Gastfriend, and Jellinek (1986) treated 18 children diagnosed with ADD with desipramine for 4 to 52 weeks. Initial dose was 10 or 25 mg of desipramine, and the dose was titrated weekly. Dose at time 4-weeks ranged from 0.7 to 4 mg/kg/day (mean 2.0 ± 0.9 mg/kg/day); at later follow-up, doses were significantly higher, ranging from 1.3 to 6.3 mg/kg/day. Improvement at follow-up time (mean time at follow-up,

22.9 ± 15.9 weeks) was also significantly greater than at time 4 weeks. Although there was sufficient time for tolerance to medication to have developed, it was not observed.

Biederman et al. (1989a, 1989b) reviewed earlier work in this area and studied the efficacy of desipramine in treating 42 children and 20 adolescents diagnosed with attention deficit disorder with hyperactivity (N = 60) or without hyperactivity (N = 2). Sixty-nine percent of their subjects had responded poorly to earlier treatment with stimulants. The subjects were randomly assigned to a 6-week, double-blind, parallel groups, placebo-controlled protocol. Desipramine was titrated upward to an average daily dose of 4.6 mg/kg ± 0.2 mg/kg, a relatively high dose. This high dose was selected because of inconsistent findings in studies using lower doses of desipramine in subjects with ADD (Biederman et al., 1989a). Patients treated with desipramine had statistically significant improvement in symptoms rated on the Conners Abbreviated Parent and Teacher Questionnaires, compared with subjects receiving placebo (P = .0001). The patterns of improvement were similar in adolescents and children. There was no significant relationship between serum desipramine levels and clinical response, making the designation of an optimal level inappropriate. Some subjects who improved had serum levels below 100 ng/ml. About one-fourth of the patients had high levels, between 300 and 900 ng/ml; of this group 80% (12 of 15) improved (Biederman et al., 1989b).

Untoward effects were usually mild and were more frequent in subjects receiving desipramine than in the placebo group (P < .05); overall, there was no discernible relationship between serum level and untoward effects. Symptoms included dry mouth (32%), decreased appetite (29%), headache (29%), abdominal discomfort (26%), tiredness (25%), dizziness (23%), and insomnia (23%). Although no subjects developed any clinically apparent cardiovascular signs or symptoms, cardiovascular and ECG untoward effects, such as increased diastolic blood pressure, tachycardia, and conduction abnormalities, were statistically more frequent in subjects receiving desipramine. There was a suggestion that ECG changes occurred more frequently at higher serum desipramine levels. Although side effects were rated as mild, the authors noted that in 71% of patients (22 of 31) receiving desipramine and 52% of patients (16 of 31) receiving placebo, untoward effects prevented the medication from being raised to the target dose of 5 mg/kg/day (Biederman et al., 1989b). Of special interest is that in contrast to reports of rapid improvement of subjects with ADD in response to imipramine, subjects in this study required 3 to 4 weeks to show significant clinical improvement with desipramine as compared to placebo (Biederman et al., 1989b).

Biederman et al. (1989b) suggested that a steady-state serum desipramine level between 100 ng/ml and a maximum of 300 ng/ml is probably efficacious and safe for most children and adolescents but that some patients will require daily doses greater than 3.5 mg/kg/day to reach these serum levels. They estimated that optimal doses range between 2.5 and 5 mg/kg/day. The authors (Biederman et al., 1989b) recommended that the following parameters are more clinically relevant in the titration of desipramine than accepting an arbitrary maximum limit in dose (e.g., 5 mg/kg):

1. The desipramine serum level should be kept under 300 ng/ml.
2. The P-R interval on the ECG should be less that 200 msec.
3. The QRS interval on the ECG should be less than 120 msec.

Desipramine shows some promise as an alternative medication for children and adolescents diagnosed with ADHD who have unsatisfactory responses to stimulant medication. Gualtieri and his colleagues (1991) reported that desipramine improved long-term memory performance, analogous to that reported with stimulants, when used in treating children diagnosed with ADHD. Its use requires strict clinical monitoring, including ECG and serum levels, because of its pharmacokinetics and cardiotoxicity.

Coadministration of Desipramine and Methylphenidate in the Treatment of ADHD with Symptoms of Major Depressive Disorder or Comorbid MDD. Rapport et al. (1993) studied the separate and combined effects of methylphenidate and desipramine on cognitive functions in 16 hospitalized children, aged 7 years 9 months to 12 years 10 months, diagnosed with ADHD and MDD, ADHD with symptoms of MDD, or MDD with symptoms of ADHD. Following a 2-week baseline period, subjects received placebo, desipramine, three dose levels of methylphenidate (10, 15, and 20 mg), and combined methylphenidate and desipramine at each of the methylphenidate levels. Desipramine was begun at 50 mg/day and increased by 25 mg every 2 days, unless untoward effects prevented the increase, until plasma levels between 125 and 225 mg/ml were reached, because prior studies had suggested this to be the range of maximum therapeutic efficacy in prepubertal children. Methylphenidate alone improved vigilance, both drugs had positive effects on short-term memory and visual problem solving, and the combination of both drugs affected learning of higher-order relationships. The effects of these drug conditions on mood and behavior were not reported. In a separate report concerning the same subjects, Pataki et al. (1993) detailed the untoward effects of methylphenidate and desipramine alone and in combination in a subset of 13 patients. The mean final dose of desipramine during combined administration with methylphenidate was 148 mg/day (range, 75 to 300 mg/day) or 4.4 mg/kg/day (range, 2.5 to 6.6 mg/kg/day); the mean plasma desipramine level during combined administration with methylphenidate was 170 ng/ml (range, <50 to 228 ng/ml for the 11 subjects for whom it was available). As methylphenidate is reported to inhibit hepatic enzymes that metabolize tricyclics, desipramine plasma levels alone and when coadministered with methylphenidate were compared. The mean final plasma level of desipramine when administered alone was 159 ng/ml, compared with a level of 170 ng/ml when administered in combination with methylphenidate and the difference in plasma levels was not significant. On individual bases, however, the most extreme variations were a subject who received 75 mg of desipramine daily (2.9 mg/kg/day) in combination with methylphenidate and had a plasma level of 158 ng/ml and a subject who received 300 mg of desipramine daily (6.6 mg/kg/day) that resulted in a plasma level of 146 ng/day.

Untoward effects were more frequent in the combined desipramine and methylphenidate treatment than in any of the other conditions: nausea (17% versus 8% in the 40 mg/day methylphenidate group), dry mouth (42% versus 8% in the 40 mg/day methylphenidate and the desipramine alone groups), and tremor (8% versus none in any other group). The combination of desipramine and methylphenidate resulted in an increase in ventricular heat rate that was significantly greater than the other conditions; however, this increase was not in a range that would place the children at clinical risk according to the pediatric cardiologist. Three children had sinus tachycardia on ECG: all three occurred during the combined drug treatment but were not thought to be of clinical significance by the pediatric cardiologist.

The authors concluded that, clinically, the untoward effects of combined desipramine and methylphenidate treatment were not significantly greater than those for desipramine alone; untoward effects were similar to those during administration of desipramine alone, and there was no evidence that the addition of methylphenidate increased DMI levels significantly (Pataki et al., 1993).

This is a very small number of patients, and much larger samples are needed before definitive conclusions may be reached.

Desipramine in Comorbid ADHD and Chronic Motor Tic Disorder or Tourette's Syndrome. Although stimulants are the treatment of choice in ADHD, they may exacerbate tics or precipitate them de novo. Hence problems arise when children have preexisting tic disorders, or when they develop tics while being treated with stimulants. Indeed, some authorities recommend not giving stimulants to children with a family history of tics or Tourette's disorder.

Riddle and his colleagues (1988) noted that Tourette's disorder and ADHD coexist in approximately 50% of children who are referred for evaluation of Tourette's disorder and that between 20% and 50% of such patients develop worsening of their tics if treated with stimulants. The authors treated with desipramine seven children, aged 7 years to 11 years, all of whom had diagnoses of ADHD and various tic disorders (one with Tourette's disorder, three with chronic multiple tics, and two with family histories of Tourette's disorder, four of whom had developed chronic tic symptoms when previously treated with methylphenidate); five of the children had an additional diagnosis of oppositional disorder. Desipramine was begun at 25 mg daily and increased by 25 mg every 2 to 3 days to a maximum of 100 mg, or a lower level when clinical improvement was satisfactory or untoward effects prevented further increase. Four children improved "remarkably" and one child "moderately" when rated on the Clinician's Global Improvement Scale; two children were considered nonresponders. Six children showed no change in the status or severity of their tics. One child's intermittent eye-blinking became persistent after 3 weeks of desipramine; this had also occurred in this patient during a previous trial of methylphenidate (Riddle et al., 1988).

In a retrospective study of 33 children and adolescents (age range, 5 to 17 years, mean 12.0 ± 0.6 years) diagnosed with chronic motor tic disorder or Tourette's syndrome, 30 of whom had comorbid ADHD, Spencer et al. (1993a) reported that 27 (82%) of the 33 had significant improvement ($P = .0001$) in their movement disorders and 24 (80%) of the 30 with ADHD had significant improvements ($P = .0001$) in their ADHD symptoms when treated with desipramine. The average dose of desipramine was 127 ± 9.8 mg/day or 3.5 ± 0.3 mg/kg/day. Mean serum desipramine level was 132 ± 16 ng/mg for the 22 patients for whom such values had been determined. Untoward effects rash (1) and abdominal pain (1) caused two patients to withdraw prematurely from the study precluding their inclusion in analysis of data. Four patients were discontinued during the study because of untoward effects: nausea and vomiting (1), irritability and agitation (2), and worsening of a tic (1). Eight subjects (24%) had asymptomatic cardiac abnormalities including new onset of incomplete right bundle branch block (4), junctional rhythms (2), benign ectopic atrial contractions on Holter monitor (1), and an increase in the QT_c interval (1). It is unclear why none of the subjects in the study of Riddle et al. (1988) had improvement in their tic disorders, whereas subjects in the 1993 study of Spencer et al. showed very significant improvement. Although further experience is necessary to establish that desipramine is both safe and efficacious in treating children and adolescents with coexisting ADHD and tic disorder, it appears to be a potentially useful alternative treatment for children whose ADHD is of sufficient severity to necessitate pharmacological intervention and for those diagnosed with ADHD who develop tics after the initiation of stimulant therapy.

CLOMIPRAMINE HYDROCHLORIDE (ANAFRANIL)

Clomipramine is an antiobsessional drug that belongs to the class of tricyclic antidepressants. Clomipramine itself has potent inhibitory effects on the neuronal reuptake of serotonin as compared to neuronal reuptake of norepinephrine; however, its primary metabolite, desmethylclomipramine, effectively inhibits norepinephrine uptake.

Flament and colleagues (1987) studied the actions of clomipramine on peripheral measures of serotonergic and noradrenergic function in children and adolescents diagnosed with obsessive-compulsive disorder. They compared 29 such children and adolescents (mean age, 13.9 ± 2.5 years; range, 8 to 18 years) with controls and found that a high pretreatment level of platelet serotonin was a strong predictor of a favorable clinical response and that clomipramine treatment produced a very marked decrease in platelet serotonin concentration for all patients ($P < .0001$). Clomipramine treatment also produced a trend toward reduction in platelet monoamine oxidase (MAO) activity ($P = .11$) and increased peripheral noradrenergic function. The plasma level of norepinephrine in standing subjects increased significantly ($P < .008$). These data suggest that clomipramine's inhibition of serotonin uptake may be essential to its antiobsessional effect (Flament et al., 1987).

Indications in Child and Adolescent Psychiatry
    Clomipramine has been approved by the FDA for the treatment of obsessions and compulsions in patients at least 10 years of age who have been diagnosed with obsessive-compulsive disorder.

Dosage Schedule for Children and Adolescents
• Children under age 10: Not recommended.

• Children at least 10 years old and adolescents to 17 years of age: Initial dose of 25 mg/day, titrated upward to a daily maximum of 100 mg or 3 mg/kg/day, whichever is less, over the first 2 weeks. Subsequently, dosage may be increased gradually to a maximum of 200 mg/day or 3 mg/kg/day, whichever is less. After the optimal dose has been determined, clomipramine may be given in a single bedtime dose to minimize daytime sedation.

• Adolescents at least 18 years old: As above, but the maximum dose may be increased to 250 mg/day.

• Abrupt withdrawal of clomipramine may result in withdrawal symptoms similar to those that occur when the tricyclics used in treating depression are suddenly discontinued. Symptoms may include dizziness, nausea, vomiting, headache, malaise, sleep disturbances, hyperthermia, irritability, and worsening of psychiatric status. Hence a gradual tapering of the dose over a period of 10 days to 2 weeks is recommended.

Dose Forms Available
• Capsules: 25 mg, 50 mg, 75 mg

Pharmacokinetics of Clomipramine

Clomipramine has a long half-life. The mean half-life of a single 150-mg dose is 32 hours, and the mean half-life of its major metabolite, desmethylclomipramine, is 69 hours. Steady-state serum levels usually occur within 1 to 2 weeks at a given daily dosage. Children and adolescents under 15 years of age had significantly lower plasma concentrations for a given dose than did adults (package insert). Dugas et al. (1980) reported that peak plasma clomipramine levels were achieved 3 to 4 hours after ingestion in the three children they studied and reported an apparent plasma terminal half-life of 11.9 to 17.3 hours. The bioavailability of clomipramine is not significantly affected by ingestion with food, and administering it during initial titration in divided doses with meals helps to reduce gastrointestinal side effects. Clomipramine is metabolized in large part into its major bioactive metabolite, desmethylclomipramine; both compounds are ultimately metabolized into their glucuronide conjugates by the liver. The metabolites are excreted through the bile duct and the kidneys.

Untoward Effects of Clomipramine

The most significant risk of clomipramine appears to be the development of seizures. Risk for seizures is cumulative and, for doses up to 300 mg/day, increased from 0.64% at 90 days to 1.45% at 1 year. Other untoward effects that occur in children and adolescents include somnolence, tremor, dizziness, headache, sleep disorders, increased sweating, gastrointestinal effects (dry mouth, constipation, and dyspepsia), anorexia, fatigue, cardiovascular effects (postural hypotension, palpitations, tachycardia, and syncope), abnormalities of vision, urinary retention, and dysmenorrhea in females and ejaculation failure in males (package insert). Because of reports of blood dyscrasias, a complete blood cell count should be determined in patients who develop fever and sore throat during the course of treatment.

Dugas and his colleagues (1980) reported in their study of 8 children and 28 adolescents administered clomipramine for enuresis or depressive symptomatology that the incidence of untoward effects was clearly related to the clomipramine plasma concentration. Untoward effects occurred in about 15% to 20% of patients with plasma clomipramine levels below 60 ng/ml and were present in more than 90% of cases with serum levels above 90 ng/ml. Hypotension occurred only in cases with serum levels above 80 ng/ml. No discernible relationship was found between untoward effects and plasma levels of desmethylclomipramine.

REPORTS OF INTEREST

Clomipramine in the Treatment of Obsessive-Compulsive Disorder in Children and Adolescents. There are few published studies on the use of clomipramine in children and adolescents diagnosed with obsessive-compulsive disorder. Those of Flament et al. (1985, 1987) and of Leonard et al. (1989) include some children below the age of 10 years and are summarized briefly below.

Clomipramine was found to be significantly superior to placebo in a placebo-controlled, double-blind, crossover study of 19 subjects whose ages ranged from 10 to 18 years (mean, 14.5 ± 2.3 years) who were diagnosed with severe primary obsessive-compulsive disorder (Flament et al., 1985). The dose range was 100 to 200 mg/day (mean, 141 ± 30 mg/day). The experimental data suggested that clomipramine has a direct antiobsessional action that is independent of any antidepressant effect. In fact, 10 of the subjects had been previously treated with other tricyclics without significant benefit. Flament et al. (1987) increased the number of their subjects to 29 (mean age, 13.9 ± 2.5 years; range, 8 to 18 years) and reported the continued efficacy of clomipramine; the mean daily dose of clomipramine was 134 ± 33 mg/day.

Leonard et al. (1989) compared the efficacy of clomipramine and desipramine in the treatment of severe primary obsessive-compulsive disorder in 49 child and adolescent subjects (31 males and 18 females) (mean age, 13.86 ± 2.87 years; range, 7 to 19 years) in a 10-week crossover design study. Administration of clomipramine was begun at 25 mg/day for children weighing 25 kg or less and at 50 mg/day for subjects weighing more than 25 kg. Dosage was increased weekly by an amount equal to each subject's initial dose. Maximum dosage did not exceed 250 mg/day or 5 mg/kg/day. The mean dose of clomipramine at week 5 was 150 ± 53 mg/day, with a range of 50 to 250 mg/day. Clomipramine was markedly superior to desipramine in decreasing obsessive-compulsive symptoms on several rating scales. In addition, 64% of patients who improved significantly when initially on clomipramine experienced relapse following the crossover to desipramine; this was a relapse rate similar to that for placebo in the above Flament (1985) study. The most common side effects reported were dry mouth, tremor, tiredness, dizziness, difficulty sleeping, sweating, constipation, poor appetite, and weakness.

Leonard et al. (1991) reported that, of the 48 children completing the above 1989 study, 28 (58%) were still receiving maintenance clomipramine 4 to 32 months later. Twenty-six of these patients agreed to participate in a 8-month double-blind study in which desipramine was substituted for clomipramine. At the time of entry to the protocol, subjects' daily doses of clomipramine ranged from 50 to 250 mg (mean dose, 134.7 ± 58.2 mg/day or 2.4 ± 0.6 mg/kg/day). Subjects continued to receive clomipramine at their maintenance level for 3 months, at which time desipramine was substituted for clomipramine for the next 2 months. For the final 3-month period, all subjects received clomipramine. Twenty subjects completed the study. Eight of 9 patients (89%) randomly assigned to desipramine relapsed during the 2-month period whereas only 2 (18%) of 11 patients remaining on clomipramine relapsed. The authors noted that the 8 patients who relapsed on desipramine experienced symptom improvement to previous levels within 1 month after clomipramine was reinstituted. This is clinically important because it suggests that a significant percentage of children and adolescents need long-term drug treatment to prevent recurrence of obsessive-compulsive symptoms; however, if relapse occurs when an attempt to discontinue clomipramine is made, comparable clinical control can usually be regained upon reinstating clomipramine.

DeVeaugh-Geiss et al. (1992) reported a multicenter trial in which 60 children and adolescents, aged 10 to 17 years, diagnosed with obsessive-compulsive disorder were administered clomipramine in a 10-week, double-blind, fully randomized, parallel groups, placebo-controlled study. Thirty-one patients were assigned to the clomipramine group and 29 to the placebo group; except for an excess of males in the clomipramine group, they were comparable. Placebo was administered to all patients under single-blind conditions for the first 2 weeks. During the active drug stage, the initial daily dose was 25 mg of active drug or placebo; over the next 2 weeks, this dose was titrated to either 75 mg or 100 mg daily based on weight. Subsequent increases to a maximum of 3 mg/kg/day or 200 mg were permitted at the discretion of the investigator. Twenty-seven subjects in each group completed the study. Untoward effects were typical of the tricyclic antidepressants. The patients receiving clomipramine improved significantly compared with those in the placebo group. On the Yale-Brown Obsessive Compulsive Scale (Y-BOCS) the clomipramine group had a mean reduction in score of 37% and the placebo group, a reduction of 8% ($P < .05$), and on the National Institute of Mental Health (NIMH) Global Scale the groups had reductions of 34% and 6%, respectively ($P < .05$).

Evidence at the present time suggests that clomipramine is the drug of choice for children and adolescents with severe obsessive-compulsive disorder, although it has not been approved by the FDA for advertising as effective and safe in treating children under 10 years of age.

Clomipramine in the Treatment of Attention-Deficit/Hyperactivity Disorder. Garfinkel and colleagues (1983) compared the clinical efficacy of methylphenidate, desipramine, and clomipramine in a double-blind, placebo-controlled, crossover study of 12 males (mean age, 7.3 years; range, 5.9 to 11.6 years) diagnosed with attention deficit disorder who required day hospital or inpatient treatment for severe impulsiveness, attention deficit, and aggression. The mean dose of clomipramine was 85 mg/day and did not exceed 100 mg or 3.5 mg/kg/day for any subject. Methylphenidate was significantly better than the other three conditions in improving overall classroom functioning as rated on the Conners Scale by teachers ($P < .005$) and program child care workers ($P < .001$). Clomipramine, however, was significantly better than desipramine in reducing scores reflecting aggressivity, impulsivity, and depressive/affective symptoms. Based on these data, clomipramine would merit further study in treating children and adolescents with ADHD who do not respond satisfactorily to stimulant medication.

Clomipramine in the Treatment of Autistic Disorder. Gordon et al. (1993) conducted a double-blind comparison of clomipramine, desipramine, and placebo in 30 subjects, 20 males and 10 females, age range of 6 to 23 years (mean, 10.4 ± 4.11 years), diagnosed with autistic disorder to assess the efficacy of clomipramine in treating obsessive-compulsive and stereotyped motor behaviors. During the initial 2-week, single-blind, placebo washout period, 2 patients were dropped, one because of positive response and the other because of a refusal to take pills. Fourteen subjects were randomly assigned to a 10-week, double-blind, crossover comparison of clomipramine and placebo and the other 14 subjects to a similar comparison of clomipramine and desipramine. Two patients were dropped from each group—a 23-year old man on placebo because of violent outbursts, a 7-year old girl on clomipramine secondary to a grand mal seizure, and two others for extraneous reasons. The 12 patients in the clomipramine/placebo comparison group showed significantly reduced autistic behaviors ($P = .0001$), anger/uncooperativeness ($P = .0001$), hyperactivity ($P = .001$), but not speech deviance ($P = .27$) in week-5 ratings on the 14-item Autism Relevant Subscale of the Children's Psychiatric Rating Scale (CPRS) while receiving clomipramine. These subjects also had a significant improvement in obsessive-compulsive symptoms ($P = .001$) and overall improvement on the Efficacy Index of the Clinical Global Impressions Scale (CGIS) ($P = .0001$) during the period on active drug. The 12 patients in the clomipramine/desipramine comparison group improved significantly more during the period on clomipramine than during the period on desipramine on week-5 ratings on the Autism Relevant Subscale of the CPRS ($P = .0003$) and anger/uncooperativeness ($P = .008$). The two drugs were not significantly different on the hyperactivity factor, but both were better than placebo; and clomipramine showed a trend toward improvement on the speech factor compared with desipramine ($P = .08$). Obsessive-compulsive symptoms improved significantly more with clomipramine ($P = .001$), and clomipramine was superior to desipramine on the Efficacy Index of the CGIS ($P = .005$). The authors noted that self-injurious behaviors (SIB) such as hitting, kicking, biting, and pinching, which were present in 4 patients and had not responded to intensive behavioral and drug interventions in 2 cases, improved significantly in all 4 subjects during the period when they were receiving clomipramine. Untoward effects of clomipramine were usually minor, and they were not significantly different from placebo or desipramine. However, dosage of clomipramine was reduced in 1 patient because of prolongation of QT_c interval to 0.45 seconds and in another because of severe tachycardia (Gordon et al., 1993).

Five patients who continued to be maintained on clomipramine underwent a double-blind placebo substitution for 8 weeks between months 5 and 12 of maintenance therapy. Four (80%) of the five worsened during the period on placebo but regained former clinical improvement when clomipramine was reinstated (Gordon et al., 1993).

Clomipramine in the Treatment of Enuresis. Dugas et al. (1980) administered clomipramine to 10 enuretic children. A therapeutic effect was observed at plasma clomipramine concentrations of 20 to 60 ng/ml, whereas lower and higher levels were associated with lack of therapeutic efficacy or untoward effects. In a later report the sample was increased to 31 enuretic children (Morselli et al., 1983). Of the 21 who had good therapeutic outcomes, 16 (76%) had plasma steady-state clomipramine concentrations greater than 15 ng/ml, whereas only 3 of the 10 nonresponders has plasma levels this high. The plasma level differences between the responders and the nonresponders was significant ($P < .05$).

Clomipramine in the Treatment of Depressive Symptoms. Dugas et al. (1980) treated 1 boy , 8.5 years old, and 25 adolescents, 13 to 19 years old, who had significant depressive symptomatology with clomipramine. Clomipramine doses ranged from 0.24 to 2.93 mg/kg/day. Sixteen patients received other psychoactive medication simultaneously. Twelve of the 26 patients responded positively. Final diagnoses of these patients were school phobia (3), anorexia nervosa (6), manic-depressive psychosis (1), depression (5), and depressive reactions in behavior disorders or borderline personalities (11). Two patients had no therapeutic response, 1 had a minimal response, 11 had moderate improvement, 3 had "good" results, and 9 had excellent results. The patients diagnosed with anorexia responded least favorably; only 2 had a good response, whereas 4 of the 5 diagnosed with depression had excellent responses. Similar plasma levels of clomipramine were present in both responders and nonresponders; however, nonresponders had proportionally higher levels of desmethylclomipramine.

Clomipramine in the Treatment of School Phobia (Separation Anxiety). Berney et al. (1981) treated 52 children diagnosed with school refusal, which consisted of a neurotic disorder with a marked reluctance to attend school for at least 4 weeks' duration and was frequently associated with depressive features. The study was double-blind and placebo controlled and lasted for 12 weeks. Forty-six patients, aged 9 to 14 years, completed the study; 19 were on placebo and 27 were on clomipramine. Clomipramine total daily dosage was titrated slowly to 40 mg/day for 9 and 10 year olds; 50 mg/day for 11 and 12 year olds; and 75 mg/day for 13 and 14 year olds. There was no evidence that clomipramine was superior to placebo in reducing separation anxiety and neurotic behavior or being specific for depression. The authors, however, noted that they used proportionally lower doses of clomipramine than the doses used in studies reporting its efficacy in treating school phobia/separation anxiety.

Selective Serotonin Reuptake Inhibitors

The selective serotonin reuptake inhibitors (SSRIs) currently approved by the FDA for the treatment of depression in adults include fluoxetine hydrochloride (Prozac), sertraline hydrochloride (Zoloft), and paroxetine hydrochloride (Paxil). Fluvoxamine maleate (Luvox), another SSRI, and fluoxetine have recently been approved for treating OCD in adults. These SSRIs are chemically unrelated to each other or to tricyclic or tetracyclic antidepressants, or to other antidepressants currently used in clinical practice (PDR, 1995). As the term SSRI suggests, at therapeutic levels, these drugs act primarily to inhibit serotonin reuptake; they also have relatively little effect on catecholaminergic (norepinephrine) reuptake mechanisms. At least five types and several subtypes of serotonin receptors with both distinct and overlapping functions have been identified in the central nervous system (Sussman, 1994a). These SSRIs have differing specificity in the serotonin receptors whose reuptake they inhibit, which explains their efficacy in treating disorders other than depression and the fact that they have somewhat different untoward effects. SSRI antidepressants also do not have clinically significant direct effects on the adrenergic, muscarinic, or histaminergic systems resulting in fewer and less severe untoward effects than the tricyclic antidepressants. The most common untoward effects of the SSRIs parallel the symptoms caused by administration of exogenous serotonin and include headache, nausea, vomiting, diarrhea, nervousness, sleep disturbance, and sexual dysfunction (Sussman, 1994a).

SSRIs are of great interest to child and adolescent psychiatrists for several reasons: (1) Only one double-blind placebo-controlled study conducted with prepubertal children and no such studies with adolescents have shown tricyclic antidepressants to be superior to placebo in treating MDD. In that study (Preskorn et al., 1987), however, subjects receiving imipramine had their dose of imipramine adjusted by laboratory personnel to achieve plasma levels within the therapeutic range. (2) There have been several reports of sudden death in children being treated with tricyclics, leading to particular concern about their cardiotoxicity in younger patients. SSRIs have a significantly safer untoward effect profile, including decreased lethality in overdose. (3) Although significant, the untoward effects of SSRIs are more tolerable than those of tricyclic and MAOI antidepressants. (4) SSRIs may be administered once daily. (5) SSRIs appear to have potential in treating a spectrum of childhood psychiatric disorders in addition to depression including obsessive compulsive disorder with and without comorbid Tourette's disorder, ADHD, anxiety disorder, selective mutism, and eating disorders.

Because sertraline and paroxetine were approved by the FDA more recently than fluoxetine, there is very little published data concerning their use in children and younger adolescents; therefore, these drugs will be noted only briefly. It is quite likely, however, that with additional clinical experience in this age group, the SSRIs will become the agents of choice in treating depression and obsessive-compulsive disorder in children and adolescents.

FLUOXETINE HYDROCHLORIDE (PROZAC)

Fluoxetine's effect is thought to be related to its specific and selective inhibition of serotonin reuptake by central nervous system neurons. This action appears to take place at the serotonin reuptake pump, not at a neurotransmitter receptor site, and fluoxetine appears to have no significant pharmacological effect on norepinephrine or dopamine uptake (Bergstrom et al., 1988)

Several studies, including some that were placebo controlled, have found fluoxetine's therapeutic efficacy to be comparable to that of the tricyclics (imipramine, amitriptyline, and doxepine) in treating adults with major depressive disorder (for reviews see Benfield et al., 1986; Lader, 1988). Fluoxetine has also been approved for treating obsessive-compulsive disorder.

Indications for Use in Child and Adolescent Psychiatry
Fluoxetine is approved for use in older adolescents and adults for the treatment of depression and obsessive-compulsive disorder.

Dosage Schedule for Children and Adolescents
• Children and younger adolescents: Not approved.
At the present time, the safety and efficacy of fluoxetine for children and younger adolescents remains to be elucidated. Although not approved by the FDA for administration to children and younger adolescents for any indication, studies including patients is this age range are appearing in the literature with increasing frequency. Riddle et al. (1992) noted that 20 mg/day may be too high a dose for some children and suggested that an initial dose of 10 mg/day of fluoxetine is the most common starting dose given to children by most clinicians. Boulos et al. (1992) found an initial dose of 20 mg of fluoxetine too often causes unacceptable untoward effects and suggested beginning with 5 mg to 10 mg weekly the first week; they noted that some of the subjects (ranging from 16 to 24 years of age) experienced good antidepressant response on doses as low as 5 to 10 mg daily. Gammon and Brown (1993) reported the optimal dose of fluoxetine to be between 2.5 and 7.5 mg/day in 22% (7 of 32) of their subjects who were receiving a combination of methylphenidate and fluoxetine.
• Older adolescents (at least 18 years old, i.e., adult dosage): An initial morning dose of 20 mg/day is recommended; there is evidence that this may frequently be the optimal dose (Altamura et al., 1988). Food does not seem to affect significantly the bioavailability of fluoxetine. The full antidepressant action may take 4 weeks or longer to develop. If adequate clinical response does not occur after several weeks, the dosage may be increased gradually to a maximum of 80 mg/day. It is recommended that once 20 mg/day is exceeded, the medication be taken in divided portions twice daily, in the morning and at noon. If significant untoward effects develop, the dose may be lowered to 20 mg every other day.

Dose Forms Available
• Pulvules: 10 mg, 20 mg
• Liquid: 20 mg/5 ml

Pharmacokinetics of Fluoxetine

Peak plasma levels of fluoxetine at usual clinical doses occur after 6 to 8 hours. Fluoxetine is metabolized by the liver; active and inactive metabolites are excreted by the kidneys. About 95% of fluoxetine is bound to plasma proteins. The elimination half-life after chronic administration is 4 to 6 days for fluoxetine and 4 to 16 days for norfluoxetine, its active metabolite. It may take up to several weeks for steady-state plasma levels to be achieved, but once obtained they remain steady (PDR, 1995).

Contraindications for Fluoxetine Administration

Known hypersensitivity to the drug is an absolute contraindication.

Fluoxetine should not be administered to any patient who has received an MAOI within the preceding 2 weeks. Because of the long half-lives of fluoxetine and its metabolites, an MAOI should not be administered sooner than 5 weeks (35 days) after discontinuing fluoxetine; the manufacturer notes that it may be advisable to wait even longer before giving an MAOI if fluoxetine has been prescribed chronically or at high doses (PDR, 1995). The drug should be administered with caution if impaired liver function is present.

Interactions of Fluoxetine with Other Drugs

The use of fluoxetine with other psychoactive drugs has not been systematically studied as yet.

Severe reactions may occur if an MAOI and fluoxetine are administered simultaneously or sufficient time has not elapsed after stopping either of these drugs before beginning the other.

When used with tricyclic antidepressants, their plasma levels may be significantly increased.

Agitation, restlessness, and gastrointestinal symptoms have occurred when used concurrently with tryptophan.

Diazepam clearance was significantly prolonged in some patients administered both drugs.

Untoward Effects of Fluoxetine

Wernicke (1985) and Cooper (1988) have reviewed the safety and untoward effects of fluoxetine. The most frequent troublesome untoward effects are nausea, weight loss, anxiety, nervousness, insomnia, and excessive sweating. They are reported more frequently, and anticholinergic effects and sedation less frequently, than with the tricyclic antidepressants.

Many of the untoward effects may be described as behavioral activation. Riddle et al. (1990/1991) reported the behavioral side effects of fluoxetine in 24 children and adolescents of various diagnoses, age range, 8 to 16 years. Mean dose was 25.8 ± 9.0 mg/day for the 12 subjects (including the ADHD children) who developed fluoxetine-induced behavioral side effects such as restlessness, hyperactivity, insomnia, an internal feeling of excitation, subtle impulsive behavioral changes, and suicidal ideation (Riddle et al. 1990/1991; King et al. 1991). Bangs et al. (1994) documented significant memory impairment in a 14-year-old who was receiving 20 mg/day of fluoxetine for treatment of major depressive disorder. Hypomania, mania, and transient psychosis have also been reported to occur in children and adolescents treated with fluoxetine (Hersh et al., 1991; Jafri, 1991; Jerome, 1991; Boulos et al., 1992; Rosenberg et al, 1992; Venkataraman et al., 1992).

Simeon et al. (1990) reported that their depressed subjects receiving fluoxetine experienced a small but significant weight loss compared with subjects receiving placebo. As many teenagers, especially females, refuse to take tricyclic antidepressants because of frequently associated weight gain, this could be a clinically advantageous characteristic of fluoxetine.

REPORTS OF INTEREST

Fluoxetine in the Treatment of Child and Adolescent Major Depressive Disorder.   Joshi and colleagues (1989) reported on their treatment with fluoxetine of 14 patients (8 males, 6 females) ranging in age from 9 to 15 years (average age, 11.25 years) who were diagnosed with major depression by DSM-III-R (APA, 1987) criteria and who had not responded adequately to tricyclic antidepressants, had serious untoward effects from tricyclics, or could not be treated with tricyclics for medical reasons. Ten (71.4%) of the subjects responded favorably within 6 weeks to fluoxetine 20 mg administered in the morning. Side effects were limited to transient nausea and hyperactivity in one patient each and did not require discontinuation of the drug.

Simeon et al. (1990) reported a 7-week, double-blind, placebo-controlled fluoxetine treatment study of 40 adolescents, 22 females and 18 males, aged 13 to 18 years (mean age, 16 years), who met DSM-III criteria for major depression unipolar type and had baseline Hamilton Depression Scores (HAM-D) of at least 20.   In addition, the HAM-D scores of all subjects improved less than 20% during a preceding 1-week, single-blind placebo treatment protocol. Fluoxetine was begun at 20 mg/day, increased to 40 mg/day after 4 to 7 days, and increased to 60 mg/day during the second week. Further dosage changes were individually titrated.

At baseline, no significant differences were found between the groups. Thirty subjects completed the study divided equally between medication and control groups. About two-thirds of patients in each group showed moderate to marked clinical global improvement with significant improvement by week 3. With the exception of disturbances of sleep, all symptoms showed slightly greater improvement in subjects treated with fluoxetine than in those receiving placebo, but differences were not significant. Patients taking fluoxetine, however, experienced a small but significantly greater weight loss than those receiving placebo. Untoward effects were usually mild and transient, and none necessitated discontinuation of medication. Those most frequently reported were headache, vomiting, insomnia, and tremor. There were no significant differences in the effects of fluoxetine and placebo on heart rate or blood pressure. Thirty-two patients were successfully followed up 8 to 46 months later (mean, 24 months) at ages 15 to 22 years (mean, 18 years). No significant differences were found between the fluoxetine and placebo groups, or between responders and nonresponders to the initial clinical trial. Both groups showed further overall improvement; however, psychosocial functioning was still poor in more than one-third of the patients, and 50% of the subject's parents felt their children still required professional help. The authors noted that 10 patients were still depressed and 7 of these were still in treatment. About half of patients who did not respond to placebo or fluoxetine during the initial 8 weeks of treatment were thought to constitute a very high risk group and remained very disturbed at follow-up (Simeon et al., 1990).

Boulos et al. (1992) treated, with fluoxetine, 15 adolescents and young adults diagnosed with major depressive disorder who had responded unsatisfactorily to prior treatment with antidepressants, usually including tricyclics, for a minimum of 2 months at doses associated with clinical efficacy. Seven subjects were 18 years old or younger. Eleven patients completed at least 6 weeks of treatment. Of these, 64% showed at least a 50% improvement on the Hamilton Depression Rating Scale, and 73% achieved scores of much or very much improved on the Clinical Global Impression Scale. Optimal doses ranged from 5 to 40 mg daily, and several patients received other medications concurrently. Untoward effects included headache, vomiting and other gastrointestinal complaints, insomnia, tremor, sweating, dry mouth, and hair loss.

Jain et al. (1992) conducted a retrospective chart review of 31 hospitalized subjects (age range, 9 to 18 years old) whose primary diagnosis was MDD (N = 27) or bipolar disorder (N = 4) and who were treated with fluoxetine. Twelve children were also diagnosed with a disruptive behavior disorder. The initial dose of fluoxetine was 20 mg/day. Nineteen patients (64%) continued at this dose for the duration of the hospitalization. The other subjects received maximum doses of 40 mg/day (8 patients, 25%), 60 mg/day (3 patients, 9%), and 80 mg/day (1 patient, 2%); no increased benefit was noted in patients receiving doses of more than 40 mg/day. After a mean treatment duration of 35 days, 74% of patients had improved ratings on the Clinical Global Impressions Scale; 54% were rated "much" or "very much" improved. The most common untoward effects included hypomanic symptoms, e.g., pervasive silliness, increased energy and activity, racing thoughts, insomnia, and socially intrusive or obnoxious behavior (23%), irritability (19%), insomnia, (13%) and gastrointestinal complaints (13%). All 4 bipolar patients developed hypomanic symptoms. Fluoxetine was discontinued in 8 (28%) of the patients, primarily because of increased irritability and hypomanic symptoms.

Fluoxetine in the Treatment of Children and Adolescents with Obsessive-Compulsive Disorder or Obsessive-Compulsive Disorder and Tourette's Disorder. In an open clinical study, Riddle et al. (1990) treated, with fluoxetine, 10 children (5 males, 5 females) ranging in age from 8 to 15 years (average age, 12.2 years) diagnosed with obsessive-compulsive disorder only or with both obsessive-compulsive disorder and Tourette's disorder. Dosage ranged from 10 to 40 mg/day, with 80% of the patients receiving 20 mg/day; duration of treatment ranged from 4 to 20 weeks. Four of the patients with Tourette's disorder received concomitantly additional medication for treatment of their tics. Fifty percent were considered responders to fluoxetine and were rated much improved; response rates were similar in patients with obsessive-compulsive disorder alone and in those with both diagnoses. The most common untoward effect was behavioral agitation/activation, characterized by increased motor activity and pressured speech. It occurred in 40% of the patients and usually started within the first few days; symptoms were most severe during the first 2 to 3 weeks but remained until medication was discontinued. No significant changes in blood pressure, pulse, weight, laboratory tests, or ECG were observed (Riddle et al., 1990).

Riddle and his colleagues (1992) reported a randomized, 20-week, double-blind, placebo-controlled, fixed-dose study with crossover after 8 weeks of fluoxetine in treating 14 subjects (6 males and 8 females; age range, 8.6 to 15.6 years; mean, 11.8 ± 2.3 years) diagnosed with obsessive-compulsive disorder by DSM-III-R criteria. Subjects received 20 mg of fluoxetine or placebo. For various reasons, 13 subjects completed the first 4 weeks, 11 subjects completed the first 8 weeks, and only 6 subjects satisfactorily completed the entire 20 weeks. A comparison of between-group differences at 8 weeks was made for 13 subjects; this number of subjects was made possible by carrying the 4-week data forward to 8 weeks for the 2 subjects who dropped out during that time. The 7 subjects receiving fluoxetine showed significant decreases on the Children's Yale-Brown Obsessive Compulsive Scale (CY-BOCS) total score (mean decrease, 44%;

P = .003), obsessions score (mean decrease, 54%; P = .009), and compulsions score (mean decrease, 33%; P = .005), and on the Clinical Global Impression for Obsessive Compulsive Disorder (CGI-OCD) (mean decrease, 33%, P = .0004). The 6 subjects on placebo also showed reduction in their obsessive-compulsive symptomatology on the CY-BOCS of 27% and on the CGI-OCD of 12%, but these reductions were not significant. When the two groups were compared, the improvement of subjects on fluoxetine was significantly greater than those on placebo on the CGI-OCD (P = .01) but not on the CY-BOCS (P = .17). The most frequently reported untoward effects were insomnia, fatigue, motoric activation, and nausea. Preexisting chronic motor tics worsened in two subjects; however, fluoxetine was continued and the tics subsided to negligible levels over the subsequent 2 years. A subject with comorbid diagnoses of MDD, separation anxiety, and oppositional disorder developed suicidal ideation, which resolved after fluoxetine was discontinued. The authors noted that 20 mg/day may be too high a dose for some children and that an initial dose of 10 mg/day of fluoxetine was the most common starting dose given to children by most child and adolescent psychiatrists.

Of the six subjects initially on fluoxetine who crossed over to placebo at 8 weeks, three dropped out at week 12 because of worsening of symptoms with a mean increase of 53% ± 37% in CY-BOCS scores; a fourth subject was worse at week 20 on the CY-BOCS, and the remaining two showed improvement (decrease) in their CY-BOCS scores. Although three of the four subjects who crossed over from placebo to fluoxetine had shown substantial reductions in their CY-BOCS scores during the placebo period, further reduction in these scores were present at 20 weeks. Overall, these results complement findings in adults and suggest that fluoxetine is both safe and effective in treating children and adolescents with obsessive-compulsive disorder for 20 weeks (Riddle et al., 1992).

Fluoxetine in the Treatment of Children and Adolescents with Anxiety Disorders.   Birmaher et al. (1994) treated with fluoxetine 21 patients (age range, 11 to 17 years; mean, 14 years) diagnosed with overanxious disorder (OAD) only (N = 6); OAD, social phobia, and separation anxiety disorder (SAD) (N = 5); or OAD and social phobia or SAD (N = 10), who had not responded to prior psychopharmacotherapy or psychotherapy. Subjects with a prior history of OCD, panic disorder, or current major depressive disorder were excluded. The mean fluoxetine dose after an average of 10 months (range, 1 to 31 months) on fluoxetine was 25.7 mg/day; the following distribution of doses was reported: 10 mg/day (1); 20 mg/day (15); 30 mg/day (1); 40 mg/day (2); 60 mg/day (2).

Twenty subjects (95%) showed some improvement in anxiety with 17 (81%) rated as moderately to markedly improved on the severity and improvement subscales of the Clinical Global Impression Scale (CGIS) ($P = .0001$). Importantly, in most cases, improvement did not begin until 6 to 8 weeks after initiation of fluoxetine. Although no subject fulfilled diagnostic criteria for MDD or dysthymia, 10 patients did have depressive symptoms. These symptoms also improved significantly ($P = .0001$); analysis suggested the improvements in depressive symptoms and anxiety were independent. Only a few untoward effects, which were usually mild and transient, were reported: mild headache (1), nausea (3), insomnia (1), and stomachaches (1). No significant changes in pulse, blood pressure, or ECG were found, and no subject experienced agitation, manic, or hypomanic symptoms or suicidal ideation. These data suggest that fluoxetine may be a useful treatment for children and adolescents with anxiety disorders (Birmaher et al., 1994).

Fluoxetine in the Treatment of Children and Adolescents with Attention-Deficit/Hyperactivity Disorder.   Barrickman et al. (1991) reported on 19 children and adolescents (age range, 7 to 15 years) diagnosed with ADHD who were treated for 6 weeks in an open study with fluoxetine hydrochloride. Fourteen subjects had comorbid diagnoses of either conduct disorder (N = 6) or oppositional defiant disorder (N = 8). Most subjects had prior psychopharmacologic treatment that was unsatisfactory or had untoward effects on stimulants (e.g., tics) or antidepressants (e.g., sedation). Initial daily dose was 20 mg in the morning; subsequent doses were individually adjusted. Average daily dose was 27 mg (0.6 mg/kg); range, 20 to 60 mg. Nine subjects took 20 mg/day; 8 took 40 mg/day, and 2 took 60 mg/day. Most subjects improved within 1 week after a therapeutic dose was reached. Ratings were made on a large number of standardized instruments. Eleven subjects (58%) were rated moderately or very much improved after 6 weeks; 8 had minimal improvement. Side effects were minimal and all remitted spontaneously or with dose reduction except mild sedation in one case. In particular, there were no reports of loss of appetite or significant changes in weight. Only 1 subject experienced nervousness and none had insomnia or developed suicidal ideation.

All three children diagnosed with ADHD showed worsening of ADHD symptoms on fluoxetine in the Riddle et al. (1990/1991) study of behavioral side effects of fluoxetine discussed above.

Gammon and Brown (1993) reported the use of fluoxetine augmentation of methylphenidate in an 8-week open trial with 32 patients, 9 to 17 years old, who were diagnosed with ADHD and one or more comorbid disorders, i.e., dysthymia (78%), oppositional defiant disorder (59%), major depressive disorder (18%), anxiety disorders (18%), and conduct disorder (13%), and who had inadequate therapeutic responses to methylphenidate alone. Addition of fluoxetine was begun with an initial dose of 2.5 mg/day or 5.0 mg/day for subjects under 12 years of age and 12 years of age or older, respectively. Dose was titrated upward every 3 to 4 days in increments equal to the initial dose, to a maximum of 20 mg/day. Optimal daily dose of fluoxetine at 8 weeks ranged from 2.5 to 20 mg. The majority of subjects (19 or 59%) required 20 mg/day, 6 subjects (18%) received 10 to 15 mg/day, 4 subjects 5 to 7.5 mg/day, and 3 subjects (9%) had optimal fluoxetine doses of 2.5 mg/day. No significant or lasting untoward effects were reported.

After 8 weeks of combined drug treatment, all 32 subjects showed statistically significant improvements on assessments rating attention, behavior, and affect; these improvements were also rated clinically significant in 94% (30) of the subjects. Scores on the Children's Global Assessment Scale dramatically improved ($P < .0001$). Mean scores on the Children's Depression Inventory declined from 22, which is in the clinical range for depressive symptoms, to 8, which is below that range ($P < .0001$). On the Conners Parents Rating Scale, group means improved on all 6 scales; on 5 scales improvement was significant ($P < .001$ to $P < .0001$). There was also a marked jump in student grade point average within one marking period. Parents reported substantial improvement in hyperactivity, impulsivity, anxiety, conduct, and learning problems. Augmentation with fluoxetine also produced significant further improvement in sustaining attention and concentration and helped to alleviate symptoms of anxiety, depression, irritability, and oppositionalism that had not responded adequately to methylphenidate alone. More seriously affected children showed the most significant improvements (Gammon & Brown, 1993).

Fluoxetine in the Treatment of Children Diagnosed with Elective Mutism.   Black and Uhde (1994) treated 15 subjects, age range of 6 to 11 years, who were diagnosed with elective mutism with fluoxetine in a double-blind 12-week study. During a single-blind, 2-week placebo period preceding the study, a 16th subject who responded to placebo was dropped. Three boys and three girls, mean age of 9.1 ± 2.3 years, were randomly assigned to fluoxetine. Three boys and 6 girls, mean age of 8.1 ± 1.6 years, were assigned to placebo. Fluoxetine was given at a dose of 0.2 mg/kg/day for the 1st week, increased to 0.4 mg/kg for the 2nd week, and further increased to 0.6 mg/kg for the final 10 weeks of the study. The mean maximum dose of fluoxetine was 0.60 to 0.62 mg/kg/day or 21.4 mg/day (range, 12–27 mg/day). The fluoxetine group improved more than the placebo group on 28 or 29 rating scales, but most of the differences were not significant. Both groups showed significant improvement from baseline over time in elective mutism, anxiety, and social anxiety as rated by parents, teachers, and clinicians. The fluoxetine group improved significantly more than the placebo group on parents', but not on teachers' or clinicians', ratings of mutism and clinical global improvement. This was consistent with earlier findings that children with elective mutism show improvements in the home setting before school and clinic settings. The authors noted that, although statistically significant, the improvements were modest and that the subjects continued to show serious impairments in their functioning. Untoward effects were minimal (Black & Uhde, 1994).

SERTRALINE HYDROCHLORIDE (ZOLOFT)

Sertraline hydrochloride is approved by the FDA for the treatment of depression. Safety and efficacy have not been established for its use in children.

Dosage Schedule for Children and Younger Adolescents
Not established.

Dosage Schedule for Older Adolescents and Adults
An initial daily dose of 50 mg given either in the morning or at night is recommended. Full antidepressant response may be delayed for up to several weeks in some patients. Some patients may benefit from increases to a maximum of 200 mg/day. Dose changes should be at least a week apart because of sertraline's 24-hour elimination half-life.

Dose Forms Available
• Tablets (scored): 50 mg, 100 mg

PAROXETINE HYDROCHLORIDE (PAXIL)

Paroxetine hydrochloride is approved by the FDA for the treatment of depression. Safety and efficacy have not been established for its use in children.

Dosage Schedule for Children and Younger Adolescents
Not established.

Dosage Schedule for Older Adolescents and Adults
The recommended initial daily dose is 20 mg, usually administered in the morning. Full antidepressant response may be delayed for up to several weeks. Some patients may benefit from higher doses, and paroxetine may be titrated upward with weekly increases of 10 mg recommended (package insert).

Dose Forms Available
• Tablets (scored): 20 mg, 30 mg

FLUVOXAMINE MALEATE (LUVOX)

Fluvoxamine maleate is an SSRI that belongs to a new chemical series, the 2-aminoethyl oxime ethers of aralkylketones. In in vitro studies, the drug exhibited no significant affinity for histaminergic, α- or β-adrenergic, muscarinic, or dopamine receptors (package insert).

Indications for Use in Child and Adolescent Psychiatry
Fluvoxamine is approved only for the treatment of obsessions and compulsions in adults diagnosed with obsessive-compulsive disorder. Its safety and efficacy have not been established in individuals less than 18 years old.

Dosage Schedule for Children and Adolescents
• Children and younger adolescents: Not approved.
• Older adolescents (at least 18 years old, i.e., adult dosage): An initial bedtime dose of 50 mg is recommended. The dose may be titrated upward as clinically indicated in 50-mg increments to a maximum of 300 mg to achieve maximal therapeutic response. Daily doses totaling more than 100 mg should be given in two doses; if the two doses are unequal, the larger dose should be taken at bedtime. Usual optimal doses range from 100 to 300 mg.

Dose Forms Available
• Tablets (scored): 50 mg, 100 mg

Pharmacokinetics of Fluvoxamine

Food does not significantly affect the bioavailability of fluvoxamine. In volunteers, peak plasma concentrations at steady state occurred between 3 and 8 hours after ingestion of the drug and revealed nonlinear pharmacokinetics for single doses of 100, 200, and 300 mg with higher doses resulting in disproportionately higher plasma levels, e.g., plasma levels of 88, 283, and 546 ng/ml, respectively. The mean plasma half-life at steady state for young adults taking 100 mg/day was 15.6 hours (package insert).

Contraindications for Fluvoxamine Administration

Known hypersensitivity to fluvoxamine is a contraindication. Coadministration of terfenadine or astemizole with fluvoxamine is contraindicated.

Interactions of Fluvoxamine with Other Drugs

Because of the potential of serious interaction with monoamine oxidase inhibitors (MAOIs), fluvoxamine should not be administered concomitantly for at least 2 weeks after an MAOI has been discontinued. Conversely, an MAOI should not be administered until at least 2 weeks after fluvoxamine has been discontinued. Benzodiazepines should be used with great caution, and coadministration of diazepam is not recommended. Many other potential interactions, particularly with drugs that inhibit or are metabolized by cytochrome P_{450} isoenzymes, have been reported (package insert).

Untoward Effects of Fluvoxamine

The most frequently reported untoward effects were somnolence, insomnia, dry mouth, nervousness, tremor, nausea, dyspepsia, anorexia, vomiting, abnormal ejaculation, asthenia, and sweating.

REPORT OF INTEREST

Apter et al. (1994) reported treating 20 adolescent inpatients, aged 13 to 18 years, who were diagnosed with major depressive disorder (MDD) (N = 6) or obsessive-compulsive disorder (OCD) (N = 14) with fluvoxamine in an 8-week, open-label protocol. Inclusion criteria for the 6 depressed patients included lack of response to a tricyclic antidepressant, additional symptoms of suicidality, impulsivity or affective instability, or a comorbid major psychiatric diagnosis. Four had comorbid diagnoses of both borderline personality and conduct disorders; 1 had comorbid bulimia, and the sixth was diagnosed with MDD only. Eleven of the 14 patients with OCD also had comorbid diagnoses: Tourette's syndrome (TS) (4), schizophrenia (4), and anorexia nervosa (3). All 8 subjects diagnosed with comorbid TS or schizophrenia also received haloperidol, and 3 of them additionally received benzhexol, an anticholinergic drug. Fluvoxamine was increased by 50 mg weekly until either a therapeutic result was obtained or untoward effects prevented further increase. Doses ranged from 100 to 300 mg/day (mean, 200 mg/day). Sixteen patients completed the study, and 4 dropped out because of untoward effects; for the latter 4 patients, the last ratings while on medication were used in analyzing the data.

All six patients with MDD improved significantly on the Beck Depression Inventory ($P < .0002$), but only 2 of the 4 patients with comorbid MDD and borderline personality disorder showed clinically significant decreases in impulsivity and suicidality. As a group, the 14 patients with OCD improved significantly on the Yale-Brown Obsessive Compulsive Scale (Y-BOCS) ($P < .0001$); however, 1 of the 3 patients with comorbid anorexia nervosa developed confusion and delirium and another developed hallucinations; both were dropped from the study at week 6. Of note, statistically significant improvement over baseline ratings on the Y-BOCS did not occur until week 6, and there was further improvement at week 8.

All subjects developed at least some mild untoward effects compared with baseline ratings on the Dosage Record Treatment Emergent Symptom Scale (DOTES). Fluvoxamine, like other SSRIs, initially caused some activating untoward effects such as insomnia, hyperactivity, agitation, excitement, anxiety, and hypomania. These were mild and transient in most cases; however, one patient with a family history of bipolar disorder who developed hypomania was dropped during the 5th week. Nausea, tremor, and dermatitis occurred in about 75% of subjects; in one case the drug had to be discontinued because of itchy maculopapular dermatitis. No changes in heart rate, blood pressure, ECG, or routine laboratory tests were reported. No patient showed a significant increase in ratings on the Suicide Potential or Overt Aggression Scales (Apter et al., 1994).

Other Antidepressants

TRAZODONE HYDROCHLORIDE (DESYREL)

Trazodone hydrochloride is chemically unrelated to tricyclic, tetracyclic, and other currently approved antidepressant agents. Although it is a serotonin reuptake inhibitor, it is unlike the SSRIs in that its metabolites have significant effects on other neurotransmitter systems and their receptors (Cioli et al., 1984). It is approved for the treatment of patients diagnosed with major depressive episode, both with and without prominent symptoms of anxiety. Although trazodone's antidepressant activity is not fully understood, in animals it selectively inhibits serotonin reuptake in the brain and potentiates behavioral changes induced by 5-hydroxytryptophan.

Pharmacokinetics of Trazodone. It is recommended that trazodone be ingested soon after eating. When taken in this manner, up to 20% more drug may be absorbed than when taken on an empty stomach, and maximum serum concentration is achieved more slowly (in about 2 hours rather than 1 hour) and with a lesser peak. This appears to diminish the likelihood of developing dizziness and/or lightheadedness.

Trazodone is eliminated through the liver (about 20% biliary) and the kidneys (about 75%). Elimination is biphasic: the initial half-life is between 3 and 6 hours, which is followed by a second phase with a half-life of between 5 and 9 hours.

Contraindications for Trazodone Administration. Known hypersensitivity to the drug is a contraindication.

Interactions of Trazodone with Other Drugs. Increased phenytoin levels have been reported when administered concomitantly with trazodone.

Because of lack of experience, trazodone should not be administered with MAOIs because the effects of their interaction are unknown.

Untoward Effects of Trazodone. The most common side effects include drowsiness, dizziness or lightheadedness, dry mouth, and nausea or vomiting.

Priapism, which has necessitated surgical intervention and resulted in some cases of permanent impairment of sexual functioning, has been reported (incidence, about 1:15,000). Male patients with a prolonged or inappropriate erection should be informed to immediately discontinue trazodone and contact their physician or, if it persists, to go to an emergency room.

Indications for Use in Child and Adolescent Psychiatry
  Trazodone is approved only for the treatment of major depressive disorder in individuals at least 18 years old.
  The drug is not recommended for use in the pediatric age group because its safety and effectiveness have not been established for this age range.

Dosage Schedule for Children and Adolescents
  USPDI (1992) reports the following pediatric doses guidelines when trazodone is used as an antidepressant:
• Children under 6 years old: Dosage not determined.
• Children 6 to 18 years old: Begin with 1.5 to 2 mg/kg/day in divided doses. Titrate dosage gradually at 3- to 4-day intervals to a maximum of 6 mg/kg/day.

Dose Forms Available
• Tablets: 50 mg scored, 100 mg scored
• Divided dose tablets: 150 mg and 300 mg (both tablets scored to divide into 3 equal parts)

REPORTS OF INTEREST

Trazodone in the Treatment of Children and Adolescents with Significant Aggressivity. Fras (1987) reported successfully treating a 15-year-old male hospitalized for recurrent violence with a daily dose of 200 mg of trazodone. Because of a misunderstanding, following discharge the dose was significantly decreased and at times omitted altogether. Repeated angry outbursts and threats of violence developed within 1 week and the patient became morose. Upon resumption of a daily dose of 200 mg, the patient returned to the previous stability and cooperativeness and remained so for 8 months of follow-up.

Zubieta and Alessi (1992) reported an open study of 22 inpatients (18 males and 4 females; age range, 5 to 12 years; mean age, 9 ± 2 years) with severe, treatment-refractory, behavioral disturbances. They were diagnosed with disruptive behavioral and mood disorders often with comorbidity. Six of the children continued to receive neuroleptic drugs for psychotic symptoms during the trial of trazodone. An initial dose of 50 mg of trazodone at bedtime was begun an average of 23 ± 20 days after admission. It was titrated over a period of about 1 week to the maximum dose tolerated and given three times daily. The 13 children designated as responders received a mean dose of 185 ± 117 mg/day (4.8 ± 1.7 mg/kg/day) of trazodone for a mean of 27 ± 13 days. The 7 nonresponders received a mean dose of 158 ± 70 mg/day (4.7 ± 2.0 mg/kg/day) for a mean of 24 ± 11 days. One patient was dropped from the study for severe orthostatic hypotension and a second for reported painful erections (not priapism). The other children tolerated any untoward effects that occurred. The most frequent was orthostatic hypotension (50%), but this effect diminished over a few days and did not require clinical intervention; 27% of children reported drowsiness; 9%, nervousness; and 9%, anger. Dizziness, increased fatigue, and nocturnal enuresis each occurred in one child (4.5%).

Target symptoms that improved most frequently were impulsivity, hyperactivity, "involvement in dangerous activities," cruelty to people, frequency of physical fights, arguing with adults, and losing one's temper. Symptom improvement usually occurred within a few days of the initial administration of trazodone as contrasted to the several weeks of continuous administration typically required for its antidepressant effects to occur. In a telephone follow-up 3 to 14 months later (mean, 8.8 ± 4.2 months), 9 of the 13 responders were successfully contacted. Eight of the children continued to receive a mean trazodone dose of 241 ± 128 mg/day (range, 100–800 mg/day). Trazodone was the only medication being taken at follow-up, the neuroleptics that 3 children were taking at discharge having been withdrawn within 2 months after discharge. The 9th child had an unsatisfactory response and his medication was changed to a combination of carbamazepine and pemoline. Overall, parents rated their children's improvement at 70 ± 20 (range, 50–90) on a subjective overall rating of efficacy scale ranging from 0 to 100 (Zubieta & Alessi, 1992). Trazodone appears to be a potentially useful drug in treating acute and chronic behavioral disorders that have not responded to other treatments and merits further investigation.

Ghaziuddin and Alessi (1992) noted the relationship of the expression of aggression and decreased levels of serotonin in the central nervous system and the successful use of trazodone to control aggressive behavior in adults with organic mental disorders. They administered trazodone to three boys who were 7, 8, and 9 years old with primary diagnoses of severe disruptive behavioral disorders; two of the boys were hospitalized. Trazodone was initiated at doses of 25 mg once or twice daily and increased gradually. Improvement of symptoms was noted within 7 to 10 days at a mean dose of 3.5 mg/kg/day of trazodone (about 75 mg/day). In all three cases, marked deterioration of behavior occurred upon discontinuing the medication and aggressiveness decreased to former treatment levels once medication was resumed. One boy had no reported untoward effects; one experienced mild sedation during the first week, but this remitted with no change in dosage. The third experienced spontaneous erections on 100 mg/day; because of concerns about reported priapism, dosage was reduced to 75 mg daily and behavioral control deteriorated. When 1000 mg daily of L-tryptophan (which has been subsequently withdrawn from the commercial market) was added, behavior markedly improved again. No ECG changes were noted in any of the boys. The authors note that further studies will be needed to determine the efficacy and safety of trazodone in treating aggressive children.

BUPROPION HYDROCHLORIDE (WELLBUTRIN)

Bupropion hydrochloride is an antidepressant of the aminoketone class. It is not related chemically to the tricyclics, tetracyclics, or other known antidepressants. It has been approved by the FDA for treating depression in individuals at least 18 years of age.

Indications in Child and Adolescent Psychiatry
• Children and Adolescents under age 18: Not approved for any use.
• Adolescents at least 18 years of age: Used to treat depression, especially major depressive disorder.

(continues)

(continued)

Dosage Schedule for Children and Adolescents
- Children and adolescents under 18 years of age: Not recommended.
- Adolescents at least 18 years of age: An initial dosage of 100 mg twice daily is suggested. Based on clinical response, this may be increased to 100 mg three times daily but not before day 4 of treatment. If no clinical improvement occurs within 4 weeks, dosage may gradually be increased. Because of increased risk of seizure, a dose of 150 mg should not be exceeded within a 4-hour time period. The maximum daily dosage should not exceed 450 mg.

Dose Forms Available
- Tablets: 75 mg, 100 mg

Contraindications for Bupropion Hydrochloride Administration

Known hypersensitivity to bupropion hydrochloride and seizure disorders are contraindications.

A current or prior diagnosis of bulimia or anorexia nervosa is also a contraindication because a higher incidence of seizures is reported when bupropion is administered to such patients.

Bupropion should not be administered concurrently with an MAOI. At least a 14-day period off MAOIs should precede initiation of treatment with bupropion hydrochloride.

Concurrent administration with any drug that reduces the seizure threshold is a relative contraindication.

Interactions of Bupropion Hydrochloride with Other Drugs

There are relatively few data available on this subject. Increased adverse experiences were reported when the drug was administered concomitantly with L-dopa. MAOIs may increase the acute toxicity of bupropion.

Untoward Effects of Bupropion Hydrochloride

Of particular clinical concern is the finding that seizures have been associated with about 4 (0.4%) of 1000 patients treated with bupropion at doses of 450 mg/day or less. This is about fourfold the incidence of seizures reported with other approved antidepressants, and the incidence of seizures increases with higher daily doses. Conversely, Clay et al. (1988) note that bupropion's positive effects on memory performance may be unique among antidepressants and that other antidepressants either have no effect or a negative effect on memory performance.

The most common untoward effects were reported to be agitation, dry mouth, insomnia, headache, nausea, vomiting, constipation, and tremor.

Ferguson and Simeon (1984) reported no adverse (or positive) effects on cognition on a cognitive battery in 17 children with attention deficit disorder or conduct disorders who were treated in an open trial with bupropion.

REPORTS OF INTEREST

Bupropion Hydrochloride in the Treatment of ADHD.

Simeon et al. (1986) treated 17 male subjects (age range, 7 to 13.4 years; mean, 10.4 years) with bupropion in a 14-week, single-blind, uncontrolled study. Fourteen subjects were diagnosed with ADDH; of these, 8 were additionally diagnosed with conduct disorder, undersocialized aggressive type, and 2 with overanxious disorder. Eleven of the subjects had prior drug treatment; of these, 8 had shown no improvement. Four weeks of placebo were followed by 8-weeks of bupropion and then 2 weeks of placebo. The initial dose of bupropion was 50 mg/day; this was increased to 50 mg twice daily during the 2nd week and to a maximum of 50 mg three times daily during the 3rd week. No subjects responded to the baseline placebo. On drug, 5 patients showed marked improvement, 7 moderate improvement, and 2 mild improvement on Clinical Global Improvement scale ratings. Significant improvements also occurred on the Children's Psychiatric Rating Scale (CPRS), Conners Parents and Teachers scales, and self-ratings. Although not significant, group means for all 9 cognitive test variables showed improvement. Optimal dose was 150 mg/day in 15 cases and 100 mg/day and 50 mg/day in the other 2 subjects. Untoward effects were reported to be infrequent, mild, and transient.

Clay et al. (1988) reported that bupropion hydrochloride was safe and efficacious in treating prepubertal children diagnosed with ADHD. The authors' clinical impression was that children with additional prominent symptoms of conduct disorder responded particularly well to bupropion.

Thirty prepubertal children diagnosed with ADHD were enrolled in a double-blind placebo-controlled study and individually titrated to optimal doses of bupropion (Clay et al., 1988). Optimal doses ranged from 100 to 250 mg/day (3.1 to 7.1 mg/kg/day; mean, 5.3 ± 1 mg/kg/day). Subjects receiving bupropion showed statistically significant improvement on the Clinical Global Impressions Improvement and Severity Rating scales, the Self-Rating Scale, and on digit symbol and delayed recall on the Selective Reminding Test. Improvement that did not reach significance was also reported on the Conners Parent Questionnaire and the Conners Teacher Questionnaire. The only serious side effect noted was an allergic rash in two children. Clay et al. (1988) also noted that some children who had previously not responded satisfactorily to stimulants had a good response to bupropion. On the other hand, some subjects who had never received stimulants and who did not respond well to bupropion responded well when methylphenidate was openly prescribed at a later time.

Casat et al. (1989) administered bupropion to 20 children and placebo to 10 children in a parallel-groups design, double-blind comparison study. All subjects were diagnosed with attention deficit disorder with hyperactivity. Decreases in symptom severity and overall clinical improvement were noted in physician ratings, and hyperactivity in the classroom settings was significantly decreased on the Conners Teachers Questionnaire.

Although confirmation of these findings is needed, bupropion may be an alternative treatment for ADHD that does not respond to standard therapies.

Bupropion in the Treatment of Comorbid ADHD and Chronic Motor Tic Disorder or Tourette's Syndrome. Spencer et al. (1993b) reported that bupropion exacerbated tics in four children with ADHD and comorbid Tourette's syndrome (TS). All four patients had been initially treated with stimulants during which time two patients with preexisting symptoms of ADHD and TS experienced worsening of their tics and the other two developed tics and TS. Bupropion was subsequently prescribed as a possibly effective alternative treatment for children diagnosed with ADHD who did not respond satisfactorily to stimulants or could not tolerate their untoward effects. All four children experienced an exacerbation of tics over a period ranging from almost immediately to 2 months. The tics rapidly improved to pretreatment levels when bupropion was discontinued. The authors suggest that bupropion may not be a useful alternative to stimulants in treating patients with comorbid ADHD and TS.

Monoamine Oxidase Inhibitors

There are two forms of monoamine oxidase (MAO), which are distinguished by their substrate specificity. Type A MAO deaminates or deactivates norepinephrine, serotonin, and normetanephrine; and Type B MAO deaminates dopamine and phenylethylamine (Zametkin & Rapoport, 1987).

Monoamine oxidase inhibitors (MAOIs) are primarily used in treating adults with depressive disorders that are unresponsive to antidepressant drugs of other classes. MAOIs presently FDA-approved and marketed in the United States include phenelzine sulfate (Nardil), which has been approved for use only in individuals at least 16 years of age, and tranylcypromine sulfate (Parnate), which has been approved only for adults.

MAOIs that have been used in children and adolescents include clorgyline (a selective MAO-A inhibitor), tranylcypromine sulfate and phenelzine sulfate (mixed MAO-A and MAO-B inhibitors), and L-deprenyl or selegiline hydrochloride (Eldepryl) (a selective central MAO-B inhibitor). Because of the potentially very serious drug interactions and untoward effects of MAOIs, their use in children and adolescents is not usually recommended, and only a few reports in this age group will be reviewed.

SPECIAL CONSIDERATIONS IN USING MAOIS

It is critical to have a minimum of a 2-week washout period after stopping an MAOI and beginning a tricyclic or when changing from one MAOI to another MAOI. It is also contraindicated to add a tricyclic antidepressant when an MAOI is already being used, although the reverse has been done; that is, an MAOI can be added to an ongoing treatment regimen to augment a tricyclic that has been only partially effective (Ryan et al., 1988b). If patients are on MAOIs and will be in areas that are not rapidly accessible to medical treatment, they may be given several 25-mg chlorpromazine tablets to take should they accidentally ingest tyramine and become symptomatic (Ryan et al., 1988b). Pare et al. (1982) suggested that a combination of tricyclics and MAOIs might provide a relative protection against tyramine-induced hypertension, or "cheese effect," which may occur with dietary indiscretions while taking MAOIs; however, this is not common practice at the present time.

CONTRAINDICATIONS FOR MONOAMINE OXIDASE
INHIBITOR ADMINISTRATION

Known hypersensitivity to a monoamine oxidase inhibitor, pheochromocytoma, congestive heart failure, liver disease, or abnormal liver function are contraindications.

MAOIs must not be prescribed if a tricyclic antidepressant (however, see Ryan et al., 1988b, for a different opinion), another MAOI, or buspirone hydrochloride has been taken within the preceding 2 weeks.

Other contraindications usually found more frequently in older patients also exist. In addition, the patient must not be unreliable or be unable to keep to a strict diet, i.e., avoiding foods with high tyramine or dopamine concentrations.

INTERACTIONS OF MAOIS WITH OTHER DRUGS

Ingestion of tyramine can cause a hypertensive crisis. Hence foods rich in tyramine, such as cheese, wine, beer, yeast derivatives, some beans, and others, must be avoided.

Concomitant use with tricyclic antidepressants should be avoided because hypertensive crises or severe seizures have been reported with such combinations (see Ryan et al., 1988b, for a different opinion).

Use with sympathomimetic drugs such as amphetamines, methylphenidate, cocaine, dopamine, caffeine, epinephrine, norepinephrine, and related compounds may cause a hypertensive crisis. Other drug interactions occur as well.

UNTOWARD EFFECTS OF MAOIS

MAOIs may cause significant orthostatic hypotension, dizziness, headache, sleep disturbances, sedation, fatigue, weakness, hyperreflexia, dry mouth, and gastrointestinal disturbances; other untoward effects occur as well.

REPORTS OF INTEREST

MAOIs in the Treatment of Adolescent Depression

Ryan and his colleagues (1988b) reported an open clinical trial of tranylcypromine sulfate and phenelzine sulfate, both alone and in combination with a tricyclic antidepressant, in which 23 adolescents diagnosed with major depressive disorder who had responded inadequately to tricyclic antidepressants were treated with these MAOIs. Seventy-four percent (17) had a fair to good antidepressant response; however, because of dietary noncompliance the MAOI was discontinued in 4 subjects and only 57% (13) of the subjects continued on the medication. The authors concluded that MAOIs appeared to be useful in treating some adolescents with major depression that has not responded satisfactorily to tricyclic antidepressants. During the study a total of 7 (30%) had purposeful or accidental dietary noncompliance, and the authors emphasized that only very reliable adolescents are suitable for treatment with MAOIs (Ryan et al., 1988b).

MAOIs in the Treatment of Attention-Deficit/Hyperactivity Disorder

Zametkin et al. (1985) conducted a double-blind crossover study of 14 boys (mean age, 9.2 ± 1.5 years) who were diagnosed with attention deficit disorder with hyperactivity. The authors compared dextroamphetamine with either clorgyline, a selective MAO-A inhibitor (6 subjects), or tranylcypramine sulfate, a mixed MAO-A and MAO-B inhibitor (8 subjects). Both MAOIs had immediate, clinically significant effects (in contrast to delayed effects when used as an antidepressant), which were clinically indistinguishable from those of dextroamphetamine.

Zametkin and Rapoport (1987) reported that M. Donnelly had administered 15 mg/day of L-deprenyl, a selective MAO-B inhibitor, to 14 hyperactive children with relatively little therapeutic effect. The authors suggested that the reason a type A MAOI and a mixed MAOI showed therapeutic efficacy in children with ADHD, but a type B MAOI did not, supported the hypothesis that dysregulation of the noradrenergic system is important in the etiology of ADHD (Zametkin & Rapoport, 1987).

At the present time, the use of MAOIs in the treatment of ADHD is not recommended because of necessary dietary constraints.

6

Lithium Carbonate

Introduction

At the present time, lithium carbonate is approved by the FDA only for the treatment of manic episodes of bipolar disorders and for maintenance therapy of bipolar patients with a history of mania; the drug is approved only for persons 12 years of age and older. Over the past 2 decades, however, lithium carbonate has been investigated in the treatment of many child and adolescent disorders, but especially in the treatment of children with severe aggression directed toward self or others, children with bipolar or similar disorders, and behaviorally disturbed children whose parents are known lithium responders. One major impetus for this research is that antipsychotic agents, which are frequently used to control severe behavioral disorders and sometimes mania, may cause cognitive dulling when used in sufficient dosage to control symptoms and carry significant risk of causing tardive dyskinesia when used on a long-term basis (Platt et al., 1984).

Pharmacokinetics of Lithium Carbonate

The lithium ion is readily absorbed from the gastrointestinal tract and is most commonly administered in the form of lithium carbonate (Li_2CO_3), a highly soluble salt. Peak plasma concentrations occur within 2 to 4 hours, and complete absorption takes place within about 8 hours (Baldessarini, 1990). About 95% of a single dose of lithium is excreted by the kidneys with up to two-thirds of an acute dose being excreted within 6 to 12 hours. The serum half-life is approximately 20 to 24 hours. Depletion of the sodium ion causes a clinically significant degree of lithium retention by the kidneys.

Steady-state serum lithium levels typically occur within 5 to 8 days following repeated identical daily doses of lithium carbonate. Although lithium pharmacokinetics differ considerably among individuals, they are fairly stable over time for a given person (Baldessarini & Stephens, 1970).

Vitiello et al. (1988) studied the pharmacokinetics of lithium carbonate in 9 children aged 9 to 12 years. The children had a trend toward a shorter elimination half-life of lithium and a significantly higher total renal clearance of lithium. The clinical significance of this rate is that a steady state of lithium serum levels is reached more rapidly in children than in adults, and therapeutic levels can be achieved more quickly.

Contraindications for Lithium Carbonate Administration

Administration of lithium carbonate is relatively contraindicated in individuals with significant renal or cardiovascular disease, severe debilitation, severe dehydration, or sodium depletion, because these conditions are associated with a very high risk of lithium toxicity. Patients with such disorders should be thoroughly assessed, usually in consultation with the person providing medical care, prior to beginning lithium therapy.

Adolescents who may purposely or accidentally become pregnant should not be administered lithium, particularly in early pregnancy, except under urgent circumstances. Lithium carbonate is associated with a significant increase in cardiac teratogenicity and especially with Ebstein's anomaly. A significantly increased incidence of other cardiac anomalies has also been reported. Kallen and Tandberg (1983) reported that 7% of the infants of women who used lithium in early pregnancy had serious heart defects other than Ebstein's anomaly.

Significant thyroid disease is a relative contraindication to lithium carbonate therapy; however, with careful monitoring of thyroid function and the use of supplemental thyroid preparations when necessary, it may be used when other drugs are not effective and the potential benefits outweigh the risks.

Interactions of Lithium Carbonate with Other Drugs

There are several reports that increased neuroleptic toxicity with an encephalopathic syndrome or neuroleptic malignant syndrome may occur when lithium and neuroleptics are used concomitantly, but this has usually been seen with high doses. The simultaneous use of lithium and neuroleptic agents, however, may be indicated in some cases of mania or schizoaffective psychoses, and many patients have received both a neuroleptic and lithium with no untoward effects.

Elevations in lithium serum concentration and increased risk of neurotoxic lithium effects may occur when carbamazepine and lithium are used simultaneously, because carbamazepine decreases lithium renal clearance.

Many other drugs may potentially increase or decrease serum lithium levels by influencing its absorption or excretion by the kidneys; for example, tetracyclines increase lithium levels.

Lithium Toxicity

One major difficulty associated with the administration of lithium carbonate is its low therapeutic index; lithium toxicity is closely related to serum levels and may occur at doses close to therapeutic levels. Untoward or side effects are those unwanted symptoms that occur at therapeutic serum lithium levels, whereas toxic effects occur when serum lithium levels exceed therapeutic levels.

Lithium toxicity may be heralded by diarrhea, vomiting, mild ataxia, coarse tremor, muscular weakness and fasciculations (twitches), drowsiness, sedation, slurred speech, and impaired coordination. Patients and/or their caretakers must be made familiar with the symptoms of early lithium toxicity and instructed to discontinue lithium immediately and contact their physician if such signs occur. Increasingly severe and life-threatening toxic effects, including cardiac arrhythmias and severe central nervous system difficulties such as impaired consciousness, confusion, stupor, seizures, coma, and death, may occur with further elevations in serum lithium levels.

No specific treatment for lithium toxicity is available. If signs of early lithium toxicity appear, the drug should be withheld, lithium levels determined, and the medication resumed at a lower dosage only after 24 to 48 hours. Severe lithium toxicity is life threatening and requires hospital admission, treatments to reduce the concentration of the lithium ion, and supportive measures.

Lithium's low therapeutic index and its pharmacokinetics make it necessary to administer lithium carbonate tablets or immediate release capsules in divided doses, usually three or four times daily, to maintain therapeutic serum levels without toxicity. Even controlled-release tablets must be administered every 12 hours. It is essential that a laboratory capable of determining serum lithium levels rapidly and accurately be readily available to the clinician. For accuracy and serial comparisons, determinations of serum lithium levels should be made when lithium concentrations are relatively stable, and at the same time each day. Typically, blood is drawn 12 hours after the last dose of lithium and immediately before the morning dose.

Lithium saliva levels have also been used to monitor lithium levels in children, which avoids the necessity of repeated venipunctures, an upsetting experience for some children and adolescents. Perry et al. (1984) reported that saliva lithium levels in 15 children diagnosed with undersocialized aggressive conduct disorder averaged about 2.5 times higher than serum lithium levels, with saliva/serum ratios for individual children ranging from 1.56 to 3.99. Weller et al. (1987) found that saliva lithium levels were about 1.82 times serum levels in 14 prepubertal children receiving lithium for treatment of bipolar disorder. Saliva/serum lithium ratios in these children ranged from 1.50 to 2.32. Vitiello et al. (1988) reported saliva lithium levels to be 2.84 times those of serum lithium levels in 9 children, 6 of whom were diagnosed with conduct disorder and 3 of whom were diagnosed with adjustment disorders. Saliva/serum lithium ratios in these children ranged from 2.08 to 3.88. Bernstein (1988) found that in adults the ratio of saliva lithium levels to serum lithium levels varied from 1:1 to as high as 3:1. Despite the rather marked interindividual variability in the saliva/serum ratio, it appears to be relatively constant for a given individual. Therefore, to be clinically useful, a stable saliva/serum lithium level ratio must be calculated for each patient.

Although some patients who are unusually sensitive to lithium may exhibit toxic effects at serum levels below 1 mEq/l, for most patients, mild-to-moderate toxic effects occur at serum levels between 1.5 and 2 mEq/l, and moderate-to-severe reactions occur at levels of 2 mEq/l and above. Younger subjects may be at greater risk than adults for developing untoward effects at lower serum lithium levels. Many untoward effects have been reported to occur in children at serum levels well below 1 mEq/l (Campbell et al., 1984a). The most common side effects of lithium carbonate in 36 children, aged 3 years to 13 years and diagnosed with conduct disorder (N = 24), infantile autism (N = 8), or other (N = 4) were weight gain in 44.4%, excessive sedation in 27.8%, decreased motor activity in 25%, and stomachache, vomiting, tremor, and/or irritability in 19.4% of patients (Campbell et al., 1984a).

Lithium decreases sodium reuptake by the renal tubules; hence adequate sodium intake must be maintained. This is especially important if there is significant sodium loss during illness (e.g., sweating, vomiting, or diarrhea) or because of changes in diet or elimination of electrolytes. The importance of adequate ingestion of ordinary table salt and fluids should be emphasized. Caution during hot weather or vigorous exertion has been advised, because additional salt loss and concomitant dehydration secondary to pronounced diaphoresis may cause the serum lithium levels of patients on maintenance lithium to increase and move into the toxic range. This may also be true of sweating caused by elevated body temperature secondary to infection or heat without exercise (e.g., sauna), but some evidence suggests that heavy sweating caused by exercise may result in lowered rather than elevated serum lithium levels. Jefferson et al. (1982) studied four healthy athletes who were stabilized on lithium for 1 week prior to running a 20-km race. At the end of the race, the subjects were dehydrated but their serum lithium levels had decreased by 20%. The authors found that the sweat-to-serum ratio for the lithium ion was about four times greater than that for the sodium ion. These authors concluded that strenuous exercise with extensive perspiration was more likely to decrease rather than increase serum lithium levels, and patients were more likely to require either no change or an increase, rather than a decrease, in dosage of lithium to maintain therapeutic levels. The authors do caution, however, that any conditions that significantly alter fluid and electrolyte balance, including strenuous exercise with heavy sweating, should be carefully monitored with serum lithium levels.

Untoward Effects of Lithium Carbonate

Lithium carbonate is frequently reported to have untoward effects early in the course of treatment. Most of these diminish or disappear during the first weeks of treatment.

These early untoward effects include fine tremor (unresponsive to antiparkinsonism drugs), polydipsia, and polyuria that may occur during initial treatment and persist or be variably present throughout treatment. Nausea and malaise or general discomfort may initially occur but usually subside with ongoing treatment. Weight gain, headache, and other gastrointestinal complaints such as diarrhea may also occur. Taking the lithium with meals or after meals or increasing the dosage more gradually may be helpful in controlling gastrointestinal symptoms.

Later untoward effects are often related to serum level, including levels in the therapeutic range; these include continued hand tremor that may worsen, polydipsia, polyuria, weight gain and edema, thyroid and renal abnormalities, dermatological abnormalities including acne, fatigue, leukocytosis, and other symptoms. As serum levels increase, toxicity increases and other, more severe untoward effects, discussed above under toxicity, appear.

Abnormalities in renal functioning (diminution of renal concentrating ability) and morphological structure (glomerular and interstitial fibrosis and nephron atrophy) have been reported in adults on long-term lithium maintenance. Occasional proteinuria was reported in a 14-year-old girl (Lena et al., 1978). Vetro et al. (1985) reported that after 1 year of lithium treatment, one child developed polyuria with daytime enuresis and impaired renal concentration. Other parameters of renal function did not change, and polyuria ceased within a few days after lithium was discontinued. Five other children on long-term lithium therapy showed transient albuminuria that remitted spontaneously, and discontinuation of treatment was not necessary (Vetro et al., 1985).

Lithium also may interfere with thyroid function, with decreased circulating thyroid hormones and increased thyroid-stimulating hormone. Vetro et al. (1985) reported that two children developed goiter with normal function after 1.5 to 2 years of lithium therapy.

Neuroleptic malignant syndrome has been reported in patients who were administered neuroleptic drugs and lithium simultaneously.

Dostal (1972) reported specific untoward effects of lithium in 14 retarded adolescent males that interfered with patient management, despite significant therapeutic gains. Polydipsia, polyuria, and nocturnal enuresis were so severe as to alienate staff who cared for the youngsters. These symptoms remitted within 2 weeks after discontinuing lithium (Dostal, 1972).

Premedication Work-Up and Periodic Monitoring for Lithium Treatment

ROUTINE LABORATORY TESTS

Complete Blood Cell Count with Differential

Lithium frequently causes a clinically insignificant and reversible elevation of white blood cells, with counts commonly between 10,000 and

15,000 cells/mm[3]. The lithium-induced leukocytosis characteristically shows neutrophilia (increased polymorphonuclear leukocytes) and lymphocytopenia (Reisberg & Gershon, 1979). This leukocytosis can usually be differentiated from one caused by infection, because the increase in neutrophils is in more mature forms, whereas in infection younger forms predominate. Lithium may also increase platelet counts.

Serum Electrolytes

Serum electrolyte levels should be determined in particular to verify that sodium ion levels are normal, because hyponatremia decreases lithium excretion by the renal tubules.

Pregnancy Test

Lithium crosses the placenta, and data from birth registries suggest teratogenicity with increased abnormalities, including cardiac malformations, especially Ebstein's anomaly. Lithium is relatively contraindicated during pregnancy but especially during the first trimester. Infants born to mothers taking lithium appear to be at increased risk for hypotonia, lethargy, cyanosis, and ECG changes (United States Pharmacopeial Dispensing Information [USPDI}, 1990). All females who could be pregnant should be tested prior to initiation of lithium therapy and warned that, because of lithium's teratogenic potential for the fetus, they should take care not to become pregnant while taking the medication.

Renal Function Tests

Baseline assessment of renal functioning is essential, because the kidney is the primary route of elimination of lithium. For healthy children and adolescents, a baseline serum creatinine, blood urea nitrogen (BUN) level, and urinalysis are usually adequate (Jefferson et al., 1987). If kidney disease is suspected or abnormalities are found, a more thorough evaluation including tests such as urinalysis (including specific gravity), 24-hour urine volume, and 24-hour urine for creatinine clearance and protein should be performed and the patient referred to a renal consultant if necessary.

Thyroid Function Tests

Lithium causes thyroid abnormalities primarily by decreasing the release of thyroid hormones. This causes such findings as euthyroid goiter; hypothyroidism; decreased triiodothyronine (T_3), thyroxine

(T_4), and protein-bound iodine (PBI) levels; and elevated ^{131}I and thyroid-stimulating hormone (TSH) levels in between 5% and 15% of patients receiving long-term lithium therapy (Jefferson et al., 1987). Hypothyroidism resulting from lithium treatment is thought to be related to preexisting Hashimoto's thyroiditis, suggesting that determining antithyroid antibodies as part of the work-up may be useful (Rosse et al., 1989). Recommended baseline studies include thyroxine (T_4), triiodothyronine resin uptake (T_3RU), and TSH levels.

Cardiovascular Function Tests

Various cardiac conduction and repolarization abnormalities, (e.g., bradycardia) and reversible ECG abnormalities have been reported in a large percentage of adults receiving lithium. ECG changes commonly include benign, reversible T wave changes (flattening, isoelectricity, and inversion of T waves), which are dose dependent, and an increase in the P-Q interval (Jefferson et al., 1987). It has been hypothesized that lithium's cardiotoxic effects result from its displacing and substituting for intracellular potassium. A baseline ECG should be obtained routinely in patients over age 40 or those who have any history or clinical suggestions of cardiovascular disease. Although not considered mandatory in young, healthy patients, a baseline ECG is justifiable and useful to have for comparison should cardiovascular abnormalities develop at some later time. If patients have or develop cardiac abnormalities, frequent ECG monitoring should be done and the advice of a cardiac consultant sought. In other patients it is prudent to repeat the ECG at the time of scheduled routine physical examinations.

Calcium Metabolism Tests

Lithium may increase renal calcium reabsorption, resulting in hypocalcuria (Jefferson et al., 1987). Lithium may also cause hyperparathyroidism with hypercalcemia and hypophosphatemia, with resulting decreased bone formation or density in children. If abnormal results occur, parathyroid hormone (parathormone) levels may be determined. Lithium may also replace calcium in bone formation, especially in immature bones (USPDI, 1990). A baseline calcium level should be determined in children and adolescents, but a baseline parathormone level is not usually recommended.

Electroencephalogram

Bennett el al. (1983) reported that optimal doses of lithium caused worsening of conduct-disordered children's EEGs in statistically significant numbers. Paroxysmal and focal EEG abnormalities, in particular, were increased over pretreatment EEGs. EEG worsening, however, did not correlate with clinical symptoms of toxicity, and children receiving lithium showed significantly more behavioral improvement than those receiving placebo. Although an EEG is not required as a baseline work-up for normal healthy youngsters, if EEG abnormalities or a seizure disorder is known to exist, a baseline EEG should be obtained and the EEG periodically monitored. Lithium levels should be determined the morning that the EEG is performed, to facilitate correlation of EEG changes and serum lithium levels.

PERIODIC MONITORING

Because there is little information on the long-term effects of lithium on the development and maturation of children and adolescents, periodic monitoring of thyroid, kidney, and cardiac functioning is particularly important. It is recommended that TSH, BUN, and serum creatinine levels be determined at approximately 6-month intervals. When there is a concern about renal function, 24-hour urine volume, creatinine clearance, and protein excretion should also be determined. If a suggestion of thyroid abnormality arises, T_3 and T_4 levels should also be determined (Rosse et al., 1989).

LITHIUM CARBONATE (ESKALITH, LITHANE, LITHOBID); LITHIUM CITRATE SYRUP (CIBALITH-S)

Indications in Child and Adolescent Psychiatry
   Lithium carbonate is FDA approved for the treatment of manic episodes of manic-depressive illness and maintenance therapy of manic-depressive patients with a history of mania who are at least 12 years of age. Significant normalization of manic symptomatology may require up to 3 weeks of lithium carbonate therapy; hence concomitant use of antipsychotic medication may be initially required for more rapid control of manic symptoms.

Dosage Schedule for Treating Acute Mania and Maintenance Therapy
• Children under 12 year old: Not approved for use (see below under "Reports of Interest").
• Persons 12 years of age and older: Dosage must be individually regulated according to clinical response and serum lithium levels. As noted above, the pharmacokinetics of lithium carbonate make it necessary to administer the total daily dose in smaller doses administered three or four times daily if immediate-release tablets or syrup is used, or twice daily if controlled release capsules are used, to minimize risk of reaching toxic serum levels of lithium. (More detailed information on administering, titrating, and monitoring lithium in children and adolescents is found below.)

(continues)

(continued)

Dose Forms Available
• Tablets: 300 mg
• Capsules: 300 mg
• Controlled-release tablets: 300 mg, 450 mg
• Syrup (lithium citrate): 8 mEq/5 ml (equivalent to one 300-mg tablet)

Titration of Lithium Dosage

Schou (1969) noted that early untoward effects, such as nausea, diarrhea, muscle weakness, thirst, urinary frequency, hand tremor, and a dazed feeling, may be caused by a too rapid rise in serum lithium levels. Lithium is also a gastric irritant. A low initial dose of lithium taken after meals, which slows absorption, and gradual increases in dose will often avert the development of these symptoms. When they develop, they usually subside spontaneously within a few days.

Serum lithium levels should be monitored twice weekly during the acute manic phase and until both serum level and clinical condition have stabilized. In the maintenance phase of therapy during remission, serum lithium levels and thyroid, kidney, and cardiac functions should be periodically monitored. The National Institute of Mental Health/National Institutes of Health (NIMH/NIH) Consensus Development Panel (1985) recommends that serum lithium levels be determined at intervals of 1 to 3 months and that TSH and serum creatinine values be determined every 6 to 12 months. Because there is less experience in long-term administration of lithium carbonate to children and adolescents than to adults, the author recommends monitoring at the shorter recommended intervals—that is, determining the lithium level at least bimonthly and TSH and serum creatinine levels every 6 months.

Typically, doses of approximately 1800 mg/day will achieve the serum lithium levels of between 1 and 1.5 mEq/l necessary to control symptoms during acute mania. During long-term maintenance serum lithium levels usually range between 0.6 and 1.2 mEq/l; this usually requires a divided daily dose of between 900 mg and 1200 mg (PDR, 1995). Berg et al. (1974), however, reported that a 14-year-old girl and her father, who were both diagnosed with bipolar manic-depressive disorder, required daily doses of lithium as high as 2400 mg to achieve therapeutic levels.

Kutcher et al. (1990) reported differences in lithium responsiveness in adolescents with bipolar disorder only and with comorbid personality disorder. When assessed during a period of relative euthymia following discharge from an inpatient unit, 35% (N = 7) of 20 adolescents (mean age, 17.5 years) diagnosed with bipolar disorder and having had at least one manic and one depressive episode were diagnosed with at least one comorbid personality disorder. None of the subjects diagnosed with comorbid personality disorder improved on lithium, whereas 6 of the 13 subjects with bipolar disorder only improved on lithium ($P = .05$).

The NIMH/NIH Consensus Development Panel (1985) notes that criteria for prophylactic use of lithium in children and adolescents do not yet exist, and thus the preventive use of lithium must be based on clinical judgment. The risks versus the benefits for this age range are not yet firmly established, although available data suggest the potential problems are similar to those encountered in adults (NIMH/NIH, 1985).

Use of Lithium Carbonate in Children under 12 Years Old

The therapeutic dosages of lithium carbonate used in treating children over 5 years of age with various disorders do not differ significantly from those used in treating older adolescents and adults, and the principles of administration are essentially the same (Campbell et al., 1984a). This higher dose per body weight ratio may reflect the fact that higher renal lithium clearance may occur in children and adolescents compared with adults.

Weller et al. (1986) published a guide for determining the initial total daily lithium dose for prepubertal children 6 to 12 years of age. The guide and summary of how it is used are presented in Table 6.1. Lower initial doses should be used for children diagnosed with mental retardation or organicity (central nervous system damage) (E. B. Weller, personal communication, 1990).

The purpose of this guide is to reach therapeutic serum lithium levels (0.6 to 1.2 mEq/l) as rapidly as possible using currently available tablet strengths without undue risk of reaching toxic serum levels. The authors administered lithium to 10 subjects diagnosed with manic-depressive illness and 5 subjects diagnosed with conduct disorder, following these guidelines. Thirteen of the 15 subjects had serum lithium levels in the therapeutic range after only 5 days of treatment. Side effects were reported to be minimal, primarily mild nausea, abdominal pain, polydipsia and polyuria, and increase in preexisting enuresis. Most were transient and none required discontinuation of lithium. As discussed above, some untoward effects of lithium appear to be related to too rapid increases in serum lithium level. It remains to be determined whether the use of the

Table 6.1.
Lithium Carbonate Dosage Guide for Prepubertal School-Aged Children[a,b,c]

| | Dosage (mg) | | |
Weight (kg)	8 AM	12 Noon	6 PM	Total Daily Dose
<25	150	150	300	600
25–40	300	300	300	900
40–50	300	300	600	1200
50–60	600	300	600	1500

aFrom Weller EB, Weller RA, Fristad MA. Lithium dosage guide for prepubertal children: A preliminary report. J Am Acad Child Psychiatry 1986;25;92–95.
bDose specified in schedule should be maintained at least 5 days with serum lithium levels drawn every other day 12 hours after ingestion of the last lithium dose until two consecutive levels appear in the therapeutic range (0.6–1.2 mEq/l). Dose may then be adjusted based on serum level, side effects, or clinical response. Do not exceed 1.4 mEq/l serum level.
cLower initial dose should be used for children diagnosed with mental retardation or organicity.

proposed lithium dosage guide will cause significantly more untoward effects or will increase their severity more than would a more gradual titration of lithium. In cases where very rapid control of symptoms is critical, however, it may be prove to be especially useful.

REPORTS OF INTEREST

Lithium Carbonate in the Treatment of Mood Disorders (Mania, Bipolar Disorder), Behavioral Disorders with Mood Swings, and/or Patients Whose Parent(s) Are Lithium Responders. DeLong and Aldershof (1987) reported successful treatment with lithium carbonate of 66% of 59 children diagnosed with bipolar affective disorder, 82% of 11 children with emotionally unstable character disorder; and 71% of 7 offspring of a lithium-responsive parent.

Varanka et al. (1988) treated with lithium carbonate 10 prepubertal children (9 males, 1 female) (mean age, 9 years 6 months ± 2 years; range, 6 years 9 months to 12 years 7 months). All 10 children were diagnosed with manic episode with psychotic features. Doses ranged from 1150 to 1800 mg/day (32 to 63 mg/kg/day). Therapeutic lithium levels of 0.6 to 1.4 mEq/l were reached in all cases within 3 to 5 days. Substantial improvement was observed in all of the children an average of 11 days (range, 3 to 24 days) after therapy was begun. All psychotic symptoms remitted, and mood normalized. The children became less irritable and destructive; their thought processes, motor activity, and attention spans improved remarkably. Untoward effects such as fatigue, diminished appetite, abdominal discomfort, nausea, urinary frequency, and tremor were infrequent and so mild that they did not necessitate discontinuation of lithium.

Carlson et al. (1992) reported data on 11 hospitalized children (age range, 5 years 11 months to 12 years) whom the authors thought were likely to be lithium responders. Diagnoses and symptomatology varied but included bipolar disorder (2), manic episode (3), bipolar not otherwise specified (4); disruptive behavior disorders (9), exhibited psychotic symptoms (7), and multiple placements in the seclusion room for explosive behaviors (6). Four subjects had first-degree relatives with histories of bipolar illness. Seven of the subjects participated in a double-blind, placebo-controlled protocol, whereas the other 4 received lithium on an open basis. Lithium dosage ranged from 600 to 1500 mg/day resulting in serum lithium levels ranging between 0.7 and 1.1 mEq/l. In general, positive clinical responses increased with time, and improvements in self-control, aggression, and anxiety/agitation were greater at 8 weeks than at 4 weeks in all subjects. These improvements, however, could not be distinguished from the effects of a longer time in the hospital, because the 7 children in the double-blind crossover study maintained their gains on placebo. Only 3 subjects improved sufficiently on lithium to be discharged on that drug. Three patients diagnosed with bipolar disorder or bipolar disorder NOS and one diagnosed with major depressive disorder did not have adequate therapeutic responses to lithium; however, they improved and were discharged when given an open trial of desipramine. There was no evidence that lithium caused worsening or improvement in attention, cognitive functioning, or learning performance on several rating scales (Carlson et al., 1992).

Lithium Carbonate in the Treatment of Disorders with Severe Aggression, Especially when Accompanied by Explosive Affect, Including Self-Injurious Behavior. In a double-blind placebo-controlled study of 61 treatment-resistant hospitalized children with undersocialized aggressive conduct disorder, both haloperidol and lithium were found to be superior to placebo in ameliorating behavioral symptoms (Campbell et al., 1984b). Optimal doses of lithium carbonate ranged from 500 to 2000 mg/day (mean, 1166 mg/day); corresponding serum levels ranged from 0.32 to 1.51 mEq/l (mean, 0.993 mEq/l), and saliva levels ranged from 0.81 to 5.05 mEq/l (mean, 2.515 mEq/l). The authors noted that lithium caused fewer and milder untoward effects than did haloperidol and that these effects did not appear to interfere significantly with the children's daily routines. There was also a suggestion that lithium was particularly effective in diminishing the explosive affect and that other improvements followed (Campbell et al., 1984b).

Vetro et al. (1985) treated 17 children, aged 3 years to 12 years, who were hospitalized for hyperaggressivity, active destruction of property, severely disturbed social adjustment, and unresponsiveness to discipline. Ten of the children had not responded to prior pharmacotherapy including haloperidol and concomitant individual and family therapy. Lithium carbonate was titrated slowly over 2 to 3 weeks to achieve serum levels in the therapeutic range (0.6 to 1.2 mEq/l). Mean serum lithium level was 0.68 mEq/l ± 0.30 mEq/l. The authors reported that 13 of the children improved enough that their abilities to adapt to their environment could be described as good, and their aggressivity had been reduced to tolerable levels. Three of the four cases that did not improve had poor compliance in taking the medication at home. The authors also noted that these children usually required continuous treatment with lithium for longer than 6 months.

DeLong and Aldershof (1987) reported that rage, aggressive outbursts, and, interestingly, encopresis responded favorably to lithium pharmacotherapy in children with behavioral disorders associated with a variety of neurological and medical diseases, including mental retardation.

Lithium Carbonate in the Treatment of ADHD.   Greenhill et al. (1973) and DeLong and Aldershof (1987) reported that lithium was not effective or worsened symptoms in the treatment of children with earlier equivalent diagnoses of ADHD.

7

Antianxiety Drugs

Benzodiazepines

Benzodiazepines, introduced into clinical practice in the early 1960s, were the most frequently prescribed drugs in the United States for the 12 years prior to 1980; in 1978 alone, 68 million prescriptions for benzodiazepines were written for about 10 million individuals; more than half of these were for diazepam (Ayd, 1980). Greenblatt, Shader, and Abernethy (1983) noted that by 1980 the trend toward increasing use of the benzodiazepines had reversed, perhaps subsequent to publicity about abuse of and addiction to the benzodiazepines. The abuse and addiction potential of the benzodiazepines continues to be of concern, and in 1989 New York state began requiring all prescriptions for benzodiazepines to be written on triplicate forms, as for other controlled drugs. It should be noted, however, that many experts think that compared to other drugs of abuse, the dangers of benzodiazepines have been "greatly exaggerated" (Simeon & Ferguson, 1985). The American Psychiatric Association (APA) Task Force on Benzodiazepines in a summary statement noted that "overall, the APA Task Force found that benzodiazepines, when prescribed appropriately, are therapeutic drugs with relatively mild toxic profiles and low tendency for abuse" (Salzman, 1990, p. 62). Benzodiazepines are poor self-reinforcers of use and tend to be taken alone for pleasure rarely. An exception to this occurs among substance abusers. Benzodiazepine abuse is very frequent among alcoholics; cocaine, narcotic, and methadone abusers frequently abuse benzodiazepines as well. These groups use benzodiazepines to "augment the euphoria (narcotics and methadone users), to decrease anxiety and withdrawal symptoms (alcoholics), or to ease the 'crash' from cocaine-induced euphoria" (Salzman, 1990, p. 62).

Surprisingly little is known about the use of benzodiazepines in child and adolescent psychiatric disorders. In their important 1974 monograph, Greenblatt and Shader, after reviewing the use of benzodiazepines in children and adolescents, stated, "At present it is doubtful that the benzodiazepines have a role in the pharmacotherapy of psychoses or in the treatment of emotional disorders in children" (p. 88).

Werry concluded that if pharmacotherapy is necessary for certain childhood sleep disturbances, including insomnia, night waking, night terrors, and somnambulism, "probably" benzodiazepines are indicated and that they are "possibly" indicated for some kinds of anxiety (Rapoport et al., 1978b).

In 1983, Coffey and her colleagues reported that benzodiazepines appeared to be prescribed to both older adolescents and adults for relief of anxiety and tension, muscle relaxation, sleep disorders, and seizures. In children, however, they were used primarily for treatment of sleep and seizure disorders and were used much less commonly for their anxiolytic and muscle relaxant qualities.

More recently, the literature concerning their use in children has been reviewed by Campbell, Green, and Deutsch (1985) and by Simeon and Ferguson (1985). Most published reports in the literature appeared in the 1960s and were open studies. Many of the studies were comprised of diagnostically heterogeneous subjects; results were discrepant. Diazepam and chlordiazepoxide were the drugs most frequently employed.

At the present time, the psychiatric conditions occurring in childhood for which there is the most convincing rationale for the use of a benzodiazepine as the drug of choice are sleep terror disorder (pavor nocturnus) and sleepwalking disorder (somnambulism); however, these conditions are not usually treated with pharmacotherapy unless they are unusually frequent or severe. Both sleep terror disorder and sleepwalking disorder usually occur "during the first third of the major sleep period (the interval of nonrapid eye movement [NREM] sleep that typically contains EEG δ activity, sleep stages 3 and 4)" (APA, 1987, pp. 310–311). Because benzodiazepines decrease stage 4 sleep, they theoretically might be of therapeutic value in these conditions. Conversely, benzodiazepines are theoretically contraindicated in treating sleep disturbance in psychosocial dwarfism (psychosocially determined short stature), because they would further compromise nocturnal secretion of growth hormone, which occurs maximally during sleep stages 3 and 4, slow-wave sleep (Green, 1986). Reite et al. (1990) suggested that either 2 mg of diazepam or 0.125 mg of triazolam at bedtime may decrease the frequency of night terrors or somnambulism in children with severe cases.

Coffey and her colleagues (1983) have emphasized that the infant has an immature liver and that the newborn's capacity for hydroxylation, demethylation, and especially glucuronide conjugation is limited until about 5 months of age, when the necessary liver enzymes reach and begin to exceed adult capacities. During childhood and until pubescence, enzyme activity levels may exceed those of adults, causing the rate of metabolism to exceed that in adults and necessitating more frequent administration of benzodiazepines than in adolescents and adults (Coffey et al., 1983).

If a benzodiazepine is used as a hypnotic, consideration of the drug's serum half-life is important. For example, flurazepam (Dalmane), temazepam (Restoril), and triazolam (Halcion) are used for treating sleep disorders. Flurazepam is a long-acting benzodiazepine with a half-life (for it and its metabolites) of 47 to 100 hours. The manufacturer notes that this pharmacokinetic profile may explain the clinical observation that flurazepam is increasingly effective on the second or third night of use and, similarly, that after discontinuing the drug, both sleep latency and total wake time may still be decreased. Hence flurazepam appears to be most useful in persons with both significant daytime anxiety and insomnia. In contrast, temazepam and triazolam, also effective hypnotics, are short-acting benzodiazepines with a relatively rapid onset of action and half-lives of 9.5 to 12.4 hours (temazepam) and of 1.5 to 5.5 hours (triazolam). These data suggest that triazolam is the drug of choice for sleep onset insomnia and is preferable in terms of reduced risk of any unwanted daytime sedation. The manufacturer of triazolam reports that all benzodiazepines used to induce sleep can cause an anterior-grade amnesia in which the person may not recall events occurring for several hours after taking the drug; triazolam is more likely than other benzodiazepines to cause such amnesia if a person is awakened before the drug has been metabolized sufficiently and/or excreted to eliminate the effect. Because many travelers, especially on long flights, may take medication to induce sleep and subsequently are awakened before the effects of the drug wears off, this phenomenon has commonly been called "traveler's amnesia"; triazolam should not be used in such situations. Also, because of triazolam's short half-life, there can be a withdrawal effect resulting in increased awakeness during the last third of the night and subsequent increased daytime anxiety or nervousness.

Wysowsky and Barash (1991) compared postmarketing adverse behaviorial reactions of triazolam and temazepam reported through the FDA's spontaneous reporting system. Triazolam was associated with significantly more frequent reports of confusion than temazepam (133 versus 2), of amnesia (109 versus 3), of bizarre behavior (59 versus 2), of agitation (58 versus 4), and of hallucinations (40 versus 1); overall, the incidence was quite small because, during the period of comparison, 13.5 million prescriptions were written for triazolam and 19.1 million prescriptions were written for temazepam. The authors noted that adverse reactions to triazolam tended to occur at higher doses (0.25 mg and higher) and in the elderly.

Klein et al. (1980) suggested that a supplemental low dose of a benzodiazepine (e.g., diazepam 5 mg) might be useful in treating residual anticipatory anxiety in school-phobic youngsters whose separation anxiety had been alleviated by treatment with imipramine.

Simeon and Ferguson (1985) reported that some overly inhibited children may show lasting behavioral improvement following brief (not exceeding 4 to 6 weeks) treatment with a benzodiazepine. They attributed the improvement to an interaction between disinhibition facilitated by the medication and social learning. Consistent with this finding, they noted that children and adolescents with impulsivity and aggression who were under significant environmental stress should not be treated with benzodiazepines, because the disinhibition could result in worsening of behavior (Simeon & Ferguson, 1985).

Most of the literature suggests that benzodiazepines usually worsen symptoms in psychotic children. In studies comparing dextroamphetamine, placebo, and chlordiazepoxide or diazepam in treating hyperactive children, chlordiazepoxide and diazepam were both less effective than dextroamphetamine, and placebo was rated better than diazepam (Zrull et al., 1963, 1964).

CONTRAINDICATIONS FOR BENZODIAZEPINE ADMINISTRATION

Known hypersensitivity to benzodiazepines and acute narrow-angle glaucoma are usually considered absolute contraindications.

Persons predisposed to substance abuse or alcoholism should be prescribed benzodiazepines with caution because they may cause physical and psychological dependence and also interact additively with sedative or hypnotic drugs.

Adolescents who are likely to become pregnant or who are known to be pregnant should rarely if ever be prescribed benzodiazepines, because there are suggestions of increased risk for congenital malformations. Also, maternal abuse of benzodiazepines may cause a withdrawal syndrome in the newborn (Rall, 1990). Simeon and Ferguson (1985) conclude that benzodiazepines are relatively contraindicated in children and adolescents with significant impulsivity, aggressiveness, and environmental stress (negative disinhibiting drug effects may occur).

INTERACTIONS OF BENZODIAZEPINES WITH OTHER DRUGS

The most clinically important drug interactions of the benzodiazepines are associated with additive effects when combined with other sedative or hypnotic drugs, including alcohol (ethanol). Phenothiazines, narcotics, barbiturates, MAOIs, tricyclic antidepressants, and cimetidine (Tagamet) have been reported to potentiate benzodiazepines. The rate of absorption of benzodiazepines and the resulting central nervous system depression are both increased by ethanol (Rall, 1990). Benzodiazepines are relatively safe drugs, and even large overdoses are infrequently fatal unless taken in combination with other drugs (Rall, 1990).

Flumazenil (Romazicon) is a benzodiazepine receptor antagonist that is specific for the reversal of the sedative effects of benzodiazepines; it does not reverse hypoventilation or respiratory suppression caused by benzodiazepines. The manufacturer does not recommend its use in children because no clinical studies have been done in this age group to determine risks, benefits, or dosage. In cases of overdose of adolescents and adults, flumazenil is administered intravenously in doses of 0.2 mg (2 ml) over a 30-second period. If the desired level of consciousness is not obtained, a second dose of 0.3 mg may be administered over 30 seconds, and additional doses of 0.5 mg over 30 seconds at 1-minute intervals to a maximum of 3 mg. Only rarely do patients benefit from higher doses. Resedation may occur because flumazenil has a relatively short half-life compared with many benzodiazepines; in such cases additional flumazenil may be administered. Risk of precipitating seizures is of particular concern in patients who have taken benzodiazepines on a long-term basis or in patients who show evidence of concomitant tricyclic antidepressant overdose.

UNTOWARD EFFECTS OF BENZODIAZEPINES

The most common untoward effects of benzodiazepines are manifestations of their being central nervous system depressants: oversedation, fatigue, drowsiness, ataxia, and confusion progressing to coma may occur at high doses. When anxiety is the target symptom, benzodiazepines should be administered in divided doses to minimize sedation.

"Paradoxical reactions," episodes of marked dyscontrol and disinhibition, have been reported in children and adolescents. Symptoms have included acute excitation, increased anxiety, increased aggression and hostility, rage reactions, loss of all control and "going wild," hallucinations, insomnia, and nightmares.

USE OF BENZODIAZEPINES IN CHILD AND ADOLESCENT PSYCHIATRY

In general psychiatry, the benzodiazepines are indicated in the management of anxiety disorders or for the short-term relief of symptoms of anxiety and the short-term treatment of some sleep disorders. They are also used to treat acute symptoms of alcohol withdrawal. Several manufacturers note that they are usually not indicated for anxiety or tension associated with the everyday stresses of life. The effectiveness of benzodiazepines in treatment lasting more than 4 months has not been assessed by systematic clinical studies.

At the present time, there are no specific clinical guidelines for treating any of the childhood psychiatric disorders with benzodiazepines. If used, manufacturers' clinical recommendations for children should not be exceeded. Table 7.1 gives usual daily dosages for some benzodiazepines, an estimate of the serum half-life of the parent compound and/or its significant active metabolites, the youngest age for which the FDA has approved their use for any purpose, and, when available, suggested dosages for their use in child and adolescent psychiatric disorders.

It is recommended that the need for benzodiazepines be reassessed frequently and that they be discontinued within a relatively short period, usually within a few weeks.

Because of the relative paucity of information available on the use of benzodiazepines in children and young adolescents, most of the available studies are reviewed below, although many are older, uncontrolled studies or case reports.

CHLORDIAZEPOXIDE (LIBRIUM)

Reports of Interest

Chlordiazepoxide in the Treatment of Behaviorally Disordered Children and Adolescents of Various Diagnoses. Krakowski (1963) treated 51 emotionally disturbed children and

Table 7.1.
Some Representative Benzodiazepines

Benzodiazepine (Trade Name) (Estimated Serum Half-Life)	Minimum Age Approved for Any Use	Usually Daily Dosage
Alprazolam (Xanax) (12 to 15 hr)	18 years	See text
Chlordiazepoxide (Librium) (24 to 48 hr)	6 years	5 mg 2 to 4 times/day; maximum 30 mg/day
Clonazepam (Klonopin) (18 to 50 hr)	Not specified	See text
Clorazepate (Tranxene) (about 48 hr)	9 years	For children 9 to 12 years old, maximum initial dose of 7.5 mg twice daily. Maximum weekly increase, 7.5 mg. Maximum total dose, 60 mg.
Diazepam (Valium) (30 to 60 hr)	6 months	0.1–0.3 mg/kg per day for infants and younger children. 1 to 2½ mg 3 to 4 times per day for older children and adolescents; titrate as needed and tolerated
Estazolam (ProSom) (10 to 24 hr)	18 years	1 mg to 2 mg at bedtime
Flurazepam (Dalmane) (47 to 100 hr)	15 years	15 to 30 mg at bedtime
Lorazepam (Ativan) (12 to 18 hr)	12 years	1 to 6 mg/day
Oxazepam (Serax) (5.7 to 10.9 hr)	6 years	Not established for children 6 to 12 years old; adolescents' usual dose is 10 mg 3 times daily to maximum of 30 mg 4 times daily
Quazepam (Doral) (73 hours)	18 years	7.5 mg to 15 mg at bedtime
Temazepam (Restoril) (9.5 to 12.4 hr)	18 years	15 to 30 mg at bedtime
Triazolam (Halcion) (1.5 to 5.5 hr)	18 years	0.125 to 0.25 mg at bedtime. See text also.

adolescents, aged 4 years to 16 years, with chlordiazepoxide. Criteria for inclusion were the presence of anxiety (especially with coexisting hyperactivity), irritability, hostility, impulsivity, and insomnia. Nine children had concurrent individual therapy, and 7 received other medications, mainly antiepileptics. Chlordiazepoxide was administered initially in divided doses totaling 15 mg and individually titrated. Maintenance dosage for periods of up to 10 months ranged from 15 to 40 mg/day (mean, 26 mg/day). Twelve patients

(23.5%) showed complete remission of psychiatric symptoms, and 22 (43.1%) improved moderately. Children with adjustment disorders were particularly likely to improve; specifically, 11 of 18 with conduct disorders, 2 of 3 with habit disturbances, and all 4 with neurotic traits showed marked or moderate remission of symptoms. Of 12 mentally deficient patients, 3 improved moderately and 3 improved markedly. Untoward effects were relatively infrequent and included drowsiness, fatigue, muscular weakness, ataxia, anxiety, and depression. These effects were alleviated to a satisfactory degree by dosage reduction in all but one case.

Kraft and coworkers (1965) prescribed chlordiazepoxide to 130 patients (99 males, 31 females) who ranged in age from 2 to 17 years (112 were between 7 and 14 years of age). The most common diagnoses were primary behavior disorder (50), school phobia (18), adjustment reaction of adolescence (17), and chronic brain damage (14). Most subjects had marked hyperactivity and neurotic traits. Dosage ranged from 20 to 130 mg/day and was administered in divided doses; 94 subjects (72%) received 40 mg or more daily. Moderate or marked improvement occurred in 53 subjects (40.8%). Forty subjects (30.8%) had either no or insignificant improvement, and 37 (28.5%) worsened. The diagnostic group showing the greatest improvement was school phobia (77%). Only 38% of the primary behavior disorder subjects and 41.2% of the adolescent adjustment disorder subjects improved to a moderate or marked degree. Of those with organic brain damage, 50% worsened, 28.6% showed minimal or no benefit, and none had an excellent response. Across diagnoses, symptoms of hyperactivity, fears, night terrors, enuresis, reading and speech problems, truancy, and disturbed or bizarre behavior were moderately or markedly improved in 40.8% of the 130 subjects. The authors concluded that chlordiazepoxide was effective in decreasing anxiety and "emotional overload" (Kraft et al., 1965). The authors also reported that 22 of the 130 had untoward effects of sufficient severity to interfere with treatment results and that 14 other subjects had milder untoward effects that were transient or responded to a lowering of the dose.

Breitner (1962) administered chlordiazepoxide, 20 to 50 mg/day, to more than 50 juvenile delinquents between 8½ and 24 years of age. He reported that the drug produced cooperativeness, released tension, created a feeling of well-being, and made the subjects more accessible to psychotherapy.

D'Amato (1962) treated 9 children, aged 8 years to 11 years who were diagnosed with school phobia, with 10 to 30 mg/day of chlordiazepoxide for from 5 to 30 days. The children were also seen in psychotherapy. Only 1 child did not attend school regularly after the 2nd week of treatment. The author compared these 9 children with 11 other children aged 5 years to 12 years, also diagnosed with school phobia, whom she had treated over the 6 preceding years with psychotherapy only. Only 2 of these 11 children returned to school within 2 weeks, and 9 remained out of school for 1 month or longer. The author thought that this strongly suggested that chlordiazepoxide was an effective adjunct to psychotherapy in mobilizing children with school phobia to return to school.

Petti and his colleagues (1982) treated, with chlordiazepoxide, 9 boys aged 7 years to 11 years who had failed to respond to 3 weeks of hospitalization and treatment with placebo. Subjects' diagnoses were conduct disorder (5, three of whom had borderline features), personality disorder (3, one of whom had borderline features), and schizophrenia (1). Verbal IQs on the Wechsler Intelligence Scale for Children (WISC) ranged from 71 to 110. Target symptoms were anxiety, depression, impulsivity, and explosiveness. The initial dose of chlordiazepoxide was 15 mg, administered in divided doses. Optimal dose was determined by individual titration and ranged from 15 to 120 mg/day (0.58 to 5.28 mg/kg/day). Children's ratings on optimal dose were compared with baseline ratings. Marked improvement was noted in 2 boys, improvement in 4, and no change or worsening in 3. The major improvements were increased verbal production, increased rapidity of thought associations, and a shift from blunted affect or depressed mood to a more animated appearance and feeling subjectively better. The authors noted that chlordiazepoxide had the most positive effect on children who were withdrawn, inhibited, anergic, depressed, or anxious. The child with schizophrenia had worsening of psychotic symptoms, and two children with severe impulsive aggressiveness had worsening of behavior; the authors suggest that chlordiazepoxide's use may be contraindicated in such children (Petti et al., 1982).

DIAZEPAM (VALIUM)

Reports of Interest

Diazepam in the Treatment of Children and Adolescents with Various Psychiatric Diagnoses.   Lucas and Pasley (1969), in one of the few double-blind placebo-controlled studies of benzodiazepines in this age group, administered diazepam to 12 subjects 7 to 17 years old (mean, 12.3 years) who were diagnosed as psychoneurotic (N = 10) or with schizophrenia (N = 2). All subjects were inpatients or in a daycare program. Target symptoms included moderate-to-high anxiety levels, highly oppositional behavior, poor peer relationships, and aggression. The initial dose of diazepam was 2.5 mg twice daily. The drug was increased until a satisfactory therapeutic response or untoward effects occurred. The maximum dose achieved was 20 mg/day. The study lasted 16 weeks, during which four sequences of drug and placebo were randomly used. Subjects were rated on 10 items: hyperactivity, anxiety and tension, oppositional behavior, aggressiveness, impulsivity, relationship to peers, relationship to adults, need for limit setting, response to limit setting, and participation in program. There was no significant difference between diazepam and placebo on any item for the 9 patients who completed the study (the 2 patients with schizophrenia and 1 other patient dropped out). However, when scores on all 10 items were combined, diazepam scored significantly better than placebo ($P < .05$). Clinically, though, the difference was not very apparent. Eleven of the 12 children participated in the study long enough to be rated on a global rating scale. Five subjects showed no change, 2 were somewhat more anxious, and 4 were definitely worse, with increased anxiety and deterioration in their behavior on diazepam compared with placebo. From this study and their clinical experience with diazepam, the authors concluded that diazepam was not clinically effective in reducing anxiety or acting-out behavior in children and young adolescents. Older adolescents appeared to react similarly to adults, and diazepam was thought to be useful in treating their anxiety.

Diazepam in the Treatment of Enuresis.   Kline (1968) administered diazepam or placebo to 50 children and adolescents, aged 3 years to 15 years with nightly enuresis, in a double-blind study. Organic uropathy and mental retardation were exclusion criteria. Initially, 5 mg of diazepam was given in the morning and 10 mg at night. This was increased up to a total of 25 mg if no positive response occurred at a lower dosage. If the child had at most two wet nights weekly at time 4 weeks, he or she continued on the same condition for a total of 12 weeks, when the code was broken. If the subject had three or more wet nights nightly at time 4 weeks, diazepam was given on an open basis for weeks 5 through 12. After the code was broken, it was determined that at time 4 weeks the 28 children who were assigned to diazepam improved significantly more than those assigned to placebo ($P < .05$). Of the 28 on the drug, 22 became dry, 2 were wet one or two nights per week, 3 continued to wet six or seven nights per week, and 1 worsened. Only 1 subject of the 22 on placebo became dry. The others were unchanged, except for 1 who worsened. Of 21 children on placebo at time 4 weeks who were doing poorly and were switched to known diazepam, 12 became dry (Kline, 1968). Diazepam, with its relatively low toxicity, may be a useful alternative to tricyclic antidepressants in those cases of enuresis in which pharmacological intervention is clinically indicated.

Diazepam in the Treatment of Sleep Disorders. In an open study, three children with somnambulism and pavor nocturnus and four children with insomnia were treated with 2 to 5 mg of diazepam near bedtime; all seven responded favorably (Glick et al., 1971). However, no controlled study of benzodiazepines in these disorders has yet been published.

ALPRAZOLAM (XANAX)

REPORTS OF INTEREST

Alprazolam in the Treatment of Pavor Nocturnus. Cameron and Thyer (1985) successfully treated a 10-year-old girl with severe nightly attacks of pavor nocturnus with alprazolam. Initially 0.5 mg of alprazolam was given at bedtime for 1 week; the dose was increased to 0.75 mg nightly for the next 4 weeks, and then the medication was tapered off. Attacks of night terrors ceased on the first night and had not recurred once at follow-up 9 months later.

Alprazolam in the Treatment of Anxiety Disorders. Pfefferbaum et al. (1987) used alprazolam to treat anticipatory and acute situational anxiety and panic in 13 patients, aged 7 to 14 years, who were being treated for concomitant cancer. Treatment was begun 3 days prior to and continued through the day of the stressful procedures. This study was conducted under an Investigational New Drug permit and maximum dosage allowed was 0.02 mg/kg/dose or 0.06 mg/kg/day; the higher dosage reported was on a single child for whom the FDA granted permission to increase doses incrementally by 0.25 mg to a maximum or 0.05 mg/kg/dose or 0.15 mg/kg/day. Initial doses were 0.005 mg/kg or lower and were titrated upward based on efficacy while monitoring untoward effects. Total daily dose ranged from 0.375 to 3 mg (0.003 to 0.075 mg/kg/day). Subjects were rated on four scales measuring anxiety, distress, and panic. The subjects' improvement was statistically significant ($P <$ .05) on three scales and reached borderline significance on the fourth scale. Untoward effects were minimal, mild drowsiness being the most frequently reported.

Simeon and Ferguson (1987) administered alprazolam openly to 12 children and adolescents, aged 8.8 to 16.5 years (mean, 11.5 years), who were diagnosed with overanxious and/or avoidant disorder. After a 1-week placebo baseline period, to which none of the subjects responded, alprazolam was titrated individually over a 2-week period to maximum daily dosages ranging from 0.50 to 1.5 mg. The total period of active treatment with alprazolam was 4 weeks. Seven of the 12 showed at least moderate improvement on several rating scales; no child worsened. Ratings by clinicians showed significant improvement of anxiety, depression, and psychomotor excitation; parents reported significant improvement of anxiety and hyperactivity on questionnaires, and teachers reported significant improvement on an anxious-passive factor. Improvement in the subjects' sleep problems was frequently reported by parents. The few untoward effects were mild and transient. Ferguson and Simeon (1984) reported no adverse effects of alprazolam on cognition or learning at therapeutically effective doses.

Simeon and Ferguson (1987) also noted that the subjects who responded best to alprazolam and who continued on it improved after the drug was stopped had good premorbid personalities and prominent symptoms of inhibitions, shyness, and nervousness. Patients with poor premorbid personalities and poor family backgrounds tended to develop negative symptoms of disinhibition such as increased aggressiveness and impulsivity, especially at higher doses, and relapsed following drug withdrawal.

Simeon et al. (1992) reported a double-blind placebo-controlled study of alprazolam in 30 children and adolescents (23 males and 7 females; age range, 8.4 to 16.9 years; mean, 12.6 years) who had primary diagnoses of overanxious disorder (N = 21) or avoidant disorder (N = 9). Clinical impairment ranged from moderate to severe.

Placebo was administered for 1 week and was followed by random assignment to a 4-week period of either placebo or alprazolam. Medication was tapered with placebo substitution during the fifth week. During the sixth week all subjects received only placebo. Patients who weighed under 40 kg received an initial dose of 0.25 mg of alprazolam; heavier patients were given an initial dose of 0.5 mg of alprazolam. The maximum daily dosage permitted was 0.04 mg/kg. Medication was increased at 2-day intervals until optimal dose was achieved. At completion of the active drug phase, the average daily maximum dose was 1.57 mg (range, 0.5 to 3.5 mg). Untoward effects were few and minor, e.g., dry mouth and feeling tired, and at these doses did not appear to interfere with academic performance.

There was a strong treatment effect in both groups. At the time of completion of the double-blind period, alprazolam was superior to placebo based on clinical global ratings, but the differences were not significant. There were strong individual responders in both groups. After tapering off medication and the final week of placebo, there was a slight relapse with recurrence of original symptoms among the subjects on alprazolam, whereas subjects on placebo showed no further change or continued to improve. The authors noted that doses employed were relatively low and were administered for only 4 weeks and suggested that higher doses and longer trials be investigated in the future. They also recommended that alprazolam be tapered more gradually over a period of several weeks.

Klein and Last (1989) reported Klein's unpublished data from a clinical trial of alprazolam in children and adolescents whose separation anxiety disorder did not respond to psychotherapy. Alprazolam was clinically effective when administered to 18 subjects, aged 6 years to 17 years for 6 weeks, in daily doses of 0.5 to 6 mg/day (mean, 1.9 mg/day). Parents and the psychiatrist judged that more than 80% of the subjects improved significantly, whereas 65% of the subjects rated themselves as improved.

CLONAZEPAM (KLONOPIN)

Clonazepam is approved for use alone or as an adjunct in treating various seizure disorders.

REPORTS OF INTEREST

Clonazepam in the Treatment of Panic Disorder. In an open clinical trial, Kutcher and MacKenzie (1988) treated 4 adolescents (3 females and 1 male; average age, 17.2 years; range, 16 to 19 years) who were diagnosed with panic disorder by DSM-III criteria with a fixed dose of clonazepam (0.5 mg twice daily). Average ratings on the Hamilton Anxiety Rating Scale fell from 32 at baseline, to 7.5 at 1 week, and to 5.7 after 2 weeks. The number of panic attacks fell from an average of three per week to 0.5 per week after 1 week and to 0.25 per week after 2 weeks. One adolescent complained of initial drowsiness that resolved within 4 days; no other untoward effects were reported. At follow-up examinations 3 to 6 months later, all 4 patients continued to take clonazepam with improved functioning in school and interpersonal relations.

Clonazepam in the Treatment of Childhood Anxiety Disorders. Graae et al. (1994) treated 15 subjects (8 males, 7 females;

age range, 7 to 13 years; mean, 9.8 ± 2.1 years) who were diagnosed with various anxiety and comorbid disorders with clonazepam in a double-blind, placebo-controlled, crossover study of 8 weeks' duration. Diagnoses included separation anxiety disorder (N = 14), overanxious disorder (N = 6), social phobia (N = 5), oppositional disorder (N = 3), avoidant disorder (N = 2), conduct disorder (N = 1), and attention-deficit hyperactivity disorder (N = 1). Clonazepam was initiated with a 0.25-mg dose at breakfast time and increased by 0.25 mg every third day to reach a dose of 1.0 mg/day. Subsequent increments of 0.25 mg were made every other day until a dose of 2 mg/day was reached unless untoward effects or compliance issues prevented it. After 4 days at a maximum of 2 mg/day, clonazepam was tapered to reach zero by the end of the 4-week period.

Three boys dropped out during the period on active medication, 2 because of serious disinhibition—including marked irritability, tantrums, aggressivity, and self-injurious behavior—and the other because of noncompliance. Nine children were rated as clinically improved (5 had good/marked improvement and 4 had some/moderate improvement), and 3 children showed no improvement of symptoms of anxiety or overall funtioning while on clonazepam. Although there was no statistically significant difference between periods on clonazepam and placebo for the 12 subjects, the authors thought that individual patients made significant clinical improvements while on clonazepam. The most common untoward effects of clonazepam were drowsiness, irritability or lability, and oppositional behavior. Overall, 10 (83%) of the children had untoward effects during the period on clonazepam compared with 7 (53%) while on placebo; the difference, however, was not statistically significant. Disinhibition occurred only while on clonazepam, and the 2 boys who dropped out because of this effect were not included in the data analysis. It was suggested that a slower dosage increase might reduce some untoward effects, including disinhibition (Graae et al. 1994).

Clonazepam in the Treatment of Obsessive-Compulsive Disorder.   Ross and Piggot (1993) treated, with clonazepam, a 14-year-old male who had been hospitalized with severely disabling obsessive-compulsive disorder (OCD). The patient had not responded adequately to prior trials of clomipramine, thioridazine, alprazolam, fluoxetine, or diazepam, either alone or in various combinations. Clonazepam was begun at an initial dose of 0.5 mg twice daily and increased to 1.0 mg twice daily after 1 week. Behavior began to improve after 2 weeks, and he was able to be discharged on that dose after 11 weeks.

Leonard et al. (1993) reported the use of clonazepam as an augmenting agent in a 20 year old who had severely disabling obsessive-compulsive disorder with onset at age 7. He was treatment resistant to prior trials of clomipramine, desipramine, fluoxetine, fluvoxamine, and buspirone augmentation, either alone or in various combinations. He experienced marked clinical improvement with at least 75% reduction in symptom severity on a combination of 60 mg/day of fluoxetine and 4 mg/day of clonazepam, which had been maintained for about 1 year. The authors suggested that clonazepam might be an efficacious and safe augmentation agent to specific serotonin reuptake inhibitors in treating obsessive-compulsive disorder in children and adolescents.

Azaspirodecanediones

BUSPIRONE HYDROCHLORIDE (BUSPAR)

Buspirone hydrochloride is relatively new drug with anxiolytic properties that is not pharmacologically related to the benzodiazepines or barbiturates. Buspirone has a high affinity for 5-HT$_{1A}$ serotonin receptors, which is associated with anticonflict activity in animals and predicts clinical anxiolytic activity (Sussman, 1994b). It does not appear to have significant affinity for benzodiazepine receptors or to affect γ-aminobutyric acid (GABA) binding (PDR, 1995). Buspirone does not have cross-tolerance with the benzodiazepines, does not suppress panic attacks, and lacks anticonvulsant activity (Sussman, 1994b); hence it does not block the withdrawal syndrome that may occur when benzodiazepines and other common sedative hypnotic drugs are abruptly discontinued. At therapeutic doses it is less sedating than the benzodiazepines. In addition, no evidence of physical or psychological dependence or a withdrawal syndrome has been reported, and it appears to have low abuse potential even by individuals at increased risk for drug dependency. It is not classified as a controlled (Schedule II) substance.

Buspirone has been approved by the FDA for advertising as clinically effective for the management of anxiety disorders or the short-term relief of the symptoms of anxiety. It has been reported that, unlike benzodiazepines, which have an immediate anxiolytic effect, buspirone may take as long as 1 to 2 weeks for its antianxiety effect to develop fully (Sussman, 1994b). Symptom improvement may continue for at least 4 weeks with psychic symptoms of anxiety improving sooner than somatic symptoms of anxiety (Feighner & Cohen, 1989).

Indications in Child and Adolescent Psychiatry
   Buspirone is approved only for treatment of anxiety disorders and the short-term relief of anxiety in individuals at least 18 years old. Its safety and efficacy in children and adolescents remain to be determined.

Dosage Schedule for Treating Anxiety
- Children and adolescents: Not approved. Coffey (1990), however, has cautiously suggested the following doses if a clinician elects to use buspirone in this age group:
- Prepubescent children: An initial dose of 2.5 mg to 5 mg with increases of 2.5 mg every 3 to 4 days to a maximum of 20 mg/day.
- Adolescents: An initial dose of 5 to 10 mg with increases of 5 to 10 mg every 3 to 4 days to a maximum of 60 mg/day.
- Persons 18 years old and older: Initiate treatment with 5 mg three times daily. Titrate to optimal therapeutic response by increases of 5 mg every 2 to 3 days to a maximum daily dose of 60 mg. Usual optimal doses in clinical trials were 20 to 30 mg/day in divided doses.

Dose Forms Available
- Tablets (scored): 5 mg, 10 mg

Pharmacokinetics of Buspirone Hydrochloride

Peak plasma levels occurred between 40 and 90 minutes after an acute oral dose of buspirone. Average elimination half-life after single doses of 10 to 40 mg of buspirone is usually between 2 and 3 hours.

Contraindications for Buspirone Hydrochloride Administration

Known hypersensitivity to buspirone is a contraindication. It is recommended that buspirone not be used concomitantly with monoamine oxidase inhibitors.

Interactions of Buspirone Hydrochloride with Other Drugs

The knowledge of the effects of concomitant administration of buspirone and other drugs is very limited; hence buspirone should be used cautiously with other drugs. There are reports that patients receiving MAOIs have developed elevated blood pressure when given buspirone.

Untoward Effects of Buspirone Hydrochloride

The untoward effects most frequently reported by adults taking buspirone include dizziness (12%), drowsiness (10%), nausea (8%), headache (6%), insomnia (3%), and lightheadedness (3%). Of note, however, drowsiness and insomnia were reported to occur with approximately equal frequency in subjects taking placebo; hence these effects may not have been related to buspirone per se (PDR, 1995).

Reports of Interest

Simeon (1991) reported the use of buspirone in 13 adolescents, age range of 12 to 20 years, mean of 16 years, with various diagnoses who had shown unsatisfactory response to previous drug treatment. Diagnoses were anxiety and/or depressive disorder (N = 5), ADD and/or conduct disorder (N = 4), obsessive-compulsive disorder (N = 2), and psychosis (N = 2). Daily dose of buspirone ranged from 10 to 40 mg (mean, 25 mg) and was either given alone or with other medications. Ratings 1 to 4 months after buspirone was begun showed clinical global improvement that was marked in 7 cases, moderate in 3 cases, mild in 2 cases, and none in 1 case. Improvements were reported in mood (N = 9), anxiety (N = 6), social interaction (N = 6), sleep (N = 4), aggression (N = 3), concentration (N = 3), and irritability (N = 1). Correlations of improvement with diagnoses were not reported.

Buspirone Hydrochloride in the Treatment of Mixed Anxiety Disorders in Children and Adolescents. Simeon et al. (1994) treated 15 children (10 males, 5 females; age range, 6 to 14 years, mean age, 10 years) who were diagnosed with separation anxiety disorder (5), overanxious disorder (2), comorbid separation anxiety and overanxious disorders (4), separation, overanxious, and avoidant disorders (1), separation, overanxious, and obsessive-compulsive disorders (1), and overanxious disorder and ADHD (2). Subjects were rated moderately to severely impaired on the Clinical Global Impression Scale (CGI). A single-blind placebo was administered for the initial 2 weeks. This was followed by 4 weeks of buspirone, which was begun at 5 mg daily and increased weekly by 5-mg increments, if clinically indicated, to a maximum of 20 mg/day. Optimal daily dose ranged from 5 mg twice daily to 10 mg twice daily; mean dose was 18.6 mg/day. No subjects improved significantly on placebo. After 4 weeks on buspirone, subjects' ratings on the CGI showed marked improvement (3), moderate improvement (10), and minimal improvement (2). Repeated measures of multivariate analysis of mean (MANOVA) showed a statistically significant treatment effect after 2 weeks on medication ($P < .016$), which increased to $P < .001$ after both 3 and 4 weeks on medication. There were also significant improvements on several rating scales as reported by parents, teachers, and subjects themselves. Untoward effects included nausea or stomach pain (5), headache (4), and occasional sleepwalking, sleeptalking, or nightmares and daytime tiredness (8) and seemed to occur following dosage increases. These were mild and transient, and none required cessation of therapy.

Buspirone Hydrochloride in the Treatment of Overanxious Disorder with School Phobia. Kranzler (1988) reported a single case study in which a 13-year-old adolescent diagnosed with overanxious disorder, school refusal, and intermittent enuresis was administered buspirone. A previous trial of desipramine yielded some improvement but was discontinued at the patient's request because of untoward effects. Buspirone was begun at 2.5 mg three times daily. At doses of 5 mg three times daily, some drowsiness occurred, particularly in the morning. Dosage was eventually stabilized at 5 mg twice daily. Scores on the Hamilton Anxiety Rating Scale dropped from 26 to 15 and stabilized, with improvement in phobic anxiety, insomnia, depressed mood, cardiovascular symptoms, and anxious behavior. The enuresis did not improve.

Buspirone Hydrochloride in the Treatment of Social Phobia and Mixed Personality Disorder. Zwier and Rao (1994) reported treating with buspirone a hospitalized 16-year-old male diagnosed with social phobia and schizotypal personality disorder. Buspirone was begun at 5 mg/day and increased to 20 mg in increments of 5 mg every 3 days. Scores on the Hamilton Anxiety Rating Scale fell from a predrug level of 5 to 0 at day 12 of treatment, at which time the patient was discharged. Over the subsequent year, buspirone was tapered to 5 mg/day. The patient maintained his gains, and his mild psychotic symptoms had resolved.

Buspirone Hydrochloride in the Treatment of Aggression. Quaison and her colleagues (1991) treated a hospitalized 8-year-old boy diagnosed with conduct and attention-deficit/hyperactivity disorders with buspirone hydrochloride. Dosage was begun at 5 mg three times per day and titrated gradually to 15 mg three times a day. By day 10 there was a notable decrease in his aggressive and assaultive behavior and the need for timeouts or seclusion ceased altogether.

Ratey and coworkers (1989, 1991) reported that buspirone hydrochloride in doses of 15 to 45 mg/day was useful in treating 20 developmentally disabled and mentally retarded adults (age range, 18 to 63 years) for symptoms of anxiety, aggression, and self-injurious behaviors. The decrease in aggressive behavior was independent of anxiety effects. The authors hypothesized that buspirone reduced aggression through its interaction with the serotonergic systems and that, at low dosage levels (although not necessarily at the higher doses of 30 to 60 mg/day used for its anxiolytic-antidepressant effects) buspirone may act as a serotonin agonist, especially in brains with low serotonin activity. However, it remains to be seen if buspirone hydrochloride will be efficacious and safe when its use is extended downward in age.

Buspirone Hydrochloride in the Treatment of Autistic Disorder. Realmuto et al. (1989) treated four autistic children, 9 to 10 years of age, with buspirone 5 mg administered three times daily for 4 weeks, followed by a week-long washout period and 4 weeks of 10 mg twice daily of either fenfluramine or methylphenidate. Two of the four children showed decreased hyperactivity while on buspirone. None of the children experienced adverse untoward effects from buspirone.

8

Other Drugs

Antihistamines

Diphenhydramine (Benadryl) and hydroxyzine (Atarax, Vistaril) are the antihistamines most frequently used in treating emotionally disordered children and adolescents. Chronologically, they were also among the earliest drugs used in child and adolescent psychopharmacotherapy, and they remain among the safest medications yet employed.

CONTRAINDICATIONS FOR ANTIHISTAMINE ADMINISTRATION

Known hypersensitivity to antihistamines is an absolute contraindication for their prescription.

Premature and newborn infants are especially sensitive to the stimulating effects of antihistamines, and overdose may case hallucinations, convulsions, or death. Because antihistamines may be secreted in breast milk, nursing mothers should also avoid taking antihistamines.

Narrow-angle glaucoma, stenosing peptic ulcer, pyloroduodenal obstruction, and symptomatic prostatic hypertrophy or bladder-neck obstruction are relative contraindications. The anticholinergic effects of antihistamines and the additional atropine-like effect of diphenhydramine hydrochloride may cause drying and thickening of bronchial secretions; hence they should be used with caution in patients with clinical symptoms of asthma or poorly controlled asthma.

INTERACTIONS OF ANTIHISTAMINES WITH OTHER DRUGS

Diphenhydramine and hydroxyzine have potentiating effects when used in conjunction with other central nervous system depressants such as alcohol, narcotics, nonnarcotic analgesics, barbiturates, hypnotics, antipsychotics, and anxiolytics.

Monoamine oxidase inhibitors prolong and intensify the drying effect (an anticholinergic action) of antihistamines.

DIPHENHYDRAMINE (BENADRYL)

Diphenhydramine has been used for more than 40 years to treat psychiatrically disturbed children (Effron & Freedman, 1953). Although such use is still not approved for advertising by the FDA, it is reviewed here because some child psychiatrists continue to find it clinically effective.

Fish (1960) reported that diphenhydramine is most effective in behavioral disorders associated with anxiety and hyperactivity, but that it also could be useful in moderately (not severely) disturbed children with organic or schizophrenic (including autistic) disorders. A later study of 15 children, however, found no significant difference in behavioral improvement between diphenhydramine in doses of 200 to 800 mg/day and placebo (Korein et al., 1971).

Diphenhydramine is also effective as an anxiolytic, reducing anxiety before producing drowsiness or lethargy, in children up to about 10 years of age. However, it shows a marked decrease in efficacy when administered to older children; they respond like adults with untoward effects of malaise or drowsiness. Thus for older children, diphenhydramine is useful primarily as a bedtime sedative for insomnia and/or nighttime anxiety (Fish, 1960).

Diphenhydramine has also been used to treat children with insomnia and/or children who wake up after falling asleep and have marked difficulty falling asleep again. Russo et al. (1976) compared diphenhydramine and placebo administered to 50 children, aged 2 to 12 years, who had difficulty falling asleep or problems with night awakenings. Diphenhydramine 1 mg/kg was significantly better than placebo in decreasing sleep-onset latency and decreasing the number of awakenings over a 7-day trial period. Total sleeping time, however, was not significantly increased. Side effects were minimal.

Dosage Schedule for Treatment of Children and Adolescents
- Premature and newborn infants: Use is contraindicated.
- Infants over 20 pounds (9.1 kg) and older children: Begin with 25-mg doses and titrate upward with 25-mg increases for optimal response. A maximum dose of 300 mg/day or 5 mg/kg/day, whichever is less, is recommended.
- Maximum activity occurs in about 1 hour, and the effects last about 4 to 6 hours; thus the drug is usually administered three to four times daily.

(continues)

(continued)

- Young children appear to tolerate a higher dose per unit of weight than do adolescents and adults. Fish (1960) found a dose range of from 2 to 10 mg/kg/day, with an average daily dose of 4 mg/kg, to be most effective in treating her behaviorally disturbed youngsters.

Dose Forms Available
- Capsules: 25 mg, 50 mg
- Elixir: 12.5 mg/5 ml
- Injectable preparations: 10 mg/ml, 50 mg/ml

Untoward Effects of Diphenhydramine

The most frequent untoward effects are anticholinergic effects and sedation. Children do seem more tolerant of the sedative effects of diphenhydramine, but the clinician should still be alert to any cognitive dulling that may interfere with learning. Young children may sometimes be excited rather than sedated by diphenhydramine. It is cautioned that overdose may cause hallucinations, convulsions, or death, particularly in infants and young children.

HYDROXYZINE HYDROCHLORIDE (ATARAX), HYDROXYZINE PAMOATE (VISTARIL)

Hydroxyzine is an antihistamine that is absorbed rapidly from the gastrointestinal tract. Its clinical effects usually become evident within 15 to 30 minutes after oral administration. It has been used widely as a preanesthetic medication in children and adolescents because it produces significant sedation with minimal circulatory and respiratory depression. It also produces bronchodilation; decreases salivation; has antiemetic, antiarrhythmic, and analgesic effects; and produces a calming, tranquilizing effect (Smith & Wollman, 1985).

Use in Child and Adolescent Psychiatry

One manufacturer stated that "hydroxyzine has been shown clinically to be a rapid-acting true ataraxic with a wide margin of safety. It induces a calming effect in anxious, tense, psychoneurotic adults and also in anxious, hyperkinetic children without impairing mental alertness" (PDR, 1990, p. 1858); this statement has been deleted from the current PDR (PDR, 1995). Hydroxyzine is approved for the symptomatic relief of anxiety and tension associated with psychoneurosis and as an adjunct in organic disease states in which anxiety is manifested. Its efficacy for periods longer than 4 months has not been demonstrated by systematic clinical studies.

Although not specifically indicated in the manufacturer's labeling, the sedation caused by hydroxyzine (as with diphenhydramine) has been utilized in the short-term treatment of insomnia and frequent night awakening in children.

Untoward Effects of Hydroxyzine

The most common untoward effects of hydroxyzine are sedation and dry mouth.

Dosage Schedule for Treating Children and Adolescents
- Children under 6 years old: Medication should be titrated individually and administered four times daily to a maximum of 50 mg/day.
- Children 6 years of age and older and adolescents: Medication should be titrated individually and administered three or four times daily to a maximum of 100 mg/day.

Dose Forms Available
- Tablets (hydroxyzine hydrochloride): 10 mg, 25 mg, 50 mg, 100 mg
- Capsules (hydroxyzine pamoate): 25 mg, 50 mg, 100 mg
- Syrup (hydroxyzine hydrochloride): 10 mg/5 ml
- Oral suspension (hydroxyzine pamoate) 25 mg/5 ml
- Intramuscular injectable (hydroxyzine hydrochloride): 25 mg/ml and 50 mg/ml

---

Antiepileptic Drugs

The use of antiepileptic drugs for treatment of psychiatric disorders in children and adolescents was reviewed by Stores in 1978. He concluded that "while some of the antiepileptic drugs show possibilities as psychotropic agents, their use in children with nonepileptic conditions such as behavior or learning disorders of childhood cannot be justified except as a carefully controlled research exercise" (p. 314).

At the present time, most clinical interest in the off-label use of antiepileptic drugs to treat psychiatric disorders in children and adolescents is focused on carbamazepine and valproic acid (valproate); their safety and efficacy in treating these disorders remains to be elucidated. Carbamazepine and valproic acid are being used with increasing frequency to treat many psychiatric and neuropsychiatric disorders that have failed to respond satisfactorily to more standard therapies. Both drugs have been used independently and as adjunctive agents to treat adults and children with bipolar disorder and mania as mood stabilizers and to treat patients with aggressiveness directed either toward self or others, and behavioral dyscontrol. Some mentally retarded persons with concomitant affective symptomatology and disordered behavior have also shown significant clinical benefit from these drugs allowing decrease or cessation of antipsychotic drugs. Further research is necessary to determine which specific disorders, which symptoms, and which patients or subgroups of patients are most likely to respond well, e.g., patients with various abnormal EEG findings; patients who are mentally retarded or have other evidence of abnormal central nervous system functioning compared with affectually or behaviorally disordered patients without signs of central nervous system dysfunction. It will also be important to ascertain further the untoward effects in children and adolescents when these drugs are used for off-label indications rather than to treat seizure disorders. Both have rare but potentially fatal untoward effects and must be used cautiously and monitored carefully.

CARBAMAZEPINE (TEGRETOL)

Evans et al. (1987) attribute the increased interest in carbamazepine's use in child and adolescent psychiatry in part to both the increased awareness of the serious untoward long-term complications of neuroleptic drugs and the finding that the untoward effects of carbamazepine are less formidable than initially thought. In particular, the serious blood dyscrasias, agranulocytosis, and aplastic anemia are very rare. The risk of developing these disorders when treated with carbamazepine is 5 to 8 times that of the general population; agranulocytosis occurs in about 6 per million and aplastic anemia in about 2 per million of the untreated general population (PDR, 1995).

Indications for Use in Child and Adolescent Psychiatry

Carbamazepine is approved for use in patients at least 6 years of age for the treatment of various seizure types. Patients diagnosed with partial seizures with complex symptomatology (psychomotor or temporal lobe) tend to benefit the most from carbamazepine, but patients with generalized tonic-clonic (grand mal) seizures or a mixed seizure pattern may also improve. Absence (petit mal) seizures are not controlled by carbamazepine. Patients with trigeminal and glossopharyngeal neuralgias have shown reduction in pain when treated with carbamazepine. There are no approved psychiatric indications for carbamazepine.

Dosage Schedule for Children and Adolescents
The following are doses recommended for treatment of epilepsy. It is recommended that carbamazepine be taken with meals.
- Children under 6 years of age: Not recommended.
- Children 6 through 12 years of age: Begin with a dose of 100 mg twice daily (or 50 mg four times daily if suspension is used). The dose may be increased weekly by increments of 100 mg as clinically indicated to obtain optimal response. Daily doses of 300 mg or more should be administered in three or four doses. The daily dose should usually not exceed 1000 mg. Usual maintenance daily dose is 400 to 800 mg.
- Patients more than 12 years old: Begin with a dose of 200 mg twice daily (or 100 mg four times daily if suspension is used). The dose may be increased weekly by increments of 200 mg as clinically indicated to obtain optimal response. Daily doses of 400 mg or more should be administered in three or four doses. The daily dose should usually not exceed 1200 mg. Usual maintenance daily dose is 800–1200 mg. Usual therapeutic carbamazepine plasma levels are 4 μg/ml to 12 μg/ml.

Dose Forms Available
- Tablets: 200 mg
- Chewable tablets: 100 mg
- Suspension: 100 mg/5 ml

Contraindications for Carbamazepine Administration

Known hypersensitivity to carbamazepine or tricyclic antidepressants, a history of previous bone marrow depression, and the ingestion of an MAOI within the previous 14 days are absolute contraindications.

Interactions of Carbamazepine with Other Drugs

Carbamazepine has been reported to decrease the serum half-lives of haloperidol, phenytoin, theophylline, and other drugs.

Carbamazepine serum levels are markedly reduced by the simultaneous use of phenobarbital, phenytoin, or primidone.

Increased lithium serum concentrations and increased risk of neurotoxic lithium effects may occur when carbamazepine and lithium are used simultaneously, because carbamazepine decreases lithium renal clearance.

Recently, the FDA advised that carbamazepine could lose up to one third of its potency if stored under humid conditions such as in a bathroom. Supplies should be kept tightly closed and in a dry location.

Untoward Effects of Carbamazepine

The most frequently reported untoward effects are dizziness, drowsiness, unsteadiness, nausea, and vomiting. These occur especially if treatment is not begun with the low doses recommended. As noted above, aplastic anemia and agranulocytosis, although rare, have been reported. Hence, a complete baseline hematologic evaluation must be done and complete blood cell count with differential and platelets monitored closely throughout treatment.

REPORTS OF INTEREST

Although approved only for treating certain kinds of seizure disorders and neuralgias, carbamazepine has been used to treat many psychiatric disorders. In adults, perhaps the best known of these is the treatment of lithium-resistant bipolar disorder. There is evidence that carbamazepine has acute antimanic and antidepressive effects as well as longer-term prophylactic action in treating bipolar disorder (Post, 1987). Post (1987) notes that more severe and dysphoric mania and a rapidly cycling course, variables associated with a poor response to lithium, appear to correspond to better responses to carbamazepine. It has been suggested that the efficacy of carbamazepine in psychiatric disorders may be secondary to its hypothesized ability to inhibit limbic system kindling. Kessler et al. (1989) reported that three psychotic adults improved markedly when carbamazepine was substituted for their neuroleptic medication and suggested criteria to identify affectively ill patients who may have a primary or superimposed organic mood disorder and who might benefit from carbamazepine.

There are many reports, particularly in the European literature, of the use of carbamazepine on an open basis to treat children and adolescents with psychiatric disorders; however, few placebo-controlled studies have been published. In 1988 Pleak and his colleagues noted that carbamazepine was so frequently chosen to treat aggressive children and adolescents who did not respond satisfactorily to standard treatments that it had become "somewhat of a 'vogue' medication" (p. 502).

Remschmidt (1976) reviewed data from 28 clinical trials—7 double-blind and 21 open studies—with a total of more than 800 nonepileptic child and adolescent subjects who were treated with carbamazepine. Positive clinical results were found for target symptoms of hyperactivity or hypoactivity, impaired concentration, aggressive behavioral disturbances, and dysphoric mood disorders. In addition to these behavioral effects, Remschmidt suggested that these patients also experienced positive mood changes, increased initiative, and decreased anxiety.

Groh (1976) reported on 62 nonepileptic children treated with carbamazepine for various abnormal behavioral patterns. Of the 27 who showed improvement, most had a "dysphoric or dysthymic syndrome," the most important features of which were emotional lability and moodiness, which were thought to cause most of the other behavioral abnormalities.

Kuhn-Gebhart (1976) reported symptom improvement in a large number of nonepileptic children who were treated with carbamazepine for a wide variety of behavioral disorders. The author reported that 30 of the last 50 patients treated showed good or very good responses, 10 had discernible improvement, 9 had no change in behavior, and 1 deteriorated. The author noted that the more abnormal the EEGs of these nonepileptic patients, in general, the better the response; that many of the good responders came from stable homes; and that poorer results were more frequent in subjects from unfavorable homes.

Puente (1976) reported an open study in which carbamazepine was administered to 72 children with various behavioral disorders who did not have evidence of neurological disease. Fifty-six children completed the study. The usual optimal dose was 300 mg/day (range, 100 to 600 mg/day). Carbamazepine was given for an average of 12 weeks (range, 9 to 23 weeks). Twenty symptoms were rated on a severity scale at the beginning and end of the treatment. Individual symptoms were present in as many as 55 and in as few as 2 of the 56 children. Over the course of treatment, a decrease in symptom expression of 70% or more occurred in 17 of 20 symptoms in at least 60% of the subjects. Interestingly, all 6 children (100%) with night terrors responded positively, as did 16 (94%) of the 17 children with other sleep disturbances. Anxiety, present in 47 children, improved in 34 (72%). Enuresis improved in 8 of 9 children (89%), and aggressiveness, present in 46 children, improved in 32 (70%). The most frequent untoward effects were transient drowsiness (20%), nausea and vomiting (4%), and urticaria (4%).

Pleak and his colleagues (1988) reported that adverse behavioral and neurological reactions developed in 6 of their 20 male subjects, aged 10 to 16, who were diagnosed with various disorders but primarily with ADHD and conduct disorder, and who were participating in an ongoing protocol evaluating the efficacy of carbamazepine in treating severe aggressive outbursts in child and adolescent inpatients. The untoward effects included a severe manic episode in a 16-year-old, hypomania in a 10-year-old, and increased irritability, impulsivity, and aggressiveness and/or worsening of behavior in 2 subjects aged 14 and 15. Two 11-year-old boys developed EEG abnormalities, with sharp waves and spikes; 1 of these boys improved behaviorally but had his first two absence seizures in several years. The authors caution that patients must be monitored carefully for the development of adverse neuropsychiatric untoward effects. Three additional cases of carbamazepine-induced mania have been reported in children (Reiss & O'Donnell, 1984; Myers & Carrera, 1989). Myers and Carrera (1989) speculated that when adverse behavioral effects such as irritability, insomnia, agitation, talkativeness, and prepubescent hypersexuality occur with carbamazepine administration, they may sometimes be symptoms of an unrecognized hypomania or mania.

Kafantaris et al. (1992) reported an open pilot study in which 10 children (9 male, 1 female; age range 5.25 to 10.92 years, mean 8.27 years), diagnosed with conduct disorder and hospitalized for symptoms of explosive aggressiveness, were treated with carbamazepine. Five of the subjects had previously failed to respond to a trial of lithium. After a 1-week baseline period, carbamazepine was administered in three divided doses beginning at a total of 200 mg/day and titrated to a maximum of 800 mg/day, or a serum level of 12 μg/ml over a period of from 3 to 5 weeks. Optimal dose range was 600 to 800 mg/day (mean, 630 mg/day) with serum levels from 4.8 to 10.4 μg/ml (mean, 6.2 μg/ml). Target symptoms of aggressiveness and explosiveness declined significantly on all measures compared with baseline ratings. On the Global Clinical Consensus Ratings, 4 subjects were rated as markedly improved, 4 as moderately improved, 1 as slightly improved, and 1 as not improved. Three of the lithium nonresponders showed marked improvement, and 1 showed moderate improvement; the 5th did not respond to either drug. Untoward effects during regulation and at optimal dose included fatigue (2 of 10 cases) and blurred vision (2 of 10), and dizziness (1 of 10). Untoward effects above optimal dose included diplopia (2 of 10), mild ataxia (2 of 10), mild dysarthria (1 of 10), headache (2 of 10), and lethargy (1 of 10). One child experienced worsening of preexisting behavioral symptoms and loosening of associations, which were thought to be manifestations of behavioral toxicity. Overall, the untoward effects were transient and were decreased to tolerable levels or eliminated by reduction in dose. White blood cell counts remained within normal limits, although 4 children had reductions from baseline determinations.

Evans et al. (1987) have reviewed the use of carbamazepine in treating children and adolescents with psychiatric disorders including hyperkinesis, aggression, impulsivity, and emotional lability. They noted the lack of systematic, well-controlled studies. These authors also addressed the important issue of the behavioral toxicity of carbamazepine and noted that, in their clinical experience in treating hyperactive and conduct-disordered children with carbamazepine, untoward effects on mood and behavior such as irritability, aggressiveness, increased hyperactivity, emotional lability, angry outbursts, and insomnia commonly occurred and sometimes resembled the target symptoms for which the drug was being prescribed.

VALPROIC ACID (DEPAKENE), DIVALPROEX SODIUM (VALPROIC ACID AND SODIUM VALPROATE) (DEPAKOTE)

Indications for Use in Child and Adolescent Psychiatry
Valproic acid is approved for use alone or in combination with other drugs in treating patients with simple and complex absence seizures or as an adjunctive agent in patients with multiple type seizures, which include absence seizures.
Valproic acid is not approved for use in treating any psychiatric disorder.

Dosage Schedule for Children and Adolescents
An initial daily dose of 15 mg/kg is recommended. Weekly increases of 5–10 mg/kg/day until seizures are controlled or untoward effects prevent further increases are recommended. The maximum recommended daily dose is 60 mg/kg. Amounts greater than 250 mg/day should be administered in divided doses.
Plasma levels of total valproate between 50 and 100 μg/ml are usually considered to be the therapeutic range.
Administration of valproic acid with food does not affect the total amount absorbed and may be helpful in patients who develop gastrointestinal irritation.

Dose Forms Available (Valproic Acid)
• Capsules: 250 mg
• Syrup: 250 mg/5 ml

Dose Forms Available (Divalproex Sodium)
• Sprinkle capsules: 125 mg
• Tablets (delayed release): 125 mg, 250 mg, 500 mg

Pharmacokinetics of Valproic Acid

Peak plasma concentration usually occurs between 1 and 4 hours after ingestion, and plasma half-life is between 6 and 16 hours. The drug dissociates to the valproate ion, which is the active agent, in the gastrointestinal tract.

Contraindications for Valproic Acid Administration

Valproic acid can cause severe hepatotoxicity and should not be administered to persons with hepatic disease or significant liver dysfunction. It should not be administered to persons with known hypersensitivity to the drug.

Because valproic acid has been reported to cause teratogenic effects in the fetus, it should be administered with caution to women who may become pregnant, and they should be warned to notify their physician immediately should they become pregnant.

Interactions with Other Drugs

Valproate may potentiate the action of central nervous system depressants such as alcohol and benzodiazepines. Coadministration with clonazepam may induce absence seizures in patients with a history of absence type seizures. Other drug interactions have been reported.

Untoward Effects of Valproic Acid

The most serious side effect of valproic acid is hepatic failure, which can be fatal; it occurs most frequently within the first 6 months of treatment. Children under 2 years of age are at increased risk; the risk of hepatotoxicity decreases considerably as patients become progressively older. Hence, liver function must be monitored carefully and frequently, especially during the first 6 months.

Nausea, vomiting, and indigestion may occur early in treatment with valproic acid and usually are transient. Sedation may occur, and untoward psychiatric effects such as emotional upset, depression, psychosis, aggression, hyperactivity, and behavioral deterioration have been reported. Thrombocytopenia and other hematologic abnormalities have been reported. Many other untoward effects have been reported.

Reports of Interest

Valproic Acid in the Treatment of Adolescents Diagnosed with Mania.   West et al. (1994) treated with valproate, on an open basis, 11 adolescents (9 males and 2 females; age range, 12 to 17 years; mean, 14.5 years) who were diagnosed with bipolar disorder (5 were manic type and 6 were mixed type) and hospitalized for acute mania. Seven patients had comorbid diagnoses of ADHD. All of the patients had unsatisfactory responses to antipsychotic drugs alone (N = 5) or in combination with lithium (N = 6). Valproate was added to the medications already being prescribed and was begun at a dose of 250 mg twice daily and titrated upward based on clinical response and untoward effects. Optimal doses ranged from 500 to

2000 mg/day (mean, 1068 mg/day), and serum levels ranged from 38 to 94 μg/ml (mean, 74 μg/ml). Length of inpatient valproate administration ranged from 6 to 26 days with a mean of 17 days. Three patients showed marked improvement with virtual or complete remission of manic symptoms, 6 patients improved moderately with significant reduction of symptoms, and 2 showed only slight improvement. The only untoward effects reported were sedation in 2 patients.

Valproic Acid in the Treatment of Children and Adolescents Diagnosed with Mental Retardation and Mood Disorders

Kastner et al. (1990) reported treating with valproic acid 3 patients, a 16-year-old moderately retarded male and 13-year-old and 8-year-old profoundly retarded girls, all of whom also had symptoms of mood disorder. These symptoms included self-injurious behaviors such as face gouging and head banging, irritability, aggressiveness, hyperactivity, sleep disturbance, and paroxysms of crying. All had unsatisfactory responses to several trials of other medications. All three patients showed excellent response to valproic acid and at follow-up had maintained their gains for 7 to 10 months. Maintenance doses were 2700 mg/day (serum level, 109 μg/ml) for the 16 year old, 3000 mg/day (serum level, 75 μg/ml) for the 13 year old, and 1500 mg/day (serum level, 111 μg/ml) for the 8 year old. The authors noted that the serum levels were high or just above the typical therapeutic upper range and that no hepatic abnormalities developed in their patients.

In a 2-year prospective study, Kastner et al. (1993) administered valproic acid to 21 patients diagnosed with mental retardation who also had behavioral symptoms of irritability, sleep disturbance, aggressive or self-injurious behavior, and behavioral cycling that were interpreted as symptomatic of an affective disorder. Eighteen patients completed the study (two could not be followed up and one developed acute hyperammonemia and was dropped from the study). Twelve of the patients completing the study were 18 years old or younger; the degree of their retardation ranged from moderate to profound. Valproic acid was titrated upward until symptoms remitted or untoward effects prevented further increase to plasma levels between 50 and 125 μg/ml. Patients' ratings on the Clinical Global Impression of Severity (CGI-S) scale after 2 years on medication were significantly improved ($P < .001$) from ratings at baseline. Patients with a diagnosis of epilepsy or a suspicion of seizures correlated with a positive response ($P < .005$). Of note, 9 of the 10 patients who were receiving neuroleptic drugs at the beginning of the study were no longer being prescribed these drugs at the study's completion.

PHENYTOIN, DIPHENYLHYDANTOIN (DILANTIN)

Contraindications for Phenytoin Administration

Known hypersensitivity to the phenytoin or a related drug is an absolute contraindication.

Interactions of Phenytoin with Other Drugs

Acute alcohol intake may increase serum phenytoin levels, whereas chronic alcohol use may decrease levels.

Tricyclic antidepressants may precipitate seizures in susceptible patients, necessitating increased phenytoin doses.

Specific drugs have been reported to increase, decrease, or either increase or decrease phenytoin levels. Obtaining serum phenytoin levels may help clarify the situation when necessary. Some drugs increasing phenytoin levels are alcohol (when acutely ingested), benzodiazepines, phenothiazines, salicylates, and methylphenidate. Some drugs decreasing phenytoin levels are carbamazepine, alcohol (with chronic abuse), and molindone.

Interactions of phenytoin and phenobarbital, valproic acid, and sodium valproate are unpredictable, and serum levels of the drugs involved may either increase or decrease.

Use of Phenytoin in Child and Adolescent Psychiatry

REPORTS OF INTEREST

Three double-blind placebo-controlled studies that treated children and adolescents with phenytoin (diphenylhydantoin) reported that it was not significantly better than placebo.

Lefkowitz (1969) reviewed some of the earlier literature in which phenytoin was administered, primarily on an open basis, to nonepileptic children with psychiatric disorders, with discrepant results. Lefkowitz compared the efficacy of placebo and phenytoin in treating disruptive behavior in male juvenile delinquents (mean age, 14 years 11 months; range, 13 years to 16 years 3 months) in a residential treatment center. Each group contained 25 subjects. Phenytoin or placebo was administered in doses of 100 mg twice daily for 76 days. Both groups showed marked reductions in disruptive behavior. Phenytoin, however, was not significantly better than placebo on any of 11 behavioral measures. In fact, placebo was significantly more efficacious than phenytoin in diminishing distress, unhappiness, negativism, and aggressiveness. The author suggested that mild toxic effects of phenytoin, such as insomnia, irritability, quarrelsomeness, ataxia, and gastric distress, may have accounted for the superiority of placebo.

Looker and Conners (1970) administered phenytoin to 17 children and adolescents (mean age, 9.1 years; range, 5.5 years to 14.5 years) who had severe temper tantrums and suspected minimal brain dysfunction. Eleven subjects had normal EEGs, 3 had mildly abnormal EEGs, and 3 had abnormal EEGs, but no subject had clinical seizures. Subjects were placed on a 9-week, double-blind, placebo-controlled, crossover protocol, and phenytoin was titrated to achieve blood levels of at least 10 µg/ml; 12 of the 13 subjects who had final blood levels determined had adequate levels to suppress epileptic discharge. Scores on the Continuous Performance Test, the Porteus Maze Test, parent questionnaires for all subjects, and school questionnaires for 11 subjects showed no statistically significant differences between phenytoin and placebo. The authors noted, however, that there appeared to be some individual subjects who responded positively and rather dramatically to phenytoin.

Conners and colleagues (1971) treated 43 particularly aggressive or disturbed delinquent males (mean age, 12 years; range, 9 to 14 years) living in a residential training school with phenytoin (200 mg/day), methylphenidate (20 mg/day), or placebo administered for 2 weeks in a double-blind protocol. Although the authors noted some limitations in their study, they found no significant difference between drugs and placebo on ratings by cottage parents, teachers, clinicians, and scores on the Rosenzweig Picture Frustration Test and Porteus Maze Test.

Overall, although there are individual patients without seizure disorder who appear to benefit from phenytoin, as yet there is no convincing evidence from double-blind placebo-controlled studies attesting to the effectiveness of phenytoin prescribed for psychiatric symptoms.

Opiate Antagonists

Opiate antagonists have been investigated in the treatment of mentally retarded persons with self-injurious behavior (for review see Sokol and Campbell, 1988) and in the treatment of autistic disorder. Deutsch (1986) has given a theoretical rationale for the use of opiate antagonists in the treatment of autistic disorder.

NALTREXONE (TREXAN)

Contraindications for Naltrexone Administration

The main contraindications are hypersensitivity, any liver abnormalities, and the concomitant use of any opiate-containing substances, legal or illegal.

Interactions of Naltrexone with Other Drugs

Serious adverse effects may occur if naltrexone is administered to individuals taking opioids.

Use of Naltrexone in Child and Adolescent Psychiatry

Naltrexone, a long-acting, potent, opiate antagonist, is a potentially useful agent in a subgroup of autistic children who have elevated endorphin (opioid peptides) levels.

REPORTS OF INTEREST

Naltrexone in the Treatment of Autistic Disorder

Campbell et al. (1989) administered naltrexone on an open basis to 10 hospitalized children aged 3.42 to 6.5 years (mean age, 5.04 years). The study lasted 6 weeks. Following a 2-week baseline, single doses of 0.5, 1, and 2 mg/kg/day were administered at 1-week intervals. Ratings were made 1, 3, 5, 7, and 24 hours after each dose, and 1 week after the last dose. Subjects showed diminished withdrawal at all three dose levels. Verbal production was increased at 0.5 mg/kg/day, and stereotypies were reduced following the 2-mg/kg/day dose. Symptoms such as aggressiveness and "self-aggressiveness" showed little improvement. The major untoward effect was mild sedation, which occurred in 70% of the subjects. Laboratory measurements including liver function tests and ECGs showed no significant change from baseline. Overall, raters considered 80% of the children to be positive responders for some symptoms (Campbell et al., 1989).

Campbell et al. (1990) subsequently conducted a double-blind placebo-controlled study of naltrexone in 18 children, aged 3 years to 8 years, diagnosed with autistic disorder. The study consisted of a 2-week placebo baseline phase, random assignment to placebo or naltrexone for 3 weeks, and a posttreatment 1-week placebo phase. The initial naltrexone dose was 0.5 mg/kg/day; this was increased to 1 mg/kg/day if no adverse effects occurred. Nine children received naltrexone; the optimal dose was 1 mg/kg/day. Six subjects receiving naltrexone were rated moderate (5) or marked (1) in improvement on Clinical Global Consensus Ratings, whereas only 1 child on placebo achieved a moderate rating and none was markedly improved. The difference was significant ($P = .026$). In contrast, no reduction in symptoms occurred on the Children's Psychiatric Rating Scale or Clinical Global Impressions. Naltrexone did not appear to effect discrimination learning in an automated laboratory. The authors also reported that overall symptom reduction seemed better in older autistic children than in younger ones.

Although there are case studies and open studies with some encouraging data, the 1993 report of Campbell et al.—an 8-week double-blind study in which 41 hospitalized children, 2.9 to 7.8 years of age (mean, 4.9 years), diagnosed with autistic disorder, were treated with naltrexone or placebo—did not support the efficacy of naltrexone in this population. All of their subjects received placebo during the first 2 weeks while baseline data were obtained. Following this phase, subjects were randomly assigned to naltrexone or placebo for the next 3 weeks; during the final week all subjects again received placebo. Twenty-three patients were assigned to the naltexone group and 18 to the placebo group. The initial dose was 0.5 mg/kg/day of either placebo or active drug given in the morning; dose was increased to 1.0 mg/kg/day after 1 week and maintained at that level, because untoward effects were minimal and did not require a reduction in dose. Naltrexone did not improve the core symptoms of autism. The only significant finding was a modest decrease in hyperactivity on three different measures. It did not improve discriminate learning significantly more than placebo. Naltrexone was not better than placebo in reducing self-injurious behavior, but 6 of 8 subjects who had a severity rating of mild or above on the Aggression Rating Scale who received naltrexone experienced rebound (increase) in symptoms during the final placebo period; only one child in the placebo group exhibited worsening of self-injurious behavior during that time. The authors concluded that it remains to be determined whether naltrexone is efficacious in treating moderate-to-severe self-injurious behavior and that its use cannot be recommended as a first-line treatment for patients diagnosed with either autistic disorder or self-injurious behavior.

β-Adrenergic Blockers

PROPRANOLOL (INDERAL)

Although initially used primarily in controlling hypertension, angina pectoris, various cardiac arrhythmias, and other medical disorders, there has been considerable interest in propranolol's use in general psychiatry.

Propranolol is a nonselective β-adrenergic receptor blocking agent and is the most frequently used drug in this class. Propranolol and other β-adrenergic blocking agents reduce peripheral autonomic tone, thereby lessening somatic symptoms of anxiety such as palpitations, tremulousness, perspiration, and blushing. There is some evidence that the β-adrenergic blocking agents significantly reduce these peripheral, autonomic, physical manifestations of anxiety but may not affect the psychological (emotional) symptoms of anxiety (Noyes, 1988). Noyes (1988) concludes from his review of the literature that β-blockers are relatively weak anxiolytics compared with benzodiazepines and should be used for generalized anxiety disorder, primarily in patients for whom the use of benzodiazepines is contraindicated.

In adults, propranolol has been investigated in treating anxiety disorders, including generalized anxiety, performance anxiety (stage fright), social phobia, posttraumatic stress disorder, panic disorder and agoraphobia, and episodic dyscontrol and rage outbursts (Hayes & Schulz, 1987; Noyes, 1988). It has also been used in treating schizophrenia. Propranolol is effective in the treatment of some antipsychotic-induced akathisias (Adler et al., 1986).

Contraindications for Propranolol Administration

Known hypersensitivity to propranolol is an absolute contraindication.

Patients with bronchospastic diseases, cardiovascular conditions, diabetes, hyperthyroidism, or other medical disorders should have their medical status carefully reviewed (consultation with the physician providing care for the medical condition is recommended) before prescribing propranolol. Gualtieri and his colleagues (1983) have cautioned that propranolol is contraindicated in children and adolescents with a history of cardiac or respiratory disease, those who have hypoglycemia, or those who are being medicated with a monoamine oxidase inhibitor. Because significant depression has been reported as an untoward effect, propranolol is not recommended for children and adolescents who are already depressed.

Interactions of Propranolol with Other Drugs

Propranolol may interact with many drugs. Three interactions among those most likely to be seen in child and adolescent psychiatric practice are: (a) if used concomitantly with chlorpromazine, plasma levels of both drugs are increased over what they would be if used separately; (b) alcohol slows the rate of absorption of propranolol; and (c) phenytoin, phenobarbital, and rifampin accelerate propranolol clearance.

Untoward Effects of Propranolol

There are few reports of untoward effects in children or adolescents who received propranolol for psychiatric indications. Of greatest concern have been cardiovascular effects, which are detailed below. Propranolol has also been reported to cause significant depression of mood, manifested by insomnia, lethargy, weakness, and fatigue. Vivid dreams, nightmares, and gastrointestinal symptoms have also been reported.

Use of Propranolol in Child and Adolescent Psychiatry

There are few reports on the use of these drugs in psychiatrically disturbed children and adolescents.

REPORTS OF INTEREST

Propranolol in the Treatment of Children and Adolescents with Brain Dysfunction, Uncontrolled Rage Outbursts, and/or Aggressiveness. Williams et al. (1982) administered propranolol to 30 subjects (11 children, 15 adolescents, and 4 adults) with organic brain dysfunction and uncontrolled rage outbursts who had not responded to other treatments. The subjects had various psychiatric diagnoses, including 15 with diagnoses of both conduct disorder, unsocialized, aggressive type, and attention deficit disorder with hyperactivity; 7 with comorbid diagnoses of conduct disorder, unsocialized, aggressive type, and attention deficit disorder without hyperactivity; 3 with conduct disorder only; 3 with intermittent explosive disorders; and 2 with pervasive developmental disorders. Thirteen had IQs in the retarded range, and 8 had borderline IQs. The authors reported that 80% of their subjects demonstrated moderate to marked improvement on follow-up examination between 2 and 30 months (mean, 8 months) later. Optimal dosages of propranolol ranged from 50 to 960 mg/day (mean, 160 mg/day). All untoward effects were transient and reversible with dosage reduction. Most of the patients were additionally treated with other medication: 13 subjects received anticonvulsants; 6, antipsychotics; and 3, stimulants; 21 had ongoing psychotherapy (Williams et al., 1982).

Kuperman and Stewart (1987) treated openly with propranolol 16 subjects whose mean age was 13.4 years (8 patients were 4 to 14 years old, 4 were between 14 and 17, and 4 were 18 to 24 years old). Seven subjects were diagnosed with conduct disorder, undersocialized aggressive type, 5 had infantile autism with varying degrees of mental retardation, 2 had moderate mental retardation only, 1 had borderline intellectual functioning, and 1 had attention deficit disorder. All subjects exhibited significant physically aggressive behavior that had not responded adequately to behavior therapy and/or psychotropic medication. Propranolol was begun at 20 mg twice daily and increased by 40 mg every fourth day until symptom improvement occurred or standing systolic blood pressure fell below 90 mm Hg, diastolic blood pressure fell below 60 mm Hg, or resting pulse fell below 60 beats per minute. The average dose of propranolol was 164 ± 55 mg/day. Ten patients (62.5%) were rated moderately or much improved, based on concurrence of ratings by parents, teachers, and clinicians. Responders and nonresponders did not differ significantly regarding age, sex, IQ, vital signs, or dosage. The authors noted that, although not significant, 6 of their 8 patients who were mentally retarded responded favorably, which is consistent with earlier findings in adults that suggest aggressive patients with suspected central nervous system damage respond best. Nonresponders as a group tended to develop bradycardia, which may have prevented them from reaching potentially therapeutic doses of propranolol. The authors additionally noted that before considering propranolol a therapeutic failure, a patient should receive the maximum therapeutic dose tolerated for at least 1 month. When propranolol is discontinued, it should be tapered gradually over a 2-week period to avoid rebound tachycardia (Kuperman & Stewart, 1987).

Two 12-year-old boys treated with propranolol for episodic dyscontrol and aggressive behavior showed marked improvement (Grizenko & Vida, 1988). Dosage was begun at 10 mg three times daily and was gradually increased to 50 mg three times daily.

Famularo et al. (1988) reported that 11 children (mean age, 8½ years old) diagnosed with posttraumatic stress disorder (PTSD), acute type, had significantly lower scores on an inventory of PTSD symptoms during the period when they were receiving propranolol, compared with scores before and after the drug. Dosage was begun at 0.8 mg/kg/day and administered in three divided doses; it was increased gradually over 2 weeks to approximately 2.5 mg/kg/day. Untoward effects prevented raising dosage to this level in only three cases. Propranolol was maintained at this level for 2 weeks and then tapered and discontinued over a 5th week. The authors emphasized that their subjects had presented in agitated, hyperaroused states and that propranolol might be useful during this particular stage of the disorder (Famularo et al., 1988).

At present, although there are some encouraging initial data, the use of propranolol and the β-blockers in children and adolescents must be further investigated. In particular, propranolol's use in anxiety disorders remains to be elucidated.

PINDOLOL (VISKEN)

Pindolol is a synthetic, nonselective β-adrenergic receptor blocking agent that has sympathomimetic activity at therapeutic doses but does not possess quinidine-like membrane stabilizing activity (packet insert). It is approved for use in treating hypertension, but its safety and effectiveness have not been established in children.

REPORT OF INTEREST

Buitelaar et al. (1994a) conducted a double-blind placebo-controlled comparison of pindolol and methylphenidate in 52 subjects, age range of 6 to 13 years, diagnosed with ADHD. Treatment periods were of 4 weeks' duration. For the first 3 days, a morning dose of 10 mg of methylphenidate or 20 mg of pindolol or placebo was given. This was increased to 10 mg twice daily of methylphenidate or 20 mg twice daily of pindolol or placebo for the remainder of the period. Subjects were rated on various Conners scales by parents and teachers. After 4 weeks, teachers rated students receiving methylphenidate as significantly better on impulsivity/hyperactivity, inattentiveness, and conduct than subjects receiving either pindolol or placebo. Parental ratings did not show a significant difference between pindolol and methylphenidate on improvements in impulsivity/hyperactivity or conduct, although both were better than placebo. The authors thought that the main effect of pindolol was to improve behavioral symptoms and conduct and that the drug was only modestly effective in treating ADHD.

Untoward effects of pindolol were of particular concern and limit the potential usefulness of this drug in children. Paresthesias were reported in 10% of children during treatment with pindolol and none while receiving placebo or methylphenidate ($P = <.05$). Although hallucinations and nightmares were not significantly more frequent in children on pindolol, they were of significantly greater intensity ($P < .01$) and caused so much distress that the children's daily functioning was effected adversely. These adverse effects totally remitted within 1 day after discontinuation of pindolol. The authors note that some children may be particularly sensitive to these distressing untoward effects, further limiting the usefulness of pindolol in ADHD, and requiring the clinician to be very cautious whenever prescribing pindolol to children (Buitelaar et al. 1994a, 1994b).

α-Adrenergic Agonists

CLONIDINE HYDROCHLORIDE (CATAPRES), CLONIDINE (CATAPRES-TRANSDERMAL THERAPEUTIC SYSTEM)

Clonidine is a centrally acting antihypertensive agent. The only therapeutic indication that has been approved by the FDA for advertising is treatment of hypertension in older adolescents and adults; its safety and efficacy in children have not been established. Clonidine, an α_2-noradrenergic receptor agonist (stimulating agent), acts preferentially on presynaptic α_2-neurons to inhibit endogenous release of norepinephrine in the brain (Hunt et al., 1991). The authors note that the positive results in their studies with children diagnosed with ADHD suggest that the norepinephrine system may be important in causing behavioral and cognitive abnormalities, in at least some children with ADHD.

Pharmacokinetics of Clonidine

Peak plasma levels of clonidine occur between 3 and 5 hours after ingestion, and plasma half-life is between 12 and 16 hours (package insert). Leckman et al. (1985), however, give different pharmacokinetic values for children and adolescents, stating that clonidine's half-life is about 8 to 12 hours in adolescents and adults, whereas in prepubertal children it is considerably shorter, approximately 4 to 6 hours. Between 40% and 60% of the drug is excreted unchanged by the kidneys within 24 hours after oral ingestion, and about 50% is metabolized by the liver (package insert).

Contraindications for Clonidine Administration

Significant cardiovascular disease and known allergic reactions to clonidine are relative contraindications. If clonidine is used in patients with such conditions, careful and frequent monitoring is required.

Children and adolescents with depressive symptomatology, past history of depression, or family history of mood disorder should not be given clonidine (Hunt et al., 1990).

Interactions of Clonidine with Other Drugs

Tricyclic antidepressants may decrease the effects of clonidine, necessitating higher doses.

The central nervous system depressive effects of alcohol, barbiturates, and other drugs may be enhanced by simultaneous administration with clonidine.

Interactions with additional drugs have been reported.

Untoward Effects of Clonidine

Hunt et al. (1991) note that sedation is the most frequent and troublesome untoward effect of clonidine in treating children. Cardiovascular untoward effects, including hypotension, were not usually clinically significant. Clonidine worsened or induced depressive symptomatology in about 5% of children (Hunt et al., 1991). Levin et al. (1993) reported the onset of precocious puberty in two 7-year-old girls with mild mental retardation who were being treated with clonidine for aggressivity; of note, discontinuation of clonidine halted the progression of puberty in both cases. Many other untoward effects have been reported in patients on clonidine (PDR, 1995).

Indications in Child and Adolescent Psychiatry
There are no FDA-approved uses of clonidine in the treatment of psychiatrically disturbed children and adolescents. However, clonidine has been investigated in treating children and adolescents diagnosed with attention-deficit-hyperactivity disorder and/or Tourette's disorder who have not responded to standard treatments for these disorders. Studies of these uses and the doses employed by the researchers are summarized below for each of these conditions.

Dose Forms Available
• Tablets (single scored): 0.1 mg, 0.2 mg, 0.3 mg
• Transdermal Therapeutic System: Programmed delivery by skin patch of 0.1 mg, 0.2 mg, or 0.3 mg daily for 1 week.
    Because of possible rebound phenomena, clonidine should be tapered gradually when discontinued.

Hunt et al. (1990) recommend beginning clonidine administration with bedtime doses to utilize the usual initial sedative effect to facilitate sleep. Sedation is most severe during the first 2 to 4 weeks after which tolerance usually develops (Hunt et al., 1991). Because of its short serum half-life, clonidine is usually administered 3 to 4 times daily and at bedtime. Hunt et al. (1990) have reported that some children have shown a loss of therapeutic effect or withdrawal symptoms when it is administered less frequently; transdermal patches eliminate this difficulty.

When a transdermal patch was used in treating subjects diagnosed with ADHD, Hunt (1987) found that its efficacy wore off and that it had to be replaced in 50% of subjects after 5 days rather than the 7 days stated by the manufacturer. He also noted that, to achieve the same degree of symptom control, three of his eight subjects whose daily oral dose was 0.2 mg/day had to have their doses increased to 0.3 mg/day when clonidine was administered transdermally. Comings (1990), who has extensive clinical experience with

Tourette's patients, stated that he found that clonidine administered using a patch may work when oral clonidine is ineffective. Comings also found it convenient and useful to adjust the dose of clonidine by using scissors to cut the patch to the necessary size.

Discontinuing Medication

Clonidine should be gradually reduced over a period of 2 to 4 days to avoid a possible hypertensive reaction and other withdrawal symptomatology such as nervousness, agitation, and headache (package insert).

REPORTS OF INTEREST

Clonidine in the Treatment of Attention-Deficit/Hyperactivity Disorder. Hunt et al. (1982) reported on an open pilot study in which clonidine 3 to 4 μg/kg/day was administered orally for 2 to 5 months to four children between 9 and 14 years of age diagnosed with ADDH. Improvement was noted by parents and teachers. The authors noted that distractibility often persisted but that the children were nevertheless more able to return to and complete tasks.

Hunt et al. (1985) conducted a double-blind, placebo-controlled crossover study of 12 children (mean age, 11.6 ± 0.54 years) who were diagnosed with ADDH. Ten children completed the study. Seven subjects had previously received stimulant medication; in four cases stimulants had been discontinued because of significant untoward effects. Clonidine was begun at 0.05 mg and increased every other day until a dose of 4 to 5 μg/kg/day (about 0.05 mg four times daily) was attained. Parents, teachers, and clinicians all noted statistically significant improvements on clonidine for the group as a whole. The best responders were children who had been overactive and who were uninhibited and impulsive, which, in turn, had impaired their opportunities to use their basically intact capacities for social relatedness and purposeful activity. During the placebo period, parents, teachers, and clinicians noted significant deterioration in overall behavior for the group, with symptoms usually returning between 2 and 4 days after discontinuing the medication (Hunt et al., 1985).

The most frequent untoward effect seen in this study was sedation, occurring about 1 hour after ingestion and lasting 30 to 60 minutes. In all cases but one, tolerance to this effect developed within 3 weeks. Mean blood pressure also decreased about 10%.

Hunt et al. (1990; 1991) have reported that children diagnosed with ADHD and treated with clonidine have been maintained on the same dose for up to 5 years without diminution of clinical efficacy. However, about 20% of such children require an increase in dose after several months of treatment, probably secondary to autoinduction of hepatic enzymes (Hunt et al., 1990).

Hunt (1987) compared the efficacies of clonidine (administered both orally and transdermally) and methylphenidate in an open study of 10 children diagnosed with ADDH, all of whom had ratings by both parents and teachers of more that 1.5 SD above normal on Conners behavioral rating scales. Eight subjects (7 males, 1 female; mean age, 11.4 ± 0.6 years; range, 6.7 to 14.4 years) completed the protocol. Subjects received placebo, low-dose (0.3 mg/kg) methylphenidate, or high-dose (0.6 mg/kg) methylphenidate. Each of these conditions was randomized for a period of 1 week. All subjects then received an open trial of clonidine 5 µg/kg/day administered orally for 8 weeks. Eight subjects completed the open trial with positive results and were then switched from tablets to transdermal clonidine skin patch. Both clonidine and methylphenidate were significantly more effective than placebo, and clonidine in both dosage forms was as effective as methylphenidate (Hunt, 1987). Children reported that they felt more "normal" on clonidine than on methylphenidate. Transdermal administration was preferred to oral administration by 75% of the children and their families, partly because the embarrassment of taking pills at school was avoided but also because it was more convenient. Skin patches caused localized contact dermatitis, usually presenting with itching and erythema, in about 40% of children and at times limited their usefulness (Hunt et al. 1990).

Hunt (1987) noted that in contrast to the stimulants, clonidine appears to increase frustration tolerance but does not decrease distractibility. He noted that an additional small dose of methylphenidate may be safely added to help focus attention and that this combination frequently necessitates a much lower dose of methylphenidate than would be required if it were the only drug used (Hunt, 1987).

In a review of clonidine use in child and adolescent psychiatry, Hunt and his colleagues (1990) explained more specifically the differences between clonidine and methylphenidate in treating ADHD and their possible synergistic use in treating ADHD and suggested the subgroups of ADHD children for whom each treatment would be most useful. Stimulants (methylphenidate) improve attentional focusing and decrease distractibility, whereas clonidine decreases hyperarousal and increases frustration tolerance and task orientation. The authors found that children with ADHD who respond best to clonidine often have an early onset of symptoms, are extremely energetic or hyperactive (hyperaroused), and have a concomitant diagnosis of conduct disorder or oppositional disorder. Such children often respond to clonidine treatment with increased frustration tolerance and consequent improvement in task-orientated behavior; more effort, compliance, and cooperativeness; and better learning capacity and achievement. Clonidine also was efficacious in nonpsychotic inpatient adolescents with ADHD who were aggressive and hyperaroused (Hunt et al., 1990).

Unlike stimulants, clonidine does not directly improve distractibility; hence stimulants are preferable for mildly to moderately hyperactive children with significant deficits in distractibility and attentional focus. The combination of clonidine and methylphenidate was found to be helpful for children who were diagnosed with coexisting conduct or oppositional disorder and ADHD and who were both highly aroused and very distractible (Hunt et al., 1990). The combined use of these drugs may permit the effective dose of methylphenidate to be reduced by about 40%, making it potentially useful for ADHD patients in whom significant motor hyperactivity persists, or in whom rebound symptoms or dose-limiting side effects such as aggression, irritability, insomnia, or decrements in weight or height gain have occurred with stimulant treatment (Hunt et al., 1990).

Steingard et al. (1993) published a retrospective chart review of 54 patients, age range, 3 to 18 years (mean 10.0 ± 0.5 years), who were diagnosed with ADHD only (N = 30) or ADHD and comorbid tic disorder (N = 24) and treated with clonidine. Of note, 17 subjects in the ADHD only group had prior unsatisfactory responses to stimulant or tricyclic antidepressant medication. In the comorbid group, 9 had developed tics when treated with stimulants and 10 had unsuccessful prior trials of tricyclic antidepressants. Clonidine was initiated at a low dose and titrated upwards until a positive clinical result occurred or untoward effects prevented further increase. Mean optimal daily dose for all subjects was 0.19 ± 0.02 mg/day (range, 0.025 to 0.6 mg/day). There was no significant difference in mean daily dose between subjects with and without tics, responders and nonresponders, or subjects under and over 12 years of age. Although 72% (39) of 54 subjects were rated as improved on the Clinical Global Improvement Scale subset of items for ADHD symptoms, a significantly greater proportion ($P = .0005$) of subjects with a comorbid tic disorder (23 [96%] of 24) improved than did subjects with ADHD only (16 [53%] of 30). On Clinical Global Improvement Scale items pertinent to tics, 75% (18) of 24 showed improvement. Sedation, the most frequent untoward effect, was reported in 22 (41%) of the patients. All 7 patients whose untoward effects resulted in discontinuation of medication were in the ADHD only group; 5 were discontinued because of sedation, 1 because of increased anxiety, and 1 because a depressive episode occurred.

At present, clonidine may be regarded as a possible alternative treatment for ADHD. It may eventually prove useful in treating, in particular, a subgroup of ADHD children who do not respond well to stimulants. Clonidine may also be a useful alternative treatment for some ADHD children who have chronic tics or who develop side effects of sufficient severity as to preclude the use of stimulants (Hunt et al., 1985; Steingard et al., 1993).

Clonidine in the Treatment of Sleep Disturbances in Children and Adolescents Diagnosed with ADHD.   Wilens et al. (1994) reported their experience in using the sedation that clonidine often produces to treat more than 100 patients diagnosed with ADHD who also had spontaneous or drug-induced sleep difficulties. The effect has allowed some children who responded very well to stimulants but could not tolerate them because of significant insomnia to be treated successfully with them. Typically, an initial dose of 0.05 mg of clonidine for patients between 4 and 17 years old was given about $\frac{1}{2}$ hour before bedtime and was increased by 0.05-mg increments to a maximum of 0.4 mg. A few very young or underweight children required only 0.025 mg, whereas a few other children required more than 0.4 mg. Patients and parents reported better sleep, and there were decreased familial conflicts around sleep activities and fewer ADHD-like symptoms after treatment. Some of the latter improvement is likely to result from the fact that clonidine is also effective in treating ADHD independently from its sleep-enhancing qualities. Clonidine should be tapered gradually when it is discontinued, even if only used at night for insomnia.

Clonidine in the Treatment of Chronic Severe Aggressiveness.   Kemph et al. (1993) treated openly with clonidine 17 outpatients (14 males and 3 females; age range, 5 to 15 years old; mean age, 10.1 years) diagnosed with conduct or oppositional defiant disorder. All subjects had a history of chronic and violent aggressiveness in multiple settings that had not responded to behavioral management. Clonidine was begun at an initial dose of 0.05 mg daily. After 2 days it was increased to 0.05 mg twice daily, and on day 5 it was increased to 0.05 mg three times daily following which it was titrated as clinically indicated on an individual basis. The maximum effective dose was 0.4 mg daily administered in divided doses. A comparison of mean baseline and follow-up scores on the rating of aggression against people and/or property scale (RAAPP) showed significant improvement on drug ($P < .0001$). Drowsiness was the major untoward effect most frequently reported; it usually occurred during the first weeks of treatment, and most patients developed tolerance to it. There were no significant changes in blood pressure or cardiovascular parameters. The authors noted that plasma γ-aminobutyric acid (GABA) levels increased significantly ($P < .01$) in 5 of the 6 children for whom it was available at follow-up, suggesting that GABA plasma levels may be correlated with childhood aggressiveness and may also be useful to verify compliance. Clonidine may be a useful agent in the control of aggression in children and adolescents and merits further study.

Clonidine in the Treatment of Autistic Disorder Accompanied by Inattention, Impulsivity, and Hyperactivity. Jaselskis et al. (1992) treated 8 males (age range, 5.0 to 13.4 years; mean, 8.1 ± 2.8 years) diagnosed with autistic disorder who also had significant inattention, impulsivity, and hyperactivity that had not responded to prior psychopharmacotherapy, e.g., methylphenidate or desipramine; they received clonidine in a double-blind, placebo-controlled, crossover protocol. Clonidine or placebo was titrated over the initial 2 weeks to a daily total of 4 to 10 μg/kg (0.15 to 0.20 mg/day) divided into three doses; this regimen was maintained for the next 4 weeks. During the 7th week, subjects were tapered off clonidine or placebo. At week 8, subjects were crossed over to the other condition for 6 weeks. Parents' ratings on the Conners Abbreviated Parent-Teacher Questionnaire showed significant improvement while their children were on clonidine. Teachers' ratings on the Aberrant Behavior Checklist were significantly better during clonidine treatment for irritability ($P = .03$), hyperactivity ($P = .03$), stereotypy ($P = 0.05$), and inappropriate speech ($P = .05$). Attention Deficit Disorder with Hyperactivity: Comprehensive Teacher's Rating Scale scores improved significantly only for oppositional behavior ($P = .05$). Although significant, improvement was modest. Clinician ratings at the end of each 6-week period showed no significant differences between clonidine and placebo. Untoward effects included significant drowsiness and hypotension requiring reduction of dosage in 3 subjects.

Clonidine in the Treatment of Tourette's Disorder.   Cohen et al. (1980) reported that clonidine was clinically effective in at least 70% of 25 patients between 9 and 50 years of age, diagnosed with Tourette's syndrome (TS), who either did not benefit from haloperidol or could not tolerate the untoward effects of that medication. Dosage was begun at 1 to 2 μg/kg/day (usually 0.05 mg/day) and gradually titrated up to a maximum of 0.60 mg/day. Most patients did best with small doses three to four times daily. Comings (1990) recommends a starting dose of 0.025 mg/day (one-fourth of a tablet) and sometimes found it necessary to administer as many as five divided doses daily for best results. He found it to be an excellent drug for the approximately 60% of his patients who responded and noted that it ameliorated oppositional, confrontative, and obsessive-compulsive behaviors and symptoms of ADHD when these were also present. In contrast, Shapiro and Shapiro (1989) noted that, in their experience, clonidine was only rarely effective in treating unselected patients with tics and Tourette's disorder.

Cohen et al. (1980) delineated five phases of treatment response to clonidine:

Phase 1: Within hours or days, patients felt calmer, less angry, and more in control.

Phase 2: About 3 to 4 weeks after initiation of clonidine (usually coinciding with a therapeutic dose of 3 to 4 μg/kg/day [0.15 mg/day]), the patient recognized progressive benefits characterized by decreased compulsive behavior, further behavioral control, and decreased phonic and motor tics.

Phase 3: A plateauing of improvement started at about the 3rd month.

Phase 4: Five or more months after beginning, an increase in dosage up to 4 to 6 μg/kg/day (0.30 mg/day) of clonidine was needed to maintain clinical improvement.

Phase 5: Further tolerance to clonidine may occur at a dose considered too high to increase further.

A review of the use of clonidine in Tourette's disorder (Leckman et al., 1982) noted discrepant results among studies. The reviewers estimated that about 50% of subjects improved meaningfully. Behavioral symptoms showed the most improvement and maximum benefit could take from 4 to 6 months. A minority of patients did not respond, and a few worsened.

Leckman et al. (1985) reported a 20-week, single-blind, placebo-controlled trial of clonidine in 13 patients, aged 9 to 16 years, diagnosed with Tourette's syndrome. This was followed by a 1-year open clinical trial. The mean dose of clonidine was 5.5 μg/kg/day (range,

3 to 8 μg/kg/day) (0.125 to 0.3 mg/day). There was significant improvement in motor and phonic tics and associated behavioral problems. Forty-six percent of subjects were unequivocal responders, and 46% responded equivocally. Of interest is the fact that 9 of the 13 patients reported by Leckman and colleagues also had an additional diagnosis of ADDH. As noted above, some children with ADHD have symptoms that respond to clonidine.

Leckman et al. (1991) reported a 12-week, double-blind, placebo-controlled trial of clonidine completed by 40 subjects (age range, 7 to 48 years; mean, 15.6 ± 10.4 years; 31 of the subjects were younger than 18 years old) diagnosed with Gilles de la Tourette's syndrome. Clonidine was titrated gradually during the first 2 weeks to a total daily dose of 4 to 5 μg/kg (maximum, 0.25 mg/day) and administered in two to four divided doses per day depending on the total dose. Mean clonidine dose at the end of the 12 weeks for the 21 subjects randomly assigned to clonidine was 4.4 ± 0.7 μg/kg/day (range, 3.2 to 5.7 μg/kg/day); clonidine serum levels, available for 19 subjects, ranged from 0.24 to 1.0 ng/ml, with a mean of 0.48 ± 0.23 ng/ml. Subjects receiving clonidine were rated as significantly more improved than those receiving placebo on the Tourette Syndrome Global Scale for motor tics ($P = .008$) and total score ($P = .05$); on the anchored CGI scale for Tourette syndrome (TS-CGI); on the Shapiro Tourette Severity Symptom Scale for decrease in "tics noticeable to others"; and on the Conners Parent Questionnaire for total score ($P = .02$) and the impulsive/hyperactive factor ($P = .01$). Untoward effects most frequently reported were sedation/fatigue (90%), dry mouth (57%), faintness/dizziness (43%), and irritability (33%). Although clonidine is not as effective in controlling tic behavior as the D_2-dopamine receptor-blocking agents haloperidol and pimozide, its more favorable untoward effect profile should prompt the clinician to consider a trial of clonidine before using antipsychotic drugs in milder cases (Leckman et al., 1991).

Bruun (1983) has provided useful guidelines for prescribing clonidine for Tourette's disorder. She suggests initiating daily dosage at 0.025 mg twice daily for small children and at 0.05 mg twice daily for older children and adolescents. Medication is titrated upward gradually with increases of no greater than 0.05 mg/week; this slow pace often prevents untoward effects from interfering with the treatment. The usual optimal daily dose is between 0.25 and 0.45 mg. Doses above 0.5 mg/day may be required, but untoward effects (e.g., drowsiness, fatigue, dizziness, headache, insomnia, and increased irritability) become more troublesome. Bruun (1983) notes that drowsiness may occur at very low doses and suggests that no further increases in dosage be made until drowsiness subsides. Some patients note a decrease in beneficial effects 4 to 5 hours after their last dose, and treatment is usually more effective for all patients with total daily dosage administered in three or four smaller doses (Bruun, 1983). Although presently not an approved treatment, there is evidence that some children and adolescents with Tourette's disorder respond favorably with significant symptom reduction when treated with clonidine. Clonidine may be regarded as a possible treatment for those youngsters with Tourette's disorder who have not responded satisfactorily or who have intolerable untoward effects to standard treatments.

GUANFACINE HYDROCHLORIDE (TENEX)

Guanfacine hydrochloride is a centrally acting antihypertensive agent with α_2-adrenoreceptor agonist properties. Peak plasma levels occur from 1 to 4 hours (mean, 2.6 hours) after ingestion. Average plasma half-life is about 17 hours; younger subjects tend to metabolize guanfacine more rapidly, however. Steady-state blood levels usually occur within 4 days. The only FDA-approved indication for guanfacine hydrochloride is the treatment of hypertension. Its use is not recommended in children under the age of 12 years because its safety and efficacy have not been proven in this age range.

Dose Forms Available
• Tablets: 1 mg, 2 mg
    Because of possible rebound phenomena, guanfacine should be tapered gradually when discontinued.

REPORTS OF INTEREST

Guanfacine in the Treatment of Attention-Deficit/ Hyperactivity Disorder

Guanfacine appears to have potential advantages over clonidine in the treatment of ADHD because it has a longer plasma half-life and appears to be less sedating (Hunt el al., 1995).

Hunt et al. (1995) treated, with guanfacine, 13 subjects (11 males, 2 females; age range, 4 to 20 years; mean, 11.1 years) who were diagnosed with ADHD. Guanfacine was begun at a dose of 0.5 mg/day and individually titrated by 0.5-mg increments every 3 days to achieve optimal clinical response to a maximum of 4 mg/day. Mean optimal dose was 3.5 mg/day (0.091 mg/kg/day). The most frequent optimal dose of 3.5 mg/day was usually administered in divided doses of 0.5 mg in the morning, at noon, and at approximately 4:00 PM, and 1.0 mg before bedtime. Parental ratings on the Conners 31-Item Parent Questionnaire at baseline and after 1 month of treatment with guanfacine showed a significant improvement on guanfacine in total average score ($P < .015$), Factor I (hyperactivity) ($P < .002$), Factor II (inattention) ($P < .004$), and Factor V (immaturity) ($P < .002$). In addition, scores on the following individual behavioral items of the Conners questionnaire were significantly improved while on guanfacine: less fidgety ($P < .002$), less restless ($P < .01$), making fewer disruptive sounds ($P < .01$), less easily frustrated ($P < .005$), less anxious ($P < .005$), less excessive energy ($P < .01$), better able to finish projects ($P < .005$), more attentive ($P < .01$), functional with less supervision ($P < .025$), were less rejected and unpopular in social groups ($P < .01$), less uncooperative ($P < .05$), and less constricted or rigid ($P < .01$). Untoward effects included significant initial tiredness on guanfacine compared with baseline ($P < .01$), which resolved within 2 weeks. Headaches and stomachaches were reported by about 25% of subjects but resolved within 2 weeks except in 1 patient. Decreased appetite occurred initially in 16% of the subjects but stabilized within 2 weeks. No subjects had clinically significant changes in blood pressure.

Guanfacine in the Treatment of ADHD and Tourette's Disorder

Chappell et al. (1995) reported an open study of 10 subjects, aged 8 to 16 years, who were diagnosed with ADHD and Tourette's syndrome and treated with guanfacine. Two subjects received other psychoactive medications concurrently. An initial bedtime dose of 0.5 mg of guanfacine was titrated upward in 0.5-mg increments every 3 to 4 days and was given in two or three divided doses. Daily doses ranged from 0.75 to 3 mg; optimal daily dose was 1.5 mg for 7 of the subjects. Although analysis of the group data did not show significant improvement in ADHD symptoms, 3 subjects had moderate and 1 had marked improvement based on ratings on the 48-item Conners' Parent Rating Scale. Group means measuring the severity of motor and phonic tics decreased in ratings by clinicians and patients themselves. The most common untoward effects were lethargy or fatigue (60%), headache (40%), insomnia (30%), and dizziness or light headednesss (20%); these symptoms usually remitted over 3 to 4 days. No children experienced clinically significant exacerbation of tics. Guanfacine may be a useful drug for some children and adolescents who have comorbid ADHD and a chronic tic disorder.

Horrigan and Barnhill (1995) administered guanfacine to 15 treatment resistant boys (age range, 7 to 17 years; mean, 13.3 years) diagnosed with ADHD. Most subjects also were diagnosed with comorbid psychiatric disorders including Tourette's disorder (N = 8) and specific developmental disorders (N = 11). Overall, the subjects had a mean of 3.46 Axis I and Axis II diagnoses. Subjects failed to respond satisfactorily to a mean of 2.0 prior medications including dextroamphetamine, methylphenidate, clonidine, imipramine, fluoxetine, carbamazepine, lithium, haloperidol, thryoid hormone, tryptophan, and biotin. Guanfacine was initiated with a 0.5-mg dose at bedtime and increased every 5 to 7 days by 0.25- to 0.5-mg increments as clinically indicated. Because the pediatric population metabolizes guanfacine more rapidly than adults, it was administered in two divided doses. After 10 weeks, the range of optimal doses was from 0.5 mg to 3 mg/day with 0.5 mg twice daily being the most frequent optimal dose. Thirteen subjects received guanfacine only; one subject additionally received lithium carbonate 1800 mg/day, and another received fluoxetine 10 mg/day.

Overall, guanfacine produced a significant clinical response. Parental ratings, made 4 to 8 weeks after the dose was stabilized on the 13 subjects who completed the study, showed a decrease on the Conner Parent-Teacher Scale (short form) of 11.1 points (from 19.9 to 8.8); on the Edelbrock CAP Inattention Subscale of 4.85 points; and on the Edelbrock CAP Overactivity Subscale of 3.23. The authors noted that the greater improvement in inattention compared with overactivity is the opposite of the pattern often seen with clonidine; they thought that this reversal might be explained by guanfacine's having a greater affinity for α-2 adrenoreceptors in the prefrontal areas compared with clonidine's having a greater affinity for the α-2 adrenoreceptors in more basal regions (Horrigan & Barnhill, 1995). One subject did not complete the trial because his mother discontinued the medication because of lack of improvement and another because he developed symptoms of overactivation/overarousal. The only other untoward effects noted were initial mild sedation in 5 boys. No patient experienced a significant change in blood pressure or pulse.

Barbiturates and Hypnotics

At the present time, the barbiturates and hypnotics have little, if any, place in treating psychiatric disorders in children and adolescents. Today, barbiturates, especially phenobarbital, are used in children and adolescents primarily for their antiepileptic properties. Behaviorally disordered children frequently may worsen when given barbiturates. As long ago as 1939, Cutts and Jasper administered phenobarbital to 12 behavior problem children with abnormal EEGs. Behavior worsened in 9 (75%), with increased irritability, impulsivity, destructiveness, and temper tantrums. The authors concluded that phenobarbital was contraindicated in the treatment of such children. For sleep disorders, diphenhydramine and benzodiazepines, which are much safer to use, are now the drugs of choice.

Clinically, barbiturates have a disinhibiting and disorganizing effect on many psychiatrically disturbed children, including psychotic children. Cognitive dulling, an untoward effect of barbiturates, is also of major concern in children and adolescents. In adults, phenobarbital was found to decrease speed of access to information in short-term memory, and short-term memory itself was highly sensitive to phenobarbital levels (MacLeod et al., 1978). The authors noted this effect could impair the ability of children and adolescents to maintain attention in the classroom and interfere with their learning new information.

Clinically, it is also important for the child and adolescent psychiatrist to remember that phenobarbital may contribute to disturbed behavior in some patients with seizure disorder in whom it is being used to control seizures. This is also the case in some younger children when phenobarbital is being used prophylactically (e.g., after febrile seizures). Some such children may show behavioral and cognitive improvement when they are switched to other antiepileptic medications.

REFERENCES

Adler L, Angrist B, Peselow E, Corwin J, Maslansky R, Rotrosen J. A controlled assessment of propranolol in the treatment of neuroleptic-induced akathisia. Br J Psychiatry 1986;149:42–45.

Adler LA, Peselow E, Rotrosen J, Duncan E, Lee M, Rosenthal M, Angrist B. Vitamin E treatment of tardive dyskinesia. Am J Psychiatry 1993;150:1405–1407.

Alexandris A, Lundell FW. Effect of thioridazine, amphetamine and placebo on the hyperkinetic syndrome and cognitive area in mentally deficient children. Can Med Assoc J 1968;98:92–96.

Allen RP, Safer D, Covi L. Effects of psychostimulants on aggression. J Nerv Ment Dis 1975;160:138–145.

Altamura AC, Montgomery SA, Wernicke JF. The evidence for 20 mg a day of fluoxetine as the optimal dose in the treatment of depression. Br J Psychiatry 1988; 153(suppl 3):109–112.

Alvir JMJ, Lieberman JA, Safferman AZ, Schwimmer JL, Schaaf JA. Clozapine-induced agranulocytosis: Incidence and risk factors in the United States. N Engl J Med 1993;329:162–167.

Aman MG, Kern RA. Review of fenfluramine in the treatment of the developmental disorders. Am Acad Child Adolesc Psychiatry 1989;28:549–565.

Aman MG, Marks RE, Turbott SH, Wilsher CP, Merry SN. Clinical effects of methylphenidate and thioridazine in intellectually subaverage children. J Am Acad Child Adolesc Psychiatry 1991a;30:246–256.

Aman MG, Marks RE, Turbott SH, Wilsher CP, Merry SN. Methylphenidate and thioridazine in the treatment of intellectually subaverage children: Effects on cognitive-motor performance. J Amer Acad Child Adolesc Psychiatry 1991b;30:816–824.

Aman MG, Singh NN. Preface. In: Aman MG, Singh NN, eds. Psychopharmacology of the developmental disabilities. New York: Springer-Verlag, 1988:v–ix.

Ambrosini PJ. Pharmacotherapy in child and adolescent major depressive disorder. In: Meltzer HY, ed. Psychopharmacology: The third generation of progress. New York: Raven Press, 1987:1247–1254.

Ambrosini PJ, Bianchi MD, Rabinovich H, Elia J: Antidepressant treatments in children and adolescents I. Affective disorders. J Am Acad Child Adolesc Psychiatry 1993;32:1–6.

American Academy of Child and Adolescent Psychiatry (AACAP). Desipramine and sudden death. Ad hoc committee on DMI [desipramine] and sudden death (J. Bie-

derman, chair). Washington, DC, 1992 Member Forum, 1992 AACAP Program, p. 8.
American Medical Association. Drug evaluations. 6th ed. Chicago: American Medical Association, 1986.
American Medical Association. Drug evaluations. Chicago: American Medical Association, 1990.
American Medical Association. Drug evaluations annual 1994. Chicago: American Medical Association, 1993.
American Psychiatric Association. Diagnostic and statistical manual of mental disorders. 2nd ed. (DSM-II). Washington, DC: American Psychiatric Association, 1968.
American Psychiatric Association. Diagnostic and statistical manual of mental disorders. 3rd ed. (DSM-III). Washington, DC: American Psychiatric Association, 1980a.
American Psychiatric Association. Diagnostic and statistical manual of mental disorders. 3rd ed, rev. (DSM-III-R). Washington, DC: American Psychiatric Association, 1987.
American Psychiatric Association. Diagnostic and statistical manual of mental disorders. 4th ed. (DSM-IV). Washington, DC: American Psychiatric Association, 1994.
American Psychiatric Association. Tardive dyskinesia: Task force report 18. Washington, DC: American Psychiatric Association, 1980b.
American Psychiatric Association. Task Force on Tardive Dyskinesia. Tardive dyskinesia: A task force report of the American Psychiatric Association. Washington, DC: American Psychiatric Association, 1992.
Amery B, Minichiello MD, Brown GL. Aggression in hyperactive boys: Response to d-amphetamine. J Am Acad Child Psychiatry 1984;23:291–294.
Anderson LT, Campbell M, Grega DM, Perry R, Small AM, Green WH. Haloperidol in the treatment of infantile autism: Effects on learning and behavioral symptoms. Am J Psychiatry 1984;141;1195–1202.
Apter A, Ratzone G, King RA, Weizman A, Iancu I, Binder M, Riddle MA. Fluvoxamine open-label treatment of adolescent inpatients with obsessive-compulsive disorder or depression. J Am Acad Child Adolesc Psychiatry 1994;33:342–348.
Arnold LE, Huestis RD, Smeltzer DJ, Scheib J, Wemmer D, Colner G. Levoamphetamine vs. dextroamphetamine in minimal brain dysfunction. Arch Gen Psychiatry 1976;33:292–301.
Ayd FJ Jr. Social issues: Misuse and abuse In: Benzodiazepines 1980: Current update. Psychosomatics 1980;21(October suppl):21–25.
Baldessarini RJ. Drugs and the treatment of psychiatric disorders. In: Gilman AF, Rall TW, Nies AS, Taylor P, eds. Goodman and Gilman's The pharmacological basis of therapeutics. 8th ed. New York: Pergamon Press, 1990:383–435.
Baldessarini RJ, Stephens JH. Clinical pharmacology and toxicology of lithium salts. Arch Gen Psychiatry 1970;22:72–77.
Ballenger JC, Carek DJ, Steele JJ, Cornish-McTighe D. Three cases of panic disorder with agoraphobia in children. Am J Psychiatry 1989;146:922–924.
Bangs ME, Petti TA, Janus M-D. Fluoxetine-induced memory impairment in an adolescent. J Am Acad Child Adolesc Psychiatry 1994;33:1303–1306.
Barrickman L, Noyes R, Kuperman S, Schumacher E, Verda M. Treatment of ADHD with fluoxetine: A preliminary trial. J Amer Acad Child Adolesc Psychiatry 1991;30:762–767.

Benfield P, Heel RC, Lewis SP. Fluoxetine: A review of its pharmacodynamic and pharmacokinetic properties, and therapeutic efficacy in depressive illness. Drugs 1986;32:481–508.

Bennett WG, Korein J, Kalmijn M, Grega DM, Campbell M. Electroencephalogram and treatment of hospitalized aggressive children with haloperidol or lithium. Biol Psychiatry 1983;12:1427–1440.

Berg I, Hullin R, Allsopp M, O'Brien P, MacDonald R. Bipolar manic-depressive psychosis in early adolescence, a case report. Br J Psychiatry 1974;125:416–417.

Bergstrom RF, Lemberger L, Farid NA, Wolen RL. Clinical pharmacology and pharmacokinetics of fluoxetine: A review. Br J Psychiatry 1988;153(suppl 3):47–50.

Berney T, Kolvin I, Bhate SR, Garside RF, Jeans J, Kay B, Scarth L. School phobia: A therapeutic trial with clomipramine and short-term outcome. Br J Psychiatry 1981;138:110–118.

Bernstein GA, Carroll ME, Crosby RD, Perwien AR, Go FS, Benowitz NL. Caffeine effects on learning, performance, and anxiety in normal school-age children. J Am Acad Child Adolesc Psychiatry 1994;33:407–415.

Bernstein JG. Handbook of drug therapy in psychiatry. 2nd ed. Littleton, MA: PSG Publishing, 1988.

Bevan P, Cools AR, Archer T. Behavioural pharmacology of 5-HT. Hillsdale, NJ: Lawrence Erlbaum, 1989.

Biederman J, Baldessarini RJ, Goldblatt A, Lapey KA, Doyle A, Hesslein PS: A naturalistic study of 24-hour electrocardiographic recordings and echocardiographic findings in children and adolescents treated with desipramine. J Am Acad Child Adolesc Psychiatry 1993;32:805–813.

Biederman J, Baldessarini RJ, Wright V, Knee D, Harmatz JS. A double-blind placebo controlled study of desipramine in the treatment of ADD: I. Efficacy. J Am Acad Child Adolesc Psychiatry 1989a;28:777–784.

Biederman J, Baldessarini RJ, Wright V, Knee D, Harmatz JS, Goldblatt A. A double-blind placebo controlled study of desipramine in the treatment of ADD: II. Serum drug levels and cardiovascular findings. J Am Acad Child Adolesc Psychiatry 1989b;28:903–911.

Biederman J, Gastfriend DR, Jellinek MS. Desipramine in the treatment of children with attention deficit disorder. J Clin Psychopharmacol 1986;6:359–363.

Birmaher B, Baker R, Kapur S, Quintant H, Ganguli R. Clozapine for the treatment of adolescents with schizophrenia. J Am Acad Child Adolesc Psychiatry 1992;31: 160–164.

Birmaher B, Greenhill LL, Cooper TB, Fried J, Maminski B. Sustained release methylphenidate: Pharmacokinetic studies in ADDH males. J Am Acad Child Adolesc Psychiatry 1989;28:568–772.

Birmaher B, Quintana H, Greenhill LL. Methylphenidate treatment of hyperactive autistic children. J Am Acad Child Adolesc Psychiatry 1988;27:248–251.

Birmaher B, Waterman GS, Ryan N, Cully M, Balach L, Ingram J, Brodsky M. Fluoxetine for childhood anxiety disorders. J Am Acad Child Adolesc Psychiatry 1994;33:993–999.

Black B, Uhde TW. Treatment of elective mutism with fluoxetine: A double-blind, placebo-controlled study. J Am Acad Child Adolesc Psychiatry 1994;33:1000–1006.

Blanz B, Schmidt MH. Clozapine for schizophrenia [letter]. J Am Acad Child Adolesc Psychiatry 1993;32:223–224.

Borison RL, Pathiraja AP, Diamond BI, Meibach RC. Risperidone: Clinical safety and efficacy in schizophrenia. Psychopharmacol Bull 1992;28:213–218.

Boulos C, Kutcher S, Gardner D, Young E. An open naturalistic trial of fluoxetine in adolescents and young adults with treatment-resistant major depression. J Child Adolesc Psychopharmacol 1992;2:103–111.

Boulos C, Kutcher S, Marton P, Simeon J, Ferguson B, Roberts N. Response to desipramine treatment in adolescent major depression. Psychopharmacol Bull 1991; 27:59–65.

Bowden CL, Sarabia F. Diagnosing manic-depressive illness in adolescents. Compr Psychiatry 1980;21:263–269.

Bradley C. The behavior of children receiving Benzedrine. Am J Psychiatry 1937;94: 577–585.

Breitner C. An approach to the treatment of juvenile delinquency. Ariz Med 1962;19: 82–87.

Brown S-LB, van Praag HM, eds. The role of serotonin in psychiatric disorders. New York: Brunner/Mazel, 1991.

Bruun R. TSA medical update: Treatment with clonidine. Tourette Syndrome Assoc Newsletter, Spring 1983.

Buitellar JK, van der Gaag RJ, Swaab-Barneveld, H, Kuipers M. A placebo-controlled comparison of methylphenidate and pinlolol in ADHD. American Academy of Child and Adolescent Psychiatry: Scientific Proceedings of the 41st Annual Meeting, New York, NY, October 25–30, 1994, New Research NR-6, 1994a;X:43.

Buitellar JK, van der Gaag RJ, Swaab-Barneveld, H, Kuipers M. Side effects of pindolol, a beta-blocker, in ADHD. American Academy of Child and Adolescent Psychiatry: Scientific Proceedings of the 41st Annual Meeting, New York, NY, October 25–30, 1994, New Research NR-7, 1994b;X:43.

Burke P, Puig-Antich J. Psychobiology of childhood depresssion. In: Lewis M, Miller SM, eds. Handbook of developmental psychopathology. New York: Plenum Press, 1990:327–339.

Burke RE, Fahn S, Jankovic J, et al. Tardive dystonia: Late-onset and persistent dystonia caused by antipsychotic drugs. Neurology 1982;32:1335–1346.

Cameron OG, Thyer BA. Treatment of pavor nocturnus with alprazolam. J Clin Psychiatry 1985;46:504.

Campbell M, Adams P, Small AM, Curren EL, Overall JE, Anderson LT, Lynch N, Perry R. Efficacy and safety of fenfluramine in autistic children. J Am Acad Child Adolesc Psychiatry 1988;27:434–439.

Campbell M, Anderson LT, Small AT, Adams P, Gonzalez NM, Ernst M. Naltrexone in autistic children: Behavioral symptoms and attentional learning. J Am Acad Child Adolesc Psychiatry 1993;32:1283–1291.

Campbell M, Anderson LT, Small AM, Locascio JJ, Lynch NS, Choroco MC. Naltrexone in autistic children: A double-blind and placebo-controlled study. Psychopharmacol Bull 1990;26:130–135.

Campbell M, Green WH, Deutsch SI. Child and adolescent psychopharmacology. Beverly Hills, CA: Sage, 1985.

Campbell M, Overall JE, Small AM, Sokol MS, Spencer EK, Adams P, Foltz RL, Monti KM, Perry R, Nobler M, Roberts E. Naltrexone in autistic children: An acute open dose range tolerance trial. J Am Acad Child Adolesc Psychiatry 1989;28: 200–206.

Campbell M, Perry R, Green WH. The use of lithium in children and adolescents. Psychosomatics 1984a;25:95–106.

Campbell M, Small AM, Green WH, Jennings SJ, Perry R, Bennett WG, Anderson L. Behavioral efficacy of haloperidol and lithium carbonate: A comparison in hospitalized aggressive children with conduct disorder. Arch Gen Psychiatry 1984b;41: 650–656.

Carlson GA, Rapport MD, Pataki CS, Kelly KL. Lithium in hospitalized children at 4 and 8 weeks: Mood, behavior and cognitive effects. J Child Psychol Psychiatry 1992;33:411–425.

Carlson GA, Strober M. Manic-depressive illness in early adolescence. J Am Acad Child Psychiatry 1978;17:138–153.

Casat CD, Pleasants DZ, Schroeder DH, Parler DW. Bupropion in children with attention deficit disorder. Psychopharmacol Bull 1989;25:198–201.

Chappell PB, Riddle MA, Scahill L, Lynch KA, Schultz R, Arnsten A, Leckman JF, Cohen DJ. Guanfacine treatment of comorbid attention deficit hyperactivity disorder and Tourette's syndrome: Preliminary clinical experience. J Am Acad Child Adolesc Psychiatry 1995;34:in press.

Chatoor I, Wells KC, Conners CK, Seidel WT, Shaw D. The effects of nocturnally administered stimulant medication on EEG sleep and behavior in hyperactive children. J Am Acad Child Psychiatry 1983;22:337–342.

Chouinard G, Jones B, Remington G, Bloom D, Addington D, MacEwan GW, Labelle A, Beauclair L, Arnott W. A Canadian multicenter placebo-controlled study of fixed doses of risperidone and haloperidol in the treatment of chronic schizophrenic patients. J Clin Psychopharmacol 1993;13:25–40.

Cioli V, Corradino C, Piccinelli D, Rocchi MG, Valeri P. A comparative pharmacological study of trazodone, etoperidone, and 1-(m-chlorophenyl)piperazine. Pharmacol Res Commun 16:85–100, 1984.

Ciraulo DA, Shader RI, Greenblatt DJ, Creelman W, eds. Drug interactions in psychiatry. Baltimore: Williams & Wilkins, 1989.

Clay TH, Gualtieri CT, Evans RW, Gullion CM. Clinical and neuropsychological effects of the novel antidepressant bupropion. Psychopharmacol Bull 1988;24: 143–148.

Clements SD. Minimal brain dysfunction in children: Terminology and identification, phase one of a three-phase project. Washington, DC: US Department of Health, Education, and Welfare, 1966. (NINDB monograph no. 3.)

Coccaro EF, Murphy DL, eds. Serotonin in psychiatric disorders. Washington, DC: American Psychiatric Press, 1990.

Coffey BJ. Anxiolytics for children and adolescents: Traditional and new drugs. J Child Adolesc Psychopharmacol 1990;1:57–83.

Coffey B, Shader RI, Greenblatt DJ. Pharmacokinetics of benzodiazepines and psychostimulants in children. J Clin Psychopharmacol 1983;3:217–225.

Cohen DJ, Detlor J, Young JG, Shaywitz BA. Clonidine ameliorates Gilles de la Tourette syndrome. Arch Gen Psychiatry 1980;37:1350–1357.

Comings DE. Tourette syndrome and human behavior. Duarte, CA: Hope Press, 1990.

Comings DE, Comings BG. Tourette's syndrome and attention deficit disorder with hyperactivity: Are they genetically related? J Am Acad Child Psychiatry 1984;23: 138–146.

Conners CK. Recent drug studies with hyperkinetic children. J Learning Disabilities 1971;4:476–483.

Conners CK, Kramer R, Rothschild GH, Schwartz L, Stone A. Treatment of young delinquent boys with diphenylhydantoin sodium and methylphenidate. Arch Gen Psychiatry 1971;24:156–160.

Conners CK, Taylor E, Meo G, Kurtz MA, Fournier M. Magnesium pemoline and dextroamphetamine: A controlled study in children with minimal brain dysfunction. Psychopharmacologia (Berlin) 1972;26:321–336. (Reprinted in Kline DF, Gettelman-Kline R, eds. Progress in drug treatment. New York, Brunner/Mazel, 1975:700–715.)

Cooper GL. The safety of fluoxetine—an update. Br J Psychiatry 1988;153(suppl 3):77–86.

Cozza SJ, Edison DL. Risperidone in adolescents [letter]. J Am Acad Child Adolesc Psychiatry 1994;33:1211.

Crumrine PK, Feldman HM, Teodori J, Handen BL, Alvin RM. The use of methylphenidate in children with seizures and attention deficit disorder. Ann Neurol 1987;22:441–442.

Cutts KK, Jasper HH. Effect of benzedrine sulfate and phenobarbital on behavior problem children with abnormal electroencephalograms. Arch Neurol Psychiatry 1939;411:1138–1145.

D'Amato G. Chlordiazepoxide in management of school phobia. Dis Nerv Sys 1962; 23:292–295.

DeGatta MF, Garcia MJ, Acosta A, Rey F, Gutierrez JR, Dominiquea-Gil A. Monitoring of serum levels of imipramine and desipramine and individuation of dose in enuretic children. Ther Drug Monit 1984;6:438–443.

DeLong GR, Aldershof AL. Long-term experience with lithium treatment in childhood: Correlation with clinical diagnosis. J Am Acad Child Adolesc Psychiatry 1987;26:389–394.

Denckla MB, Bemporad JR, MacKay MC. Tics following methylphenidate administration: A report of 20 cases. JAMA 1976;235:1349–1351.

Deutsch SI. Rationale for the administration of opiate antagonists in treating infantile autism. Am J Ment Deficiency 1986;90:631–635.

DeVeaugh-Geiss MD, Moroz G, Biederman J, Cantwell D, Fontaine R, Greist JH, Reichler R, Katz R, Landau P. Clomipramine hydrochloride in childhood and adolescent obsessive-compulsive disorder—a multicenter trial. J Am Acad Child Adolesc Psychiatry 1992;31:45–49.

Donnelly M, Rapoport JL, Potter WZ, Oliver J, Keysor CS, Murphy DL. Fenfluramine and dextroamphetamine treatment of childhood hyperactivity. Arch Gen Psychiatry 1989;46:205–212.

Donnelly M, Zametkin AJ, Rapoport JL, Ismond DR, Weingartner H, Lane E, Oliver J, Linnoila M, Potter WZ. Treatment of childhood hyperactivity with desipramine: Plasma drug concentration, cardiovascular effects, plasma and urinary catecholamine levels, and clinical response. Clin Pharmacol Ther 1986;39:72–81.

Dostal T. Antiaggressive effect of lithium salts in mentally retarded adolescents. In: Annell A-L, ed. Depressive states in childhood and adolescence. Stockholm: Almqvist & Wiksell, 1972:491–498.

Drug facts and comparisons. 49th ed. St. Louis: Facts and Comparisons, 1995.

Drug interactions and side effects index. Oradell, NJ: Medical Economics, 1995.

Dubovsky SL. Severe nortriptyline intoxication due to change from a generic to a trade preparation. J Nerv Ment Dis 1987;175:115–117.

Dugas M, Zarifian E, Leheuzey M-F, Rovei V, Durand G, Morselli PL. Preliminary observations of the significance of monitoring tricyclic antidepressant plasma levels in the pediatric patient. Ther Drug Monit 1980;2:307–314.

Duncan MK. Using psychostimulants to treat behavioral disorders of children and adolescents. J Child Adolesc Psychopharmacol 1990;1:7–20.

DuPaul GJ, Barkley RA, McMurray MB. Response of children with ADHD to methylphenidate: Interaction with internalizing symptoms. J Am Acad Child Adolesc Psychiatry 1994;33:894–903.

Effron AS, Freedman AM. The treatment of behavioral disorders in children with Benadryl. J Pediatr 1953;42:261–266.

Elia J, Borcherding BG, Rapoport JL, Kaysor CS. Methylphenidate and dextroamphetamine treatments of hyperactivity: Are there true nonresponders? Psychiatry Res 1991;36:141–155.

Elliott GR, Popper CW. Tricyclic antidepressants: The QT interval and other cardiovascular parameters [editorial]. J Child Adolesc Psychopharmacol 1990/1991;1: 187–189.

Evans RW, Clay TH, Gualtieri CT. Carbamazepine in pediatric psychiatry. J Am Acad Child Adolesc Psychiatry 1987;26:2–8.

Famularo R, Kinscherff R, Fenton T. Propranolol treatment for childhood posttraumatic stress disorder, acute type. Am J Dis Child 1988;142:1244–1247.

Feighner JP, Cohen JB: Analysis of individual symptoms in generalized anxiety—a pooled, multi-study double-blind evaluation of buspirone. Neuropsychobiology 1989;21:124–130.

Ferguson HB, Simeon JG. Evaluating drug effects on children's cognitive functioning. Progr Neuro-psychopharmacol Biol Psychiatry 1984;8:683–686.

Fish B. Drug therapy in child psychiatry: Pharmacological aspects. Compr Psychiatry 1960;1:212–227.

Fisher S. Child research in psychopharmacology. Springfield, IL: Charles C Thomas, 1959.

Fitzpatrick PA, Klorman R, Brumaghim JT, Borgstedt AD. Effects of sustained-release and standard preparations of methylphenidate on attention deficit disorder. J Am Acad Child Adolesc Psychiatry 1992;31:226–234.

Flament MF, Rapoport JL, Berg CJ, Sceery W, Kilts C, Mellström B, Linnoila M. Clomipramine treatment of childhood obsessive-compulsive disorder: A double blind controlled study. Arch Gen Psychiatry 1985;42:977–983.

Flament MF, Rapoport JL, Murphy DL, Berg CJ, Lake CR. Biochemical changes during clomipramine treatment of childhood obsessive-compulsive disorder. Arch Gen Psychiatry 1987;44:219–225.

Fleischhacker WW, Bergmann KJ, Perovich R, et al. The Hillside Akathisia Scale: A new rating instrument for neuroleptic-induced akathisia. Psychopharmacol Bull 1989;25:222–226.

Fras I. Trazodone and violence [letter]. J Am Acad Child Adolesc Psychiatry 1987; 26:453.

Frazier JA, Gordon CT, McKenna K, Lenane MC, Jih D, Rapoport JL. An open trial of clozapine in 11 adolescents with child-onset schizophrenia. J Am Acad Child Adolesc Psychiatry 1994;33:658–663.

Fritz GK, Rockney RM, Yeung AS. Plasma levels and efficacy of imipramine treatment for enuresis. J Am Acad Child Adolesc Psychiatry 1994;33:60–64.

Gadow KD. Children on medication: Vol. I. Hyperactivity, learning disabilities, and mental retardation. San Diego: College-Hill Press, 1986a.

Gadow KD. Children on medication: Vol. II. Epilepsy, emotional disturbance, and adolescent disorders. San Diego: College-Hill Press, 1986b.

Gadow KD, Nolan EE, Sverd J. Methylphenidate in hyperactive boys with comorbid tic disorder: II. Short-term behavioral effects in school settings. J Am Acad Child Adolesc Psychiatry 1992;31:462–471.

Gadow KD, Poling AG. Pharmacotherapy and mental retardation. Boston: College-Hill Press, 1988.

Gammon GD, Brown TE: Fluoxetine and methylphenidate in combination for treatment of attention deficit disorder and comorbid depressive disorder. J Child Adolesc Psychopharmacology 1993;3:1–10.

Garfinkel BD, Wender PH, Sloman L, O'Neill I. Tricyclic antidepressant and methylphenidate treatment of attention deficit disorder in children. J Am Acad Child Psychiatry 1983;22:343–348.

Gastfriend DR, Biederman J, Jellinek MS: Desipramine in the treatment of adolescents with attention deficit diosrder. Am J Psychiatry 1984;141:906–908.

Geller, B. Commentary on unexplained deaths of children on Norpramin. J Am Acad Child Adolesc Psychiatry 1991;30:682–684.

Geller B, Carr LG. Similarities and differences between adult and pediatric major depressive disorders. In: Georgotas A, Cancro R, eds. Depression and mania. New York: Elsevier, 1988:565–580.

Geller B, Cooper TB, Carr LG, Warham JE, Rodriguez A. Prospective study of scheduled withdrawal from nortriptyline in children and adolescents. J Clin Psychopharmacol 1987a;7:252–254.

Geller B, Cooper TB, Chestnut EC, Anker JA, Price DT, Yates E. Child and adolescent nortriptyline single dose kinetics predict steady state plasma levels and suggested dose: Preliminary data. J Clin Psychopharmacol 1985;5:154–158.

Geller B, Cooper TB, Chestnut EC, Anker JA, Schluchter MD. Preliminary data on the relationship between nortriptyline plasma level and response in depressed children. Am J Psychiatry 1986;143:1283–1286.

Geller B, Cooper TB, Graham DL, Fetner HH, Marsteller FA, Wells JM. Pharmacokinetically designed double-blind placebo-controlled study of nortriptyline in 6- to 12-year-olds with major depressive disorder. J Am Acad Child Adolesc Psychiatry 1992:31:34–44.

Geller B, Cooper TB, Graham DL, Marsteller FA, Bryant DM. Double-blind placebo-controlled study of nortriptyline in depressed adolescents using a "fixed plasma level" design. Psychopharmacol Bull 1990;26:85–90.

Geller B, Cooper TB, McCombs HG, Graham D, Wells J. Double-blind placebo-controlled study of nortriptyline in depressed children using a "fixed plasma level" design. Psychopharmacol Bull 1989;25:101–108.

Geller B, Cooper TB, Schluchter MD, Warham JE, Carr LG. Child and adolescent nortriptyline single dose pharmacokinetic parameters: Final report. J Clin Psychopharmacol 1987b;7:321–323.

Geller B, Fox LW, Fletcher M. Effect of tricyclic antidepressants on switching to mania and on the onset of bipolarity in depressed 6- to 12-year-olds. J Am Acad Child Adolesc Psychiatry 1993;32:43–50.

Geller B, Guttmacher LB, Bleeg M. Coexistence of childhood onset pervasive developmental disorder and attention deficit disorder with hyperactivity. Am J Psychiatry 1981;138:388–389.

Ghaziuddin N, Alessi NE. An open clinical trial of trazodone in aggressive children. J Child and Adolescent Psychopharmacology 1992;2:291–297.

Gittelman-Klein R, Klein, D. Controlled imipramine treatment of school phobia. Arch Gen Psychiatry 1971;25:204–207.

Gittelman-Klein R, Klein DF, Katz S, Saraf KR, Pollack E. Comparative effects of methylphenidate and thioridazine in hyperkinetic children: I. Clinical results. Arch Gen Psychiatry 1976;33:1217–1231.

Glick BS, Schulman D, Turecki S. Diazepam (Valium) treatment in childhood sleep disorder. Dis Nerv Sys 1971;32:565–566.

Gordon CT, State RC, Nelson JE, Hamburger SD, Rapoport JL. A double-blind comparison of clomipramine, desipramine, and placebo in the treatment of autistic disorder. Arch Gen Psychiatry 1993;50:441–447.

Graae F, Milner J, Rizzotto L, Klein RG. Clonazepam in childhood anxiety disorders. J Am Acad Child Adolesc Psychiatry 1994;33:372–376.

Green WH. Pervasive developmental disorders. In: Kestenbaum CJ, Williams DT, eds. Handbook of clinical assessment of children and adolescents. Vol. 1. New York: New York University Press, 1988:469–498.

Green WH. Psychosocial dwarfism: Psychological and etiological considerations. In: Lahey BB, Kazdin AE, eds. Advances in clinical child psychology. Vol. 9. New York: Plenum Press, 1986:245–278.

Green WH. Schizophrenia with childhood onset. In: Kaplan HI, Sadock BJ, eds. Comprehensive textbook of psychiatry. 5th ed. Baltimore: Williams & Wilkins, 1989: 1975–1981.

Green WH. The treatment of attention-deficit hyperactivity disorder with nonstimulant medications. Child Adolesc Psychiatric Clin North Am 1995;4:169–195.

Green WH, Campbell M, Hardesty AS, Grega DM, Padron-Gayol M, Shell J, Erlenmeyer-Kimling L. A comparison of schizophrenic and autistic children. J Am Acad Child Psychiatry 1984;23:399–409.

Green WH, Deutsch SI. Biological studies of schizophrenia with childhood onset. In: Deutsch SI, Weizman A, Weizman R, eds. Application of basic neuroscience to child psychiatry. New York: Plenum Medical Book, 1990:217–229.

Green WH, Deutsch SI, Campbell M, Anderson LT. Neuropsychopharmacology of the childhood psychoses: A critical review. In: Morgan DW, ed. Psychopharmacology: Impact on clinical psychiatry. St. Louis: Ishiyaku EuroAmerica, 1985:139–173.

Green WH, Padron-Gayol M, Hardesty AS, Bassiri M. Schizophrenia with childhood onset: A phenomenological study of 38 cases. J Am Acad Child Adolesc Psychiatry 1992;31:968–976.

Greenblatt DJ, Shader RI. Benzodiazepines in clinical practice. New York: Raven Press, 1974.

Greenblatt DJ, Shader RI, Abernethy DR. Current status of benzodiazepines (first of two parts). N Engl J Med 1983;309:354–358.

Greenhill LL. Attention-deficit hyperactivity disorder in children. In: Garfinkel BD, Carlson GA, Weller EB, eds. Psychiatric disorders in children and adolescents. Philadelphia: WB Saunders, 1990:149–182.

Greenhill LL, Rieder RO, Wender PH, Bushsbaum M, Zahn TP. Lithium carbonate in the treatment of hyperactive children. Arch Gen Psychiatry 1973;28:636–640.

Greenhill LL, Solomon M, Pleak R, Ambrosini P. Molindone hydrochloride treatment of hospitalized children with conduct disorder. J Clin Psychiatry 1985;46(8):20–25.

Grizenko N, Vida S. Propranolol treatment of episodic dyscontrol and aggressive behavior in children [letter]. Can J Psychiatry 1988;33:776–778.

Groh C. The psychotropic effect of Tegretol in non-epileptic children, with particular reference to the drug's indications. In: Birkmayer W, ed. Epileptic seizures—behaviour—pain. Bern: Hans Huber Publishers, 1976:259–263.

Gross MD. Imipramine in the treatment of minimal brain dysfunction in children. Psychosomatics 1973;14:283–285.

Gross MD, Wilson WC. Minimal brain dysfunction. New York: Brunner/Mazel, 1974.

Gualtieri CT, Golden R, Evans RW, Hicks RE. Blood level measurement of psychoactive drugs in pediatric psychiatry. Ther Drug Monit 1984a;6:127–141.

Gualtieri CT, Golden RN, Fahs JJ. New developments in pediatric psychopharmacology. Dev Behav Pediatr 1983;4:202–209.

Gualtieri CT, Keenan PA, Chandler M: Clinical and neuropsychological effect on desipramine in children with attention deficit hyperactivity disorder. J Clin Psychopharmacol 1991;11:155–159.

Gualtieri CT, Quade D, Hicks RE, Mayo JP, Schroeder SR. Tardive dyskinesia and other clinical consequences of neuroleptic treatment in children and adolescents. Am J Psychiatry 1984b;141:20–23.

Gualtieri CT, Wafgin W, Kanoy R, Patrick K, Shen D, Youngblood W, Mueller R, Breese G. Clinical studies of methylphenidate serum levels in children and adults. J Am Acad Child Psychiatry 1982;21:19–26.

Hamill PVV, Drizd TA, Johnson CL, Reed RB, Roche AF. NCHS growth charts, 1976. Monthly Vital Statistics Reports 1976;25(suppl 3):1–22. (Health Examination Survey Data, National Center for Health Statistics Publication [HRA] 76–1120.)

Hayes PE, Schulz SC. Beta-blockers in anxiety disorders. J Affect Disord 1987;13: 119–130.

Hayes TA, Logan Panitch M, Marker E. Imipramine dosage in children: A comment on "imipramine and electrocardiographic abnormalities in hyperactive children." Am J Psychiatry 1975;132:546–547.

Hersh CB, Sokol MS, Pfeffer CR. Transient psychosis with fluoxetine [letter]. J Am Acad Child Adolesc Psychiatry 1991;31;851.

Herskowitz J. Developmental neurotoxicology. In: Popper C, ed. Psychiatric pharmacosciences of children and adolescents. Washington, DC: American Psychiatric Press, 1987:81–123.

Holzer JF. The process of informed consent. Bull Am Coll Surgeons 1989;74(9):10–14.

Horowitz HA. Lithium and the treatment of adolescent manic depressive illness. Dis Nerv Syst 1977;38:480–483.

Horrigan JP, Barnhill LJ. Guanfacine and treatment-resistant attention-deficit hyperactivity disorder in boys. J Child Adolesc Psychopharmacol 1995;5:in press.

Huessy HR, Wright AL: The use of imipramine in children's behavior disorders. Acta Paedopsychiatrica 1970;37:194–199.

Hunt RD. Treatment effects of oral and transdermal clonidine in relation to methylphenidate: An open pilot study in ADD-H. Psychopharmacol Bull 1987;23(1):111–114.

Hunt RD, Arnsten AFT, Asbell MD. An open trial of guanfacine in the treatment of attention-deficit hyperactivity disorder. J Am Acad Child Adolesc Psychiatry 1995; 34:50–54.

Hunt RD, Capper L, O'Connell P. Clonidine in child and adolescent psychiatry. J Child Adolesc Psychopharmacol 1990;1:87–102.

Hunt RD, Cohen DJ, Shaywitz SE, Shaywitz BA. Strategies for study of the neurochemistry of attention deficit disorder in children. Schizophr Bull 1982;8:236–252.

Hunt RD, Lau S, Ryu J. Alternative therapies for ADHD. In: Greenhill LL, Osamn BB, eds. Ritalin: Theory and patient management. New York: Mary Ann Liebert, 1991:75–95.

Hunt RD, Minderaa RB, Cohen DJ. Clonidine benefits children with attention deficit disorder and hyperactivity: Report of a double-blind placebo-crossover therapeutic trial. J Am Acad Child Psychiatry 1985;24:617–629.

Jafri AB. Fluoxetine side effects [letter]. J Am Acad Child Adolesc Psychiatry 1991;31;852.

Jain U, Birmaher B, Garcia M, Al-Shabbout M, Ryan N. Fluoxetine in children and adolescents with mood disorders: A chart review of efficacy and adverse effects. J Child Adolesc Psychopharmacol 1992;2:259–265.

Jann MW. Clozapine. Pharmacotherapy 1991;11:179–195.

Jaselskis CA, Cook EH, Fletcher KE, Leventhal BL. Clonidine treatment of hyperactive and impulsive children with autistic disorder. J Clin Psychopharmacol 1992;12:322–327.

Jatlow PI. Psychotropic drug disposition during development. In: Popper C, ed. Psychiatric pharmacosciences of children and adolescents. Washington, DC: American Psychiatric Press, 1987:27–44.

Jefferson JW, Greist JH, Ackerman DL, Carroll JA. Lithium encyclopedia for clinical practice. 2nd ed. Washington, DC: American Psychiatric Press, 1987.

Jefferson JW, Greist JH, Clagnaz PJ, Eischens RR, Marten WC, Evenson ME. Effect of strenuous exercise on serum lithium level in man. Am J Psychiatry 1982;139:1593–1595.

Jerome L. Hypomania with fluoxetine [letter]. J Am Acad Child Adolesc Psychiatry 1991;30:850–851.

Jeste DV, Wyatt RJ. Understanding and treating tardive dyskinesia. New York: Guilford Press, 1982.

Johnston C, Pelham WE, Hoza J, Sturges J. Psychostimulant rebound in attention deficit disordered boys. J Am Acad Child Adolesc Psychiatry 1988;27:806–810.

Joshi PT, Capozzoli JA, Coyle JT. Low-dose neuroleptic therapy for children with childhood-onset pervasive developmental disorder. Am J Psychiatry 1988;145:335–338.

Joshi PT, Walkup JT, Capozzoli JA, Detrinis RB, Coyle JT. The use of fluoxetine in the treatment of major depressive disorder in children and adolescents. Paper presented at the 36th Annual Meeting of the American Academy of Child and Adolescent Psychiatry, October 11–15, 1989, New York.

Kafantaris V, Campbell M, Padron-Gayol MV, Small AM, Locascio JJ, Rosenberg CR. Carbamazepine in hospitalized aggressive conduct disorder children: An open pilot study. Psychopharmacol Bull 1992;28:193–199.

Kallen B, Tandberg A. Lithium and pregnancy. Acta Psychiatr Scand 1983;68:134–139.

Kaplan SL, Simms RM, Busner J. Prescribing practices of outpatient child psychiatrists. J Am Acad Child Adolesc Psychiatry 1994;33:35–44.

Kashani JH, Shekim WO, Reid JC. Amitriptyline in children with major depressive disorder: A double-blind crossover pilot study. J Am Acad Child Psychiatry 1984;23:348–351.

Kastner T, Finesmith R, Walsh K. Long-term administration of valproic acid in the treatment of affective symptoms in people with mental retardation. J Clin Psychopharmacol 1993;13:448–451.

Kastner T, Friedman DL, Plummer AT, Ruiz MQ, Henning D. Valproic acid for the treatment of children with mental retardation and mood symptomatology. Pediatrics 1990;86:467–472.

Kaufmann CA, Wyatt RJ. Neuroleptic malignant syndrome. In: Meltzer HY, ed. Psychopharmacology: The third generation of progress. New York: Raven Press, 1987:1421–1430.

Kemph JP, DeVane CL, Levin GM, Jarecke R, Miller RL. Treatment of aggressive children with clonidine: Results of an open pilot study. J Am Acad Child Adolesc Psychiatry 1993;32:577–581.

Kessler AJ, Barklage NE, Jefferson JW. Mood disorders in the psychoneurological borderland: Three cases of responsiveness to carbamazepine. Am J Psychiatry 1989;146:81–83.

King RA, Riddle MA, Chappell PB, Hardin MT, Anderson GM, Lombroso P, Scahill L. Emergence of self-destructive phenomena in children and adolescents during fluoxetine treatment. J Am Acad Child Adolesc Psychiatry 1991;30:179–186

Klein DF, Gittelman R, Quitkin F, Rifkin A. Diagnosis and drug treatment of psychiatric disorders: Adults and children. Baltimore: Williams & Wilkins, 1980.

Klein RG. Pharmacotherapy of childhood hyperactivity: An update. In: Meltzer HY, ed. Psychopharmacology: The third generation of progress. New York, Raven Press, 1987:1215–1224.

Klein RG: Thioridazine effects on the cognitive performance of children with attention-deficit hyperactivity disorder. J Child Adolesc Psychopharmacol, 1990–1991; 1:263–270.

Klein RG, Koplewicz HS, Kanner A. Imipramine treatment of children with separation anxiety disorder. Am J Acad Child Adolesc Psychiatry 1992;31:21–28.

Klein RG, Landa B, Mattes JA, Klein DF. Methylphenidate and growth in hyperactive children: A controlled withdrawal study. Arch Gen Psychiatry 1988;45: 1127–1130.

Klein RG, Last CG. Anxiety disorders in children. Newbury Park, CA: Sage, 1989.

Klein RG, Mannuzza S. Hyperactive boys almost grown up: III. Methylphenidate effects on ultimate height. Arch Gen Psychiatry 1988;45:1131–1134.

Kline AH. Diazepam and the management of nocturnal enuresis. Clin Med 1968;75: 20–22.

Klorman R, Brumaghim JT, Salzman LF, Strauss J, Borgstedt AD, McBride MC, Loeb S. Effects of methylphenidate on attention-deficit hyperactivity disorder with and without aggressive/noncompliant features. J Abnorm Psychol 1988a;97:413–422.

Klorman R, Coons HW, Brumaghim JT, Borgstedt AD, Fitzpatrick P. Stimulant treatment for adolescents with attention deficit disorder. Psychopharmacol Bull 1988b;24:88–92.

Korein J, Fish B, Shapiro T, Gehner EW, Levidon L. EEG and behavioral effects of drug therapy in children: Chlorpromazine and diphenhydramine. Arch Gen Psychiatry 1971;24:552–563.

Kraft IA, Ardall C, Duffy JH, Hart JT, Pearce P. A clinical study of chlordiazepoxide used in psychiatric disorders of children. Int J Neuropsychiatry 1965;1:433–437.

Krakowski AJ. Chlordiazepoxide in treatment of children with emotional disturbances. N Y State J Med 1963;63:3388–3392.

Krakowski AJ. Amitriptyline in treatment of hyperkinetic children. Psychosomatics 1965;6:355–360.

Kramer AD, Feiguine RJ. Clinical effects of amitriptyline in adolescent depression: A pilot study. J Am Acad Child Psychiatry 1981;20:636–644.

Kranzler HR. Use of buspirone in an adolescent with overanxious disorder. J Am Acad Child Adolesc Psychiatry 1988;27:789–790.

Kuhn-Gebhart V. Behavioural disorders in non-epileptic children and their treatment with carbamazepine. In: Birkmayer W, ed. Epileptic seizures—behaviour—pain. Bern: Hans Huber Publishers, 1976:264–267.

Kuperman S, Stewart MA. Use of propranolol to decrease aggressive outbursts in younger patients. Psychosomatics 1987;28:315–319.

Kutcher S, Boulos C, Ward B, Marton P, Simeon J, Ferguson HB, Szalai J, Katic M, Roberts N, Dubois C, Reed K. Response to desipramine treatment in adolescent depression: A fixed-dose, placebo-controlled trial. J Am Acad Child Adolesc Psychiatry 1994;33:686–694.

Kutcher SP, MacKenzie S. Successful clonazepam treatment of adolescents with panic disorder [letter]. J Clin Psychopharmacol 1988;8:299–301.

Kutcher SP, MacKenzie S, Galarraga W, Szalai J. Clonazepam treatment of adolescents with neuroleptic-induced akathisia. Am J Psychiatry 1987;144:823–824.

Kutcher SP, Marton P, Korenblum M. Adolescent bipolar illness and personality disorder. J Am Acad Child Adolesc Psychiatry 1990;29:355–358.

Lader M. Fluoxetine efficacy vs comparative drugs: An overview. Br J Psychiatry 1988:153(suppl 3):51–58.

Latz SR, McCracken JT. Neuroleptic malignant syndrome in children and adolescents: Two case reports and a warning. J Child Adolesc Psychopharmacol 1992;2: 123–129.

Leckman JF, Cohen DJ, Detlor J, Young JG, Harcherik D, Shaywitz BA. Clonidine in the treatment of Tourette syndrome: A review of data. In: Friedhoff AJ, Chase TN, eds. Gilles de la Tourette syndrome. New York: Raven Press, 1982:391–401.

Leckman JF, Detlor J, Harcherik DF, Ort S, Shaywitz BA, Cohen DJ. Short- and long-term treatment of Tourette's syndrome with clonidine: A clinical perspective. Neurology 1985;35:343–351.

Leckman JF, Hardin MT, Riddle MA, Stevenson J, Ort SI, Cohen DJ. Clonidine treatment of Gilles de la Tourette's syndrome. Arch Gen Psychiatry 1991;48:324–328.

Lefkowitz MM. Effects of diphenylhydantoin on disruptive behavior. Arch Gen Psychiatry 1969;20:643–651.

Lena B, Surtees SJ, Maggs R. The efficacy of lithium in the treatment of emotional disturbance in children and adolescents. In: Johnson FN, Johnson S, eds. Lithium in medical practice. Baltimore: University Park Press, 1978:79–83.

Leonard HL, Swedo SE, Lenane MC, Rettew DC, Cheslow DL, Hamburger SD, Rapoport JL. A double-blind desipramine substitution during long-term clomipramine treatment in children and adolescents with obsessive-compulsive disorder. Arch Gen Psychiatry 1991;48:922–927.

Leonard HL, Swedo SE, Rapoport JL, Koby EV, Lenane MC, Cheslow DL, Hamburger SD. Treatment of obsessive-compulsive disorder with clomipramine and desipramine in children and adolescents: A double-blind crossover comparison. Arch Gen Psychiatry 1989;46:1088–1092.

Leonard HL, Topol D, Bukstein O, Hindmarsh D, Allen AJ, Swedo SE. Clonazepam as an augmenting agent in the treatment of childhood-onset obsessive-compulsive disorder. J Am Acad Child Adolesc Psychiatry 1994;33:692–694.

Levin GM, Burton-Teston K, Murphy T. Development of precocious puberty in two children treated with clonidine for aggressive behavior. J Child Adolesc Psychopharmacol 1993;3:127–131.

Levkovitch Y, Kaysar N, Kronnenberg Y, Hagai H, Gaoni B. Clozapine for schizophrenia [letter]. J Am Acad Child Adolesc Psychiatry 1994;33:431.

Levy RH. Psychopharmacological interventions. In: Katz SE, Nardacci D, Sabatini A, eds. Intensive treatment of the homeless mentally ill. Washington, DC: American Psychiatric Press, 1993:129–165.

Linnoila M, Dejong J, Virkkunen M. Monoamines, glucose metabolism, and impulse control. Psychopharmacol Bull 1989;25:404–406.

Linnoila M, Gualtieri CT, Jobson K, Staye J. Characteristics of the therapeutic response to imipramine in hyperactive children. Am J Psychiatry 1979;136:1201–1203.

Looker A, Conners CK. Diphenylhydantoin in children with severe temper tantrums. Arch Gen Psychiatry 1970;23:80–89.

Lowe TL, Cohen DJ, Detlor J, Kremenitzer MW, Shaywitz BA. Stimulant medications precipitate Tourette's syndrome. JAMA 1982;247:1729–1931.

Lucas AR, Pasley FC. Psychoactive drugs in the treatment of emotionally disturbed children: Haloperidol and diazepam. Compr Psychiatry 1969;10:376–386.

MacLeod CM, Dekaban AS, Hunt E. Memory impairment in epileptic patients: Selective effects of phenobarbitol concentration. Science 1978;202:1102–1104.

Mandoki M. Clozapine for adolescents with psychosis: Literature review and two case reports. J Child Adolesc Psychopharmacol 1993;3:213–221.

Mann JJ, Marzuk PM, Arango V, McBride PA, Leon AC, Tierney H. Neurochemical studies of violent and nonviolent suicide. Psychopharmacol Bull 1989;25:407–413.

Mattes JA, Gittelman R: Growth of hyperactive children on maintenance regimen of methylphenidate. Arch Gen Psychiatry 1983;40:317–321.

McBride MC, Wang DD, Torres C. Methylphenidate in therapeutic doses does not lower seizure threshold. Ann Neurol 1986;20:428.

Meltzer, HY, ed. Psychopharmacology: The third generation of progress. New York: Raven Press, 1987.

Meyers B, Tune LE, Coyle JT. Clinical response and serum neuroleptic levels in childhood schizophrenia. Am J Psychiatry 1980;137:1459–1460.

Molitch M, Eccles AK. The effect of benzedrine sulfate on the intelligence scores of children. Am J Psychiatry 1937;94:587–590.

Molitch M, Poliakoff S. The effect of benzedrine sulfate on enuresis. Arch Pediatr 1937;54:499–501.

Molitch M, Sullivan JP. The effect of benzedrine sulfate on children taking the New Stanford Achievement Test. Am J Orthopsychiatry 1937;7:519–522.

Morselli PL, Bianchetti G, Dugas M. Therapeutic drug monitoring of psychotropic drugs in children. Pediatr Pharmacol 1983;3:149–156.

Mozes T, Toren P, Chernauzan N, Mester R, Yoran-Hegesh R, Blumensohn R, Weizman A. Clozapine treatment in very early onset schizophrenia. J Am Acad Child Adolesc Psychiatry 1994;33:65–70.

Myers WC, Carrera F III. Carbamazepine-induced mania with hypersexuality in a 9-year-old boy. Am J Psychiatry 1989;146:400.

Naruse H, Nagahata M, Nakane Y, Shirahashi K, Takesada M, Yamazaki K. A multicenter double-blind trial of pimozide (Orap), haloperidol and placebo in children with behavioral disorders, using crossover design. Acta Paedopsychiatr 1982;48:173–184.

National Institute of Mental Health/National Institutes of Health Consensus Development Panel. Mood disorders: Pharmacologic prevention of recurrences. Am J Psychiatry 1985;142:469–476.

Neppe VM, Ward NG. The evaluation and management of neuroleptic-induced acute extrapyramidal syndromes. In: Neppe VM, ed. Innovative psychopharmacology. New York: Raven Press, 1989:152–176.

New York State Department of Health. Safe, effective and therapeutically equivalent prescription drugs. 7th ed. Albany, NY: New York State Department of Health Office of Health Systems Management, 1988.

Newton JEO, Cannon DJ, Couch L, Fody EP, McMillan DE, Metzer WS, Paige SR,

Reid GM, Summers BN. Effects of repeated drug holidays on serum haloperidol concentration, psychiatric symptoms, and movement disorders in schizophrenic patients. J Clin Psychiatry 1989;50:132–135.

Noyes R. Beta-adrenergic blockers. In: Last CG, Hersen M, eds. Handbook of anxiety disorders. New York: Pergamon Press, 1988:445–459.

Nurcombe B. Malpractice. In: Lewis M, ed. Child and adolescent psychiatry: A comprehensive textbook. Baltimore: Williams & Wilkins, 1991:1127–1139.

Nurcombe B, Partlett DF. Child Mental Health and the Law. New York: Free Press, 1994:220–272.

Oxford English dictionary. Oxford; Oxford University Press, 1933.

Oxford English dictionary: A supplement to. Oxford: Oxford University Press, 1982.

Pangalila-Ratulangi EA. Pilot evaluation of Orap (Pimozide, R 6238) in child psychiatry. Psychiatr Neurol Neurochir 1973;76:17–27.

Pare CMB, Kline N, Hallstrom C, Cooper T. Will amitriptyline prevent the "cheese" reaction of monoamine oxidase inhibitors? Lancet 1982:183–186.

Pataki CS, Carlson GA, Kelly KL, Rapport MD, Biancaniello TM. Side effects of methylphenidate and desipramine alone and in combination in children. J Am Acad Child Adolesc Psychiatry 1993;32:1065–1072.

Patrick KS, Mueller RA, Gualtieri CT, Breese GR. Pharmacokinetics and actions of methylphenidate. In: Meltzer HY, ed. Psychopharmacology: The third generation of progress. New York: Raven Press, 1987:1387–1395.

Pelham WE, Bender ME, Caddell J, Booth S, Moorer SH. Methylphenidate and children with attention deficit disorder. Arch Gen Psychiatry 1985;42:948–952.

Pelham WE, Greenslade KE, Vodde-Hamilton M, Murphy DA, Greenstein JJ, Gnagy EM, Guthrie KJ, Hoover MD, Dahl RE. Relative efficacy of long-acting stimulants on children with attention deficit-hyperactivity disorder: A comparison of standard methylphenidate, sustained-release methylphenidate, sustained-release dextroamphetamine, and pemoline. Pediatrics 1990;86:226–237.

Pelham WE, Sturges J, Hoza JA, Schmidt C, Bijlsma JJ, Milich R, Moorer S. Sustained release and standard methylphenidate effects on cognitive and social behavior in children with attention deficit disorder. Pediatrics 1987;80:491–501.

Perry R, Campbell M, Adams P, Lynch N, Spencer EK, Curren EL, Overall JE. Long-term efficacy of haloperidol in autistic children: Continuous versus discontinuous drug administration. J Am Acad Child Adolesc Psychiatry 1989;28:87–92.

Perry R, Campbell M, Green WH, Small AM, DieTrill ML, Meiselas K, Golden RR, Deutsch SI. Neuroleptic-related dyskinesias in autistic children: A prospective study. Psychopharmacol Bull 1985;21:140–143.

Perry R, Campbell M, Grega DM, Anderson L. Saliva lithium levels in children: Their use in monitoring serum lithium levels and lithium side effects. J Clin Psychopharmacol 1984;4:199–202.

Pesikoff RB, Davis PC. Treatment of pavor nocturnus and somnambulism in children. Am J Psychiatry 1971;128:778–781.

Petti, TA, Fish B, Shapiro T, Cohen IL, Campbell M. Effects of chlordiazepoxide in disturbed children: A pilot study. J Clin Psychopharmacol 1982;2:270–273.

Pfefferbaum G, Overall JE, Boren HA, Frankel LS, Sullivan MR, Johnson K. Alprazolam in the treatment of anticipatory and acute situational anxiety in children with cancer. J Am Acad Child Adolesc Psychiatry 1987;26:532–535.

Physicians' desk reference (PDR). 44th ed. Oradell, NJ: Medical Economics, 1990.

Physicians' desk reference (PDR). 49th ed. Oradell, NJ: Medical Economics, 1995.

Platt JE, Campbell M, Green WH, Grega DM. Cognitive effect of lithium carbonate and haloperidol in treatment resistant aggressive children. Arch Gen Psychiatry 1984;41:657–662.

Pleak RR, Birmaher B, Gavrilescu A, Abichandani C, Williams DT. Mania and neuropsychiatric excitation following carbamazepine. J Am Acad Child Adolesc Psychiatry 1988;27:500–503.

Pliszka SR. Tricyclic antidepressants in the treatment of children with attention deficit disorder. J Amer Acad Child Adolesc Psychiatry 1987;26:127–132.

Pool D, Bloom W, Mielke DH, Roniger JJ, Gallant DM. A controlled evaluation of loxitane in seventy-five adolescent schizophrenic patients. Curr Ther Res 1976;19: 99–104.

Popper C. Medical unknown and ethical consent: Prescribing psychotropic medications for children in the face of uncertainty. In: Popper C, ed. Psychiatric pharmacosciences of children and adolescents. Washington, DC: American Psychiatric Press, 1987a.

Popper C, ed. Psychiatric pharmacosciences of children and adolescents. Washington, DC: American Psychiatric Press, 1987b.

Post RM. Mechanisms of action of carbamazepine and related anticonvulsants in affective illness. In: Meltzer HY, ed. Psychopharmacology: The third generation of progress. New York: Raven Press, 1987:567–576.

Potter WZ, Calil HM, Sutfin TA, Zavadil III AP, Jusko WJ, Rapoport J, Goodwin FK. Active metabolites of imipramine and desipramine in man. Clin Pharmacol Ther 1982;31:393–401.

Poussaint AF, Ditman KS. A controlled study of imipramine (Tofranil) in the treatment of childhood enuresis. J Pediatr 1965;67:283–290.

Preskorn SH, Bupp SJ, Weller EB, Weller RA. Plasma levels of imipramine and metabolites in 68 hospitalized children. J Am Acad Child Adolesc Psychiatry, 1989a;28:373–375.

Preskorn SH, Jerkovich GS, Beber JH, Widener P. Therapeutic drug monitoring of tricyclic antidepressants: A standard of care issue. Psychopharmacol Bull 1989b: 25:281–284.

Preskorn SH, Weller EB, Hughes CW, Weller RA, Bolte K. Depression in prepubertal children: Dexamethasone nonsuppression predicts differential response to imipramine vs. placebo. Psychopharmacol Bull 1987;23:128–133.

Preskorn SH, Weller E, Jerkovich G, Hughes CW, Weller R. Depression in children: Concentration dependent CNS toxicity of tricyclic antidepressants. Psychopharmacol Bull 1988;24:275–279.

Prien RF. Methods and models for placebo use in pharmacotherapeutic trials. Psychopharmacol Bull 1988;24:4–8.

Psychopharmacology Bulletin. Special issue: Pharmacotherapy of children. US Department of Health, Education, and Welfare, 1973. (Publication. no. [HSM] 73–9002.)

Puente RM. The use of carbamazepine in the treatment of behavioural disorders in children. In: Birkmayer W, ed. Epileptic seizures—behaviour—pain. Bern: Hans Huber Publishers, 1976:243–252.

Puig-Antich J. Major depression and conduct disorder in prepuberty. J Amer Acad Child Adolesc Psychiatry 1982;21:118–128.

Puig-Antich J. Affective disorders in children and adolescents: Diagnostic validity and psychobiology. In: Meltzer HY, ed. Psychopharmacology: The third generation of progress. New York: Raven Press, 1987:843–859.

Puig-Antich J, Perel JM, Lupatkin W, Chambers WJ, Tabrizi MA, King J, Goetz R, Davies M, Stiller RL. Imipramine in prepubertal major depressive disorders. Arch Gen Psychiatry 1987;44:81–89.

Quiason H, Ward D, Kitchen T: Buspirone for aggression [letter]. J Am Acad Child Adolesc Psychiatry 1991;30:1026.

Quinn PO, Rapoport JL. One-year follow-up of hyperactive boys treated with imipramine or methylphenidate. Am J Psychiatry 1975;132:241–245.

Rall TW. Hypnotics and sedatives; ethanol. In: Gilman AF, Rall TW, Nies AS, Taylor P, eds. Goodman and Gilman's the pharmacological basis of therapeutics. 8th ed. New York: Pergamon Press, 1990:345–382.

Rapoport JL. Clozapine and child psychiatry [editorial]. J Child Adolesc Psychopharmacol 1994;4:1–3.

Rapoport JL, Buchsbaum MS, Weingartner H, Zahn TP, Ludlow C, Mikkelsen EJ. Dextroamphetamine: Its cognitive and behavioral effects in normal and hyperactive boys and normal men. Arch Gen Psychiatry 1980a;37:933–943.

Rapoport JL, Buchsbaum MS, Zahn TP, Weingartner H, Ludlow C, Mikkelsen EJ. Dextroamphetamine: Cognitive and behavioral effects in normal prepubertal boys. Science 1978a;199:560–563.

Rapoport JL, Mikkelsen EJ. Antidepressants. In: Werry JS, ed. Pediatric psychopharmacology: The use of behavior modifying drugs in children. New York: Brunner/Mazel, 1978b:208–233.

Rapoport JL, Mikkelsen EJ, Werry JS. Antimanic, antianxiety, hallucinogenic and miscellaneous drugs. In: Werry JS, ed. Pediatric psychopharmacology: The use of behavior modifying drugs in children. New York: Brunner/Mazel, 1978c:316–355.

Rapoport JL, Mikkelsen EJ, Zavadil A, Nee L, Gruenau C, Mendelson W, Gillin JC. Childhood enuresis: Psychopathology, plasma tricyclic concentration and antienuretic effect. Arch Gen Psychiatry 1980b;37:1146–1152.

Rapoport JL, Quinn PO, Bradbard G, Riddle D, Brooks E. Imipramine and methylphenidate treatment of hyperactive boys. Arch Gen Psychiatry 1974;30:789–798.

Rapport MD, Carlson GA, Kelly KL, Pataki C. Methylphenidate and desipramine in hospitalized children: I. Separate and combined effects on cognitive function. J Am Acad Child Adolesc Psychiatry 1993;32:333–342.

Rapport MD, Denney C, DuPaul GJ, Gardner MJ. Attention deficit disorder and methylphenidate: Normalization rates, clinical effectiveness, and response prediction in 76 children. J Am Acad Child Adolesc Psychiatry 1994;33:882–893.

Ratey J, Sovner R, Parks A, Rogentine K. Buspirone treatment of aggression and anxiety in mentally retarded patients: A multiple-baseline, placebo lead-in study. J Clin Psychiatry 1991;52:159–162.

Ratey JJ, Sovner R, Mikkelsen E, Chmielinsky HE: Buspirone therapy for maladaptive behavior and anxiety in developmentally disabled persons. J Clin Psychiatry 1989:50:382–384.

Rating scales and assessment instruments for use in pediatric psychopharmacology research. Psychopharmacol Bull 1985;21:713–1124.

Realmuto GM, August GJ, Garfinkel BD. Clinical effect of buspirone in autistic children. J Clin Psychopharmacol 1989;9:122–125.

Realmuto GM, Erickson WD, Yellin AM, Hopwood JH, Greenberg LM. Clinical comparison of thiothixene and thioridazine in schizophrenic adolescents. Am J Psychiatry 1984;141:440–442.

Reisberg B, Gershon S. Side effects associated with lithium therapy. Arch Gen Psychiatry 1979;36:879–887.

Reiss AL, O'Donnell DJ. Carbamazepine-induced mania in two children: Case report. J Clin Psychiatry 1984;45:272–274.

Reite ML, Nagel KE, Ruddy JR. Concise guide to evaluation and management of sleep disorders. Washington, DC: American Psychiatric Press, 1990.

Remschmidt H. The psychotropic effect of carbamazepine in non-epileptic patients, with particular reference to problems posed by clinical studies in children with behavioural disorders. In: Birkmayer W, ed. Epileptic seizures—behaviour—pain. Bern: Hans Huber Publishers, 1976:253–258.

Remschmidt H, Schulz E, Martin PDM. An open trial of clozapine in thirty-six adolescents with schizophrenia. J Child Adolesc Psychopharmacol 1994;4:31–41.

Richardson MA, Haugland G, Craig TJ. Neuroleptic use, parkinsonian symptoms, tardive dyskinesia and associated factors in child and adolescent psychiatric patients. Am J Psychiatry 1991;148:1322–1328.

Riddle MA, Geller B, Ryan N. Another sudden death in a child treated with desipramine. J Am Acad Child Adolesc Psychiatry 1993;32:792–797.

Riddle MA, Geller B, Ryan ND. The safety of desipramine: reply [letter]. J Am Acad Child Adolesc Psychiatry 1994;33;589–590.

Riddle MA, Hardin MT, Cho SC, Woolston JL, Leckman JF. Desipramine treatment of boys with attention-deficit hyperactivity disorder and tics: Preliminary clinical experiences. J Am Acad Child Adolesc Psychiatry 1988;27:811–814.

Riddle MA, Hardin MT, King R, Scahill L, Woolston JL. Fluoxetine treatment of children and adolescents with Tourette's and obsessive compulsive disorders: Preliminary clinical experience. J Am Acad Child Adolesc Psychiatry 1990;29:45–48.

Riddle MA, King RA, Hardin MT, Scahill L, Ort SI, Chappell P, Rasmusson A, Leckman JF. Behavioral side effects of fluoxetine in children and adolescents. J Child Adolesc Psychopharmacology 1990;1:193–198.

Riddle MA, Nelson JC, Kleinman CS, Rasmusson A, Leckman JF, King RA, Cohen DJ. Sudden death in children receiving Norpramin: A review of three reported cases and commentary. J Am Acad Child Adolesc Psychiatry 1991;30:104–108.

Riddle MA, Scahill L, King RA, Hardin MT, Anderson GM, Ort SI, Smith JC, Leckman JF, Cohen DJ. Double-blind, crossover trial of fluoxetine and placebo in children and adolescents with obsessive-compulsive disorder. J Am Acad Child Adolesc Psychiatry 1992:31:1062–1069.

Rifkin A, Quitkin F, Klein DF. Akinesia: A poorly recognized drug-induced extrapyramidal behavior disorder. Arch Gen Psychiatry 1975;32:672–674.

Ritvo ER, Freeman BJ, Geller E, Yuwiler A. Effects of fenfluramine on 14 outpatients with the syndrome of autism. J Am Acad Child Psychiatry 1983;22:549–558.

Rivera-Calimlim L, Griesbach PH, Perlmutter R. Plasma chlorpromazine concentrations in children with behavioral disorders and mental illness. Clin Pharmacol Ther 1979;26:114–121.

Rivera-Calimlim L, Nasrallah H, Strauss J, Lasagna L. Clinical response and plasma levels: Effect of dose, dosage schedules, and drug interactions on plasma chlorpromazine levels. Am J Psychiatry 1976;133:646–652.

Rosenberg DR, Holttum J, Gershon S. Textbook of pharmacotherapy for child and adolescent psychiatric disorders. New York: Brunner/Mazel, 1994.

Rosenberg DR, Johnson K, Sahl R. Evolving mania in an adolescent treated with low-dose fluoxetine. J Child Adolesc Psychopharmacol 1992;2:299–306.

Ross DC, Piggott LR. Clonazepam for OCD [letter]. J Am Acad Child Adolesc Psychiatry 1993;32:470–471.

Rosse RB, Giese AA, Deutsch SI, Morihisa JM. Laboratory diagnostic testing in psychiatry. Washington, DC: American Psychiatric Press, 1989.

Rudorfer MV, Potter WZ. Pharmacokinetics of antidepressants. In: Meltzer HY, ed. Psychopharmacology: The third generation of progress. New York: Raven Press, 1987:1353–1363.

Russo RM, Gururaj VJ, Allen JE. The effectiveness of diphenhydramine HCl in pediatric sleep disorders. J Clin Pharmacol 1976;4:284–288.

Ryan ND. Heterocyclic antidepressants in children and adolescents. J Child Adolesc Psychopharmacol 1990;1:21–31.

Ryan ND, Meyer V, Dachille S, Mazzie D, Puig-Antich J. Lithium antidepressant augmentation in TCA-refractory depression in adolescents. J Acad Child Adolesc Psychiatry 1988a;27:371–376.

Ryan ND, Puig-Antich J, Cooper T, Rabinovich H, Ambrosini P, Davies M, King J, Torres D, Fried J. Imipramine in adolescent major depression: Plasma level and clinical response. Acta Psychiatr Scand 1986;73:275–288.

Ryan ND, Puig-Antich J, Cooper TB, Rabinovich H, Ambrosini P, Fried J, Davies M, Torres D, Suckow RF. Relative safety of single versus divided dose imipramine in adolescent major depression. J Am Acad Child Adolesc Psychiatry 1987;26: 400–406.

Ryan ND, Puig-Antich J, Rabinovich H, Fried J, Ambrosini P, Meyer V, Torres D, Dachille S, Mazzie R. MAOIs in adolescent major depression unresponsive to tricyclic antidepressants. J Am Acad Child Adolesc Psychiatry 1988b;27:755–758.

Safer D, Allen RP, Barr E. Depression of growth in hyperactive children on stimulant drugs. N Engl J Med 1972;287:217–220.

Safer DJ, Krager M. A survey of medication treatment for hyperactive/inattentive students. JAMA 260:2256–2258, 1988.

Sakkas P, Davis JM, Han J, Wang Z. Pharmacotherapy of NMS. Psychiatr Ann 1991; 21:157–164.

Sallee F, Stiller R, Perel JM. Pharmacodynamics of pemoline in attention deficit disorder with hyperactivity. J Am Acad Child Adolesc Psychiatry 1992;31:244–251.

Sallee F, Stiller R, Perel JM, Bates T. Oral pemoline kinetics in hyperactive children. Clin Pharmacol Ther 1985;37:606–609.

Sallee FR, Stiller RL, Perel JM, Everett G. Pemoline-induced abnormal involuntary movements. J Clin Psychopharmacol 1989;9:125–129.

Salzman C. Benzodiazepine dependency: Summary of the APA task force on benzodiazepines. Psychopharmacol Bull 1990;26:61–62.

Saraf KR, Klein DF, Gittelman-Klein R, Groff S. Imipramine side effects in children. Psychopharmacologia (Berlin) 1974;37:265–274.

Saul RC. Nortriptyline in attention deficit disorder. Clin Neuropharmacol 1985;8: 382–384.

Schmidt MH, Trott, G-E, Blanz B, Nissen G. Clozapine medication in adolescents. In: Stefania CN, Rabavilas AD, Soldatos CR, eds. Psychiatry: A world perspective. Proceedings of the VIII World Congress of Psychiatry. Amsterdam: Excerpta Medica, 1990;1:1100–1104.

Schooler NR, Kane JM. Research diagnoses for tardive dyskinesia. Arch Gen Psychiatry 1982;38:486–487.

Schou M. Lithium: Elimination rate, dosage, control, poisoning, goiter, mode of action. Acta Psychiatr Scand 1969;207(suppl):49–59.

Schroeder JS, Mullin AV, Elliott GR, Steiner H, Nichols M, Gordon A, Paulow M. Cardiovascular effects of desipramine in children. J Am Acad Child Adolesc Psychiatry 1989;28:376–379.

Shapiro AK, Shapiro E. Controlled study of pimozide vs. placebo in Tourette's syndrome. J Am Acad Child Psychiatry 1984;23:161–173.

Shapiro AK, Shapiro E. Do stimulants provoke, cause, or exacerbate tics and Tourette syndrome? Compr Psychiatry 1981;22:265–273.

Shapiro AK, Shapiro E. Tic disorders. In: Kaplan HI, Sadock BJ, eds. Comprehensive textbook of psychiatry. 5th ed. Baltimore: Williams & Wilkins, 1989:1865–1878.

Shapiro AK, Shapiro E, Eisenkraft GJ. Treatment of Gilles de la Tourette syndrome with pimozide. Am J Psychiatry 1983;140:1183–1186.

Sheard MH. Lithium in the treatment of aggression. J Nerv Ment Dis 1975;160: 108–118.

Siefen G, Remschmidt H. Behandlungsergebnisse mit clozapin bei schizophrenen jugendlichen [Clozapine in the treatment of adolescents with schizophrenia: Treatment outcome]. Zeitschrift fur Kinder-und-Jugendpsychiatrie 1986;14:245–257. (English translation by the Ralph McElroy Co., provided by the manufacturer.)

Simeon JG. Buspirone effects in adolescent psychiatric disorders. Eur Neuropsychopharmacol 1991;1:421.

Simeon JG, Dinicola VF, Ferguson HB, Copping W. Adolescent depression: A placebo-controlled fluoxetine treatment study and follow-up. Prog Neuro-psychopharmacol Biol Psychiatry 1990;14:791–795.

Simeon JG, Ferguson HB. Alprazolam effects in children with anxiety disorders. Can J Psychiatry 1987;32:570–574.

Simeon JG, Ferguson HB. Recent developments in the use of antidepressant and anxiolytic medications. Psychiatr Clin North Am 1985;8:893–907.

Simeon JG, Ferguson HB, Fleet JVW. Bupropion effects in attention deficit and conduct disorder. Can J Psychiatry 1986;31:581–585.

Simeon JG, Ferguson HB, Knott V, Roberts N, Gauthier B, Dubois C, Wiggins D. Clinical, cognitive, and neurophysiological effects of alprazolam in children and adolescents with overanxious and avoidant disorders. J Am Acad Child Adolesc Psychiatry 1992;31:29–33.

Simeon JG, Knott VJ, DuBois C, Wiggins D, Geraets I, Thatte S, Miller W. Buspirone therapy of mixed anxiety disorders in childhood and adolescence: A pilot study. J Child Adolesc Psychopharmacol 1994;4:159–170.

Sleator EK. Diagnosis. In: Sleator EK, Pelham WE Jr, eds. Attention deficit disorder. Dialogues in pediatric management. Vol. 1, No. 3. Norwalk, CT: Appleton-Century-Crofts, 1986:11–42.

Sleator EK, von Neumann A, Sprague RL. Hyperactive children: A continuous long-term placebo-controlled follow-up. JAMA 1974;229:316–317.

Small JG, Milstein V, Marhenke JD, Hall DD, Kellams JJ. Treatment outcome with clozapine in tardive dyskinesia, neuroleptic sensitivity, and treatment resistant psychosis. J Clin Psychiatry 1987;48:263–267.

Smith TC, Wollman H. History and principles of anaesthesiology. In: Gilman AF, Goodman LS, Rall TW, Murad R, eds. Goodman and Gilman's the pharmacological basis of therapeutics. 7th ed. New York: Macmillan, 1985:260–275.

Sokol MS, Campbell M. Novel psychoactive agents in the treatment of developmental disorders. In: Aman MG, Singh NN, eds. Psychopharmacology of the developmental disabilities. New York: Springer-Verlag, 1988:147–167.

Spencer EK, Kafantaris V, Padron-Gayol MV, Rosenberg CR, Campbell M. Haloperi-

REFERENCES 273

dol in schizophrenic children: Early findings from a study in progress. Psychopharmacol Bull 1992;28:183–186.

Spencer T, Biederman J, Kerman K, Steingard R, Wilens T. Desipramine treatment of children with attention-deficit hyperactivity disorder and tic disorder or Tourette's syndrome. J Am Acad Child Adolesc Psychiatry 1993a;32:354–360.

Spencer T, Biederman J, Steingard R, Wilens T. Bupropion exacerbates tics in children with attention-deficit hyperactivity disorder and Tourette's syndrome. J Am Acad Child Adolesc Psychiatry 1993b;32:211–214.

Spencer T, Biederman J, Wilens T, Steingard R, Geist D. Nortriptyline treatment of children with attention-deficit hyperactivity disorder and tic disorder or Tourette's syndrome. J Am Acad Child Adolesc Psychiatry 1993c;32:201–210.

Spitzer RL, Endicott J, Robins E. Research diagnostic criteria. Arch Gen Psychiatry 1978;35:773–782.

Sprague RL, Sleator EK. Methylphenidate in hyperkinetic children: Differences in dose effects on learning and social behavior. Science 1977;198:1274–1276.

Stanley B. An integration of ethical and clinical considerations in the use of placebos. Psychopharmacol Bull 1988;24:18–20.

Steingard R, Biederman J, Spencer T, Wilens T, Gonzalez A. Comparison of clonidine response in the treatment of attention-deficit hyperactivity disorder with and without comorbid tic disorders. J Am Acad Child Adolesc Psychiatry 1993;32:350–353.

Steingard R, Khan A, Gonzales A, Herzog DB. Neuroleptic malignant syndrome: Review of experience with children and adolescents. J Child Adolesc Psychopharmacol 1992;2:183–198.

Stores G. Antiepileptics (anticonvulsants). In: Werry JS, ed. Pediatric psychopharmacology: The use of behavior modifying drugs in children. New York: Brunner/Mazel, 1978:274–315.

Strayhorn JM, Rapp N, Donina W, Strain PS. Randomized trial of methylphenidate for an autistic child. J Am Acad Child Adolesc Psychiatry 1988;27:244–247.

Strober M, Freeman R, Rigali J. The pharmacotherapy of depressive illness in adolescents: I. An open label trial of imipramine. Psychopharmacol Bull 1990;26:80–84.

Strober M, Freeman R, Rigali J, Schmidt S, Diamond R. The pharmacotherapy of depressive illiness in adolescents: II. Effects of lithium augmentation in nonresponders to imipramine. J Am Acad Child Adolesc Psychiatry 1992;31:16–20.

Sudden death in children treated with a tricyclic antidepressant, (The) Medical Letter, 1990(June 1);32:53.

Sussman N. The potential benefits of serotonin receptor-specific agents. J Clin Psychiatry 1994a;55(suppl 1):45–51.

Sussman N. The uses of buspirone in psychiatry. J Clin Psychiatry Monograph 1994b;12(1):3–19.

Swanson JM, Lerner M, Cantwell D. Blood levels and tolerance to stimulants in ADDH children. Clin Neuropharmacol 1986;9(suppl 4):523–525.

Taylor E, Schachar R, Thorley G, Wieselberg HM, Everitt B, Rutter M. Which boys respond to stimulant medication? A controlled trial of methylphenidate in boys with disruptive behavior. Psychol Med 1987;17:121–143.

Teicher MH, Baldessarini RJ. Developmental pharmacodynamics. In: Popper C, ed. Psychiatric pharmacosciences of children and adolescents. Washington, DC: American Psychiatric Press, 1987:45–80.

Thase ME, Kupfer DJ, Frank E, Jarrett DB. Treatment of imipramine-resistant recurrent depression: II. An open clinical trial of lithium augmentation. J Clin Psychiatry 1989;50:413–417.

United States Pharmacopeial Dispensing Information (USPDI). Drug information for the health care professional. Rockville, MD: United States Pharmacopeial Convention, 1990.

Van Putten T, Marder SR. Behavioral toxicity of antipsychotic drugs. J Clin Psychiatry 1987;48(suppl 9):13–19.

Van Putten T, May PRA, Marder SR. Akathisia with haloperidol and thiothixene. Arch Gen Psychiatry 1984;41:1036–1039.

Varanka TM, Weller RA, Weller EB, Fristad MA. Lithium treatment of manic episodes with psychotic features in prepubertal children. Am J Psychiatry 1988; 145:1557–1559.

Venkataraman S, Naylor MW, King CA. Mania associated with fluoxetine treatment in adolescents. J Am Acad Child Adolesc Psychiatry 1992;31:276–281.

Verglas, GDU, Banks SR, Guyer KE. Clinical effects of fenfluramine on children with autism: A review of the research. J Autism Dev Disord 1988;18:297–308.

Vetro A, Szentistvanyi I, Pallag L, Vargha M, Szilard J. Therapeutic experience with lithium in childhood aggressivity. Pharmacopsychiatry 1985;14:121–127.

Villeneuve A. The rabbit syndrome: A peculiar extrapyramidal reaction. Can Psychiatr Assoc J 1972;17:69–72.

Vincent J, Varley CK, Leger P. Effects of methylphenidate on early adolescent growth. Am J Psychiatry 1990;147:501–502.

Vitiello B, Behar D, Malone R, Delaney MA, Ryan PJ, Simpson GM. Pharmacokinetics of lithium carbonate in children. J Clin Psychopharmacol 1988;8:355–359.

Waizer J, Hoffman SP, Polizos P, Engelhardt DM. Outpatient treatment of hyperactive school children with imipramine. Am J. Psychiatry 1974;131:587–591.

Walkup JT. Clinical decision making in child and adolescent psychopharmacology. Child Adolesc Psychiatr Clin North Am 1995;4:23–40.

Walsh BT, Giardina E-GV, Sloan RP, Greenhill L, Goldfein J. Effects of desipramine on autonomic control of the heart. J Am Acad Child Adolesc Psychiatry 1994;33: 191–197.

Weiner JM, ed. Psychopharmacology in childhood and adolescence. New York: Basic Books, 1977.

Weiner JM, ed. Diagnosis and psychopharmacology of childhood and adolescent disorders. New York: John Wiley & Sons, 1985.

Weiner JM, Jaffe SL. Historical overview of childhood and adolescent psychopharmacoloy. In: Weiner JM, ed. Diagnosis and psychopharmacology of childhood and adolescent disorders. New York: John Wiley & Sons, 1985:3–50.

Weiner N. Norepinephrine, epinephrine, and the sympathomimetic amines. In: Gilman AG, Goodman LS, Gilman A, eds. Goodman and Gilman's the pharmacological basis of therapeutics. 6th ed. New York: Macmillan, 1980:138–175.

Weiss G, Hechtman LT. Hyperactive children grown up: Empirical findings and theoretical considerations. New York: Guilford Press, 1986.

Weiss G, Kruger E, Danielson U, Elman M. Effect of long-term treatment of hyperactive children with methylphenidate. Can Med Assoc J 1975;112:159–165.

Weizman A, Weitz R, Szekely GA, Tyano S, Belmaker RH. Combination of neuroleptic and stimulant treatment in attention deficit disorder with hyperactivity. J Am Acad Child Psychiatry 1984;23:295–298.

Weller EB, Weller RA, Fristad MA. Lithium dosage guide for prepubertal children: A preliminary report. J Am Acad Child Psychiatry 1986;25:92–95.

Weller EB, Weller RA, Fristad MA, Cantwell M, Tucker S. Saliva lithium monitoring in prepubertal children. J Am Acad Child Adolesc Psychiatry 1987;26:173–175.

Weller EB, Weller RA, Preskorn SH, Glotzbach R. Steady-state plasma imipramine levels in prepubertal depressed children. Am J Psychiatry 1982;139:506–508.

Wender PH. Attention deficit hyperactivity disorder. In: Howells JG, ed. Modern perspectives in clinical psychiatry. New York: Brunner/Mazel, 1988:149–169.

Wernicke JF. The side effect profile and safety of fluoxetine. J Clin Psychiatry 1985: 46(3):59–67.

Werry JS. The safety of desipramine [letter]. J Am Acad Child Adolesc Psychiatry 1994;33:588–589.

Werry J, Aman M. Methylphenidate and haloperidol in children: Effects on attention, memory, and activity. Arch Gen Psychiatry 1975;32:790–795.

Werry J, Aman MG, Diamond E. Imipramine and methylphenidate in hyperactive children. J Child Psychol Psychiatry 1980;21:27–35.

Werry J, Weiss G, Douglas V, Martin J. Studies on the hyperactive child III: The effects of chlorpromazine upon behavior and learning ability. J Am Acad Child Psychiatry 1966;5:292–312.

Werry JS, ed. Pediatric psychopharmacology: The use of behavior modifying drugs in children. New York: Brunner/Mazel, 1978.

Werry JS, Aman MG, eds. Practitioner's guide to psychoactive drugs for children and adolescents. New York: Plenum Medical Book, 1993.

West SA, Keck PE, McElroy SL, Strakowske SM, Minnery KL, McConville BJ, Sorter MT. Open trial of valproate in the treatment of adolescent mania. J Child Adolesc Psychopharmacol 1994;4:263–267.

Whalen CK, Henker B, Swanson JM, Granger D, Kliewer W, Spencer J. Natural social behaviors in hyperactive children: Dose effects of methylphenidate. J Consult Clin Psychol 1987;55:187–193.

White L, Tursky B, Schwartz GE, eds. Placebo: Theory, research, and mechanisms. New York: Guilford Press, 1985.

Wilens, TE, Biederman J, Baldessarini RJ, Puopolo PR, Flood JG: Developmental changes in serum concentrations of desipramine and 2-hydroxydesipramine during treatment with desipramine. J Am Acad Child Adolesc Psychiatry 1992;31:691–698.

Wilens TE, Biederman J, Spencer T. Clonidine for sleep disturbances associated with attention-deficit hyperactivity disorder. J Am Acad Child Adolesc Psychiatry 1994;33:424–426.

Wilens TE, Biederman J, Baldessarini RJ, Puopolo PR, Flood JG: Electrocardiographic effects of desipramine and 2-hydroxydesipramine in children, adolescents, and adults treated with desipramine. J Am Acad Child Adolesc Psychiatry 1993a; 32:798–804.

Wilens TE, Biederman J, Geist DE, Steingard R, Spencer T. Nortriptyline in the treatment of ADHD: A chart review of 58 cases. J Am Acad Child Adolesc Psychiatry 1993b;32:343–349.

Wilens TE, Spencer T, Biederman J, Wozniak J, Conner D. Combined pharmacotherapy: An emerging trend in pediatric psychopharmacology. J Am Acad Child Adolesc Psychiatry 1995;34:110–112.

Williams DT, Mehl R, Yudofsky S, Adams D, Roseman B. The effect of propranolol on uncontrolled rage outbursts in children and adolescents with organic brain dysfunction. J Am Acad Child Psychiatry 1982;21:129–135.

Winsberg BG, Kupietz SS, Sverd J, Hungund BL, Young NL. Methylphenidate oral dose plasma concentrations and behavioral response in children. Psychopharmacology 1982;76:329–332.

Wolf DW, Wagner KD: Tardive dyskinesia, tardive dystonia, and tardive Tourette's syndrome in children and adolescents. J Child Adolesc Psychopharmacol 1993;3: 175–198.

Wysowski DK, Barash D. Adverse behavioral reactions attributed to triazolam in the Food and Drug Administration's spontaneous reporting system. Arch Intern Med 1991;151:2003–2008.

Yepes LE, Balka EB, Winsberg BG, Bialer I. Amitriptyline and methylphenidate treatment of behaviorally disordered children. J Child Psychol Psychiatry 1977; 18:39–52.

Zametkin AJ, Rapoport JL. Noradrenergic hypothesis of attention deficit disorder with hyperactivity: A critical review. In: Meltzer HY, ed. Psychopharmacology: The third generation of progress. New York: Raven Press, 1987:837–842.

Zametkin A, Rapoport JL, Murphy DL, Linnoila M, Ismond D. Treatment of hyperactive children with monoamine oxidase inhibitors. I. Clinical efficacy. Arch Gen Psychiatry 1985;42:962–966.

Zimnitzky B. A fifth case of sudden death in a child taking desipramine. New Research Poster (NR478-A). In: 1994 Annual Meeting, New Research Program and Abstracts, Philadelphia, PA, May 21–25, 1994. Washington, DC: American Psychiatric Association, 1994:181.

Zito JM, Craig TJ, Wanderling J. Pharmacoepidemiology of 330 child/adolescent psychiatric patients. J Pharmacoepidemiol 1994;3:47–62.

Zrull JP, Westman JC, Arthur B, Bell WA. A comparison of chlordiazepoxide, d-amphetamine, and placebo in the treatment of the hyperkinetic syndrome in children. Am J Psychiatry 1963;120:590–591.

Zrull JP, Westman JC, Arthur B, Rice DL. A comparison of diazepam, d-amphetamine, and placebo in the treatment of the hyperkinetic syndrome in children. Am J Psychiatry 1964;121:388–389.

Zubieta JK, Alessi NE: Acute and chronic administration of trazodone in the treatment of disruptive behavior disorders in children. J Clin Psychopharmacol 1992; 12:346–351.

Zwier KJ, Rao U. Buspirone use in an adolescent with social phobia and mixed personality disorder (cluster A type). J Am Acad Child Adolesc Psychiatry 1994;33: 1007–1011.

INDEX

Page numbers in *italics* denote figures; those followed by "t" denote tables.

Chlorpromazine—*continued*
available dose forms of, 98
bioequivalence of different preparations of, 31, 34
dosage of, 98
indications for, 98
interaction with propranolol, 236
monitoring serum levels of, 44
pharmacokinetics of, 12, 13
plasma levels of, 80–81
therapeutic window for, 95
use in persons with mental retardation, 79
use in persons with seizure disorders, 81
Cholinergic rebound, after withdrawal
of tricyclic antidepressants, 46
Cibalith-S. *See* Lithium citrate syrup
Cimetidine, interaction with benzodiazepines, 205
Circadian rhythm sleep disorder, 55t
Clinical Global Impression for Obsessive Compulsive Disorder,
171
Clinical Global Impression scale, 59,
107, 152, 162, 169, 172, 182, 217,
235
Clinical observations
of drug effects, 14
of premedication behavior, 27–28
Clinical record. *See* Documentation
Clomipramine, 70, 157–164
for attention deficit hyperactivity
disorder, 122, 161–162
for autistic disorder, 162–163
available dose forms of, 158
for depressive symptoms, 163
dosage of, 158
effects on serotonergic and noradrenergic function, 157
for enuresis, 159, 163
indications for, 122, 158
mechanism of action of, 157
for obsessive-compulsive disorder,
159–161
pharmacokinetics of, 158
developmental effects on, 12
plasma level of, 159
monitoring of, 44
for separation anxiety disorder, 163–
164
untoward effects of, 158–159

Clonazepam, 207t, 213–215
for akathisia, 85
for anxiety disorders, 213–214
interaction with valproic acid, 230
for obsessive-compulsive disorder,
214–215
for panic disorder, 213
untoward effects of, 214
Clonidine, 240–249
for aggressiveness, 245–246
for akathisia, 85
for attention deficit hyperactivity
disorder, 240, 242–245
combined with methylphenidate,
243–244
for sleep disturbances, 245
for autistic disorder, 246
available dose forms of, 241
contraindications to, 240
discontinuation of, 242
dosing schedule for, 241
drug interactions with, 240
indications for, 241
mechanism of action of, 240
pharmacokinetics of, 240
for Tourette's disorder, 246–249
transdermal patch, 241–242
untoward effects of, 241
Clorazepate, 207t
Clorgyline, 184
for adolescent depression, 185
for attention deficit hyperactivity
disorder, 186
Clozapine (Clozaril), 96t, 113–120
available dose forms of, 114
benefits of, 114
dosage of, 114
EEG monitoring of patient on, 27
indications for, 114
lack of extrapyramidal symptoms
with, 91, 114
mechanism of action of, 113–114
studies in schizophrenia, 115–120
untoward effects of, 114–116
agranulocytosis, 82, 114–115
cardiac effects, 115
seizures, 115
Cocaine abuse
benzodiazepine abuse and, 201
interaction with monoamine oxidase
inhibitors, 185
interaction with stimulants, 63